The 1984
Olympic Scientific
Congress
Proceedings
Volume 5

Sport and Aging

Series Editors:

Jan Broekhoff, PhD
Michael J. Ellis, PhD
Dan G. Tripps, PhD

University of Oregon
Eugene, Oregon

The 1984
Olympic Scientific
Congress
Proceedings
Volume 5

Sport
and
Aging

Barry D. McPherson
Editor

Human Kinetics Publishers, Inc.
Champaign, Illinois

Library of Congress Cataloging-in-Publication Data

Olympic Scientific Congress (1984 : Eugene, Or.)
   Sport and aging.

   (1984 Olympic Scientific Congress proceedings ; v. 5)
   Bibliography: p.
   1. Sports for the aged—Congress.   I. McPherson,
Barry D.   II. Title.   III. Series: Olympic Scientific
Congress (1984 : Eugene, Or.).   1984 Olympic Scientific
Congress proceedings ; v. 5.
GV565.O46 1984 vol. 5   796'.01'926   85-18124
[GV708.5]
ISBN 0-87322-012-9

Managing Editor: Susan Wilmoth, PhD
Developmental Editor: Susan Wilmoth, PhD
Production Director: Sara Chilton
Copyeditor: Eva Kingston
Typesetter: Aurora Garcia, Sandra Meier, and Yvonne Winsor
Text Layout: Gail Irwin
Cover Design and Layout: Jack Davis
Printed By: Braun-Brumfield, Inc.

ISBN: 0-87322-006-4 (10 Volume Set)
ISBN: 0-87322-012-9

Printed in the United States of America

10 9 8 7 6 5 4 3 2 1

Human Kinetics Publishers, Inc.
Box 5076, Champaign, IL 61820

Contents

Series Acknowledgments

The Congress organizers realize that an event as large and complex as the 1984 Olympic Scientific Congress could not have come to fruition without the help of literally hundreds of organizations and individuals. Under the patronage of UNESCO, the Congress united in sponsorship and cooperation no fewer than 64 national and international associations and organizations. Some 50 representatives of associations helped with the organization of the scientific and associative programs by coordinating individual sessions. The cities of Eugene and Springfield yielded more than 400 volunteers who donated their time to make certain that the multitude of Congress functions would progress without major mishaps. To all these organizations and individuals, the organizers express their gratitude.

A special word of thanks must also be directed to the major sponsors of the Congress: the International Council of Sport Science and Physical Education (ICSSPE), the United States Olympic Committee (USOC), the International Council on Health, Physical Education and Recreation (ICHPER), and the American Alliance for Health, Physical Education, Recreation and Dance (AAHPERD). Last but not least, the organizers wish to acknowledge the invaluable assistance of the International Olympic Committee (IOC) and its president, Honorable Juan Antonio Samaranch. President Samaranch made Congress history by his official opening address in Eugene on July 19, 1984. The IOC further helped the Congress with a generous donation toward the publication of the Congress papers. Without this donation it would have been impossible to make the proceedings available in this form.

Finally, the series editors wish to express their thanks to the volume editors who selected and edited the papers from each program of the Congress. Special thanks go to Barry D. McPherson of the University of Waterloo for his work on this volume.

Jan Broekhoff,
Michael J. Ellis, and
Dan G. Tripps

Series Editors

Series Preface

Sport and Aging contains selected proceedings from this interdisciplinary program of the 1984 Olympic Scientific Congress, which was held at the University of Oregon in Eugene, Oregon, preceding the Olympic Games in Los Angeles. The Congress was organized by the College of Human Development and Performance of the University of Oregon in collaboration with the cities of Eugene and Springfield. This was the first time in the history of the Congress that the event was organized by a group of private individuals, unaided by a federal government. The fact that the Congress was attended by more than 2,200 participants from more than 100 different nations is but one indication of its success.

The Congress program focused on the theme of Sport, Health, and Well-Being and was organized in three parts. The mornings of the eight-day event were devoted to disciplinary sessions, which brought together specialists in various subdisciplines of sport science such as sport medicine, biomechanics, sport psychology, sport sociology, and sport philosophy. For the first time in the Congress' history, these disciplinary sessions were sponsored by the national and international organizations representing the various subdisciplines. In the afternoons, the emphasis shifted toward interdisciplinary themes in which scholars and researchers from the subdisciplines attempted to contribute to crossdisciplinary understanding. In addition, three evenings were devoted to keynote addresses and presentations, broadly related to the theme of Sport, Health, and Well-Being.

In addition to the scientific programs, the Congress also featured a number of associative programs with topics determined by their sponsoring organizations. Well over 1,200 papers were presented in the various sessions of the Congress at large. It stands to reason, therefore, that publishing the proceedings of the event presented a major problem to the organizers. It was decided to limit proceedings initially to interdisciplinary sessions which drew substantial interest from Congress participants and attracted a critical number of high-quality presentations. Human Kinetics Publishers, Inc. of Champaign, Illinois, was selected to produce these proceedings. After considerable deliberation, the following interdisciplinary themes were selected for publication: Competitive Sport for Children and Youths; Human Genetics and Sport; Sport and Aging; Sport and Disabled Individuals; Sport and Elite Performers; Sport, Health, and Nutrition; and Sport and Politics. The 10-volume set published by Human Kinetics Publishers is rounded out by the disciplinary proceedings of Kinanthropometry, Sport Pedagogy, and the associative program on the Scientific Aspects of Dance.

Jan Broekhoff,
Michael J. Ellis, and
Dan G. Tripps

Series Editors

Preface

Driven by the demographic forces of population aging, by the increasing visibility and demands of older adults, and by changing values, norms, and opportunities concerning participation in physical activity, sport scientists are beginning to initiate research on problems, processes, and programs pertaining to the physically active middle-aged and elderly adult. The papers in this volume reflect both this emerging interest and concern and the current state of the art with respect to research on sport and aging.

Structured into four parts, the monograph illustrates the eclectic nature of research in this area. This eclecticism is partially due to the multidisciplinary nature of gerontology, to the international mix of scholars who are initiating research in this area, to the unknown scope of potential research questions, and to the variety of research methods and theoretical frameworks that are presently being used. Moreover, as with most new domains of inquiry, these early studies reveal methodological and theoretical problems unique to the study of aging cohorts and older adults. For example, some of the studies reported in the monograph utilize small samples; others constitute atheoretical, exploratory studies; only a few are concerned with women, despite the demographic fact that women comprise a majority of the elderly population; and, some describe rather than evaluate an activity program that was offered in only one setting with one group of older adults, rather than the results of replications in various settings. Nevertheless, each paper raises important research, policy, or programming questions that need to be addressed.

Each part begins with an invited keynote address that reviews and critiques theoretical and methodological concerns and the state of knowledge in a particular domain. Part I., Social Science and Health Perspectives, includes papers that address the relationship among sport participation and such issues as the quality of life, happiness, the unemployed, social change, well-being, the institutionalized, clinical health care, and voluntary association involvement. In Part II., Program Perspectives, principles, models, and programs are presented that seek to facilitate the health and well-being of older adults through exercise, sport, and physical activity. Part III., Psychological Perspectives, focuses on personality, motives, attitudes, motor fitness, cognitive processing, emotional health, and performace accuracy within sport and exercise settings. Part IV., Physiological Perspectives, includes information on the effects of training and on the physiological processes and benefits of sport and physical activity in the middle and later years of life.

In summary, the information included in this monograph represents only the starting point for gerontological research in the sport sciences. It is hoped that the inadequacies of past and current research have been revealed, and more questions than answers have been posed for the reader. Herein lies a challenge to sport scientists: That is, because of population aging and increasing longevity (especially for women), and because there is a growing propensity for older adults to engage in sport and exercise, sport scientists must initiate high-quality research concerning physical activity in the middle and later years of life. In short, our level of knowledge concerning older adults lags far behind that for younger age groups. Thus, as you read this monograph, the authors encourage you to critique their work, to pose new research questions, and to initiate research that will make this volume virtually obsolete following the 1988 Olympic Scientific Congress in Seoul.

Barry D. McPherson, Editor

The 1984
Olympic Scientific
Congress
Proceedings
Volume 5

Sport
and
Aging

PART I

Social Science and Health Perspectives

1

Sport, Health, Well-Being, and Aging: Some Conceptual and Methodological Issues and Questions for Sport Scientists

Barry D. McPherson
UNIVERSITY OF WATERLOO
WATERLOO, ONTARIO, CANADA

During the past 25 years demographers have frequently documented the decrease in birth rates and the increase in life expectancy in most modernized societies. The net outcome of these two demographic processes, a phenomenon known as "population aging," is that approximately 9% of the population in North America (between 11 and 15% in many European countries) is now comprised of people over 65 years of age. It is projected that this proportion will increase to about 12% by the year 2000 and to between 15 and 17% when the "baby boom" age cohort reaches 65 between 2010 and 2020. Moreover, it is projected that there may be as many as 390 million persons over 65 in the world by the year 2000.

As a result of population aging and the greater visibility of elderly persons, scientists in a number of disciplines are seeking to understand structural, biological, sensory, motor, behavioral, and cognitive changes and adaptations in the human organism over time. Much of this work on "individual aging" has been completed within the evolving fields of geriatrics and gerontology. In addition, an increasing number of individuals, in a variety of professions and occupations, are now required to develop policies or to provide services to meet the needs, interests, and concerns of the elderly population.

While a few sport scientists, primarily from a physiological perspective,[1] have been interested in aging processes for a number of years, aging phenomena and the elderly have not been popular research topics in the sport sciences. This is unfortunate because many practitioners are now providing activity programs for older adults and need valid research information. Therefore, because we appear to be on the threshold of a new domain of inquiry and practice, it is essential that physical activity scientists and program personnel be thoroughly familiar with the existing body of psychological, biological, and sociological knowledge concerning aging processes and the elderly.

It is important to recognize that the elderly, because of aging, historical, and cohort effects, represent a unique population. To cope with this uniqueness, gerontologists have identified and sought to resolve a number of theoretical and methodological issues related to the study of aging processes and the aged. Therefore, the major purpose of this paper is to alert physical activity scientists and practitioners to some of these conceptual and methodological issues and to identify a number of social and environmental factors that need to be controlled when studying age-related phenomena or the elderly.

The second purpose of this paper is to examine the issue of the myriad of potential interrelationships among the concepts that comprise the theme of this conference—especially as they pertain to the process of aging and the state of being old. Without considering that the relationships might change in strength or direction at different stages in the life cycle, there has been an implicit assumption, at least within the profession of physical education, that somehow the concepts of sport, health, and well-being should and do form a causal linkage. Moreover, the direction and order of the linkage is often assumed to be: sport > health > well-being.

However, there does not appear to be an overwhelming amount of valid evidence to support this trichotomous model, in general, or, indeed, even the existence of a strong relationship between "sport" and "health" or "sport" and "well-being" at any stage in the life cycle. Furthermore, little attention has been directed toward examining whether the concepts, as discrete entities or as interacting factors, can influence life chances or lifestyles across the life cycle or during the later years of life. Therefore, later sections of this paper highlight some conceptual and methodological issues that pertain to each concept, to the possible relationship between one concept and the others, and to how the concept might be operationalized when studying aging phenomena or older adults. But first, drawing upon accumulated knowledge from the field of gerontology, some general methodological issues and basic information about aging processes, about elderly persons, and about the aging population are introduced.

Aging as a Social Phenomenon

Aging is not exclusively a biological, psychological, or physiological process. Rather, there is reciprocal interaction among these processes with various social processes. More specifically, individuals with unique social characteristics pass

---

[1]A small section of the Proceedings from the 1972 (Grupe et al., 1973) and 1976 (Landry & Orban, 1978) Pre-Olympic Congresses include papers on sport or physical activity and aging. Few studies related to exercise or sport have been published in the major gerontology journals.

through stages of the life cycle within specific social contexts, historical periods, and physical environments that can significantly influence or alter one's life chances and lifestyle. Fortunately, for scientists there are some commonalities to these various experiences and patterns so that subgroups within specific age cohorts do have some common experiences, characteristics, and outcomes. However, there are often unique intercohort differences because of past experiences, historical events, or current situations that must be considered when studying aging phenomena or the elderly. For example, the unique background and the shared experiences of economic, political, historical, and social events can influence the values and lifestyle of a particular cohort and thereby differentiate a given cohort from younger or older cohorts who experience the same phenomena but at different stages in their particular life cycle (e.g., inflation, high unemployment, or the fitness boom can have a differential impact on one or more age cohorts).

There may also be unique intracohort differences, especially among the older population. It is for this reason that we should not, as in many studies to date, categorize the elderly as a single age cohort (i.e., 65 and older). In reality, there are at least two and possibly three elderly age cohorts (e.g., 55-64, 65-74, 75+), who may have different life experiences, in general, and specifically with respect to past or present physical activity involvement. Moreover, the composition of the three cohorts can vary dramatically on such important variables as: education, marital status (widowed vs. nonwidowed), health status, economic status, degree of mobility and independence, racial or ethnic background, religion, employment status, diet and nutritional status, sex ratio, amount of support provided by family and friends, fear of crime, and type of housing and place of residence. Some or all of these factors could influence the level of physical activity, health, or well-being and must be considered as possible intervening factors when attempting to explain physical activity or sport phenomena in the middle and later years of life.

Contrary to prevailing myths or assumptions, sport scientists and practitioners must recognize that only a minority of the elderly experience poor health, institutionalized living, poverty, loneliness, isolation, or senility. For those who do experience one or more of these conditions, most are among the very old (75+), and many are elderly widows. Thus, the later years should not be viewed as a period of life characterized by economic, health, psychological, social, or physical losses and problems, at least until very late in life. Rather, many of the apparent behavioral problems of the elderly reflect "ageism," "learned helplessness," or constitute "a self-fulfilling prophecy." In reality, a majority of the older population are independent individuals who live in the community rather than in institutions. As such, they are capable of participating in exercise and sport activities to varying degrees, if facilities, programs and leadership are available and if personal motivation is present. Herein lies the challenge to practitioners.

Methodological Issues and Concerns in Aging Research

With an increasing need to derive valid and more complete knowledge about physical activity patterns and outcomes in the middle and later years, serious attention needs to be directed to the unique methodological issues that pertain to the study of aging phenomena and the elderly (McPherson, 1983; Sinnott et al., 1983). These concerns must be addressed at all stages in the research process, but particular attention needs to be directed to the conceptualization of the research problem, the research design, the interpretation of data, and the generalizability of the findings. Sport scientists must not replicate the conceptual and methodological errors that characterized the early years of study in the field of gerontology. Thus, in order to enhance the quality and utility of the research process from the outset, the remainder of the paper raises a number of conceptual and methodological issues that need to be addressed and incorporated into studies of physical activity involvement during the middle and later years of life.

Aging Versus the Aged: The Process Versus the Product

With respect to physical activity, health, and well-being there is a need to understand phenomena pertaining to both the process of aging and the product of that process; namely, the status of being middle aged or elderly in a particular society or physical environment. To date, most research has been descriptive and has focused on the elderly per se, with little attempt to study physical activity phenomena from a process perspective. Hence, while we have accumulated some facts about older individuals, we know little about life-long aging processes that may influence the current situation of an elderly person or cohort. In short, there is a need for greater research emphasis on the processes than the product.

Aging, the Elderly, and the Physical Environment

In addition to the biological, psychological, and social processes that influence individual and population aging, a number of factors in the past, present, or future physical environment may influence life chances and lifestyle throughout middle and late adulthood. That is, the physical context in which individuals and cohorts age must be understood, especially with respect to current health status, health care utilization, degree of mobility and independence, and the availability of support services and programs, including those related to physical activity. Moreover, not only is the "objective" physical environment important but also the "subjective" meaning of the environment as perceived by an individual (Lawton, 1980). That is, the extent to which an environment is perceived by the elderly to be aesthetically appealing, safe, and familiar is an important element in personal lifestyle and life satisfaction, and, therefore, perhaps also in the degree to which physical activity programs and services are likely to be utilized.

To date, most studies in the area of physical activity, aging, and the aged have ignored the potential influence of such environmental factors as: geographical region, climate, seasonal migration of the retired elderly, type of housing (home, apartment, senior citizen housing, institution), quality of housing, living in an age-integrated versus an age-segregated neighborhood, rural-urban differences, and community size (Lawton, 1980; McPherson, 1983). More specifically, most research on aging phenomena and on the elderly has utilized subjects who dwell in private homes, in large middle-class urban or suburban environments, in modernized societies. Little is known about physical activity or sport involvement among aging individuals who dwell in rural settings, in small towns, in the central core of large metropolitan areas, in institutions, or in developing societies.

Aging Effects Versus Cohort Effects Versus Period Effects

People at different stages of life often exhibit not only different physical traits but different patterns of behavior in a number of social domains, including physical activity. These differences may be attributed to either changes with age within the individual as he or she matures (aging effects), to changes in behavior that may be unique to most or all members of a particular cohort because of the impact on that cohort of specific events or situations (cohort effects), or to the influence of a particular historical event (e.g., the depression, World War II) that had a more profound effect on one or more cohorts than on any other cohort (period effect). Thus, if variations between age groups are found (usually in cross-sectional studies), investigators must be able to interpret whether these variations are attributable to age changes (aging effects), to age differences (cohort effects), or to historical (period) effects (Costa & McCrae, 1982).

Research Designs

To date, most research pertaining to aging phenomena has examined either differences between age groups on a variety of variables, or changes that occur in individuals or groups as they pass through the life cycle. Typically, cross-sectional studies, using subjects from different age groups, have been utilized. These studies may or may not employ the traditional experimental design with a control group. In many instances where activity patterns across the life cycle are studied, the data are derived from secondary analyses of social surveys (e.g., McPherson & Kozlik, 1980; Canada Fitness Survey, 1982; Ministry of Tourism and Recreation, 1983). However, cross-sectional designs can only indicate *differences* between age groups at a specific point in time. They cannot be used to conclude that changes have occurred because of aging phenomena or to explain why the pattern varies by age group. Nor is this design suitable for determining whether a curvilinear relationship exists between two variables over time.

In addition, this method does not account for possible seasonal variations in emotion, interest, participation, or performance (Smith, 1979). To illustrate, data collected in February may vary from that collected in June because of seasonal variations in interests, needs, or opportunities. That is, we can never be sure that a response is stable and enduring, especially if there are changes in climate or weather. Rather, the observed pattern may represent an artifact of a single year or month when the data were collected. To illustrate, it has been found that suicide rates decline on the days surrounding special holidays, such as Christmas and one's birthday. Similarly, with respect to physical activity involvement, adults may become more or less active prior to or following festive events such as Christmas, Lent, one's wedding, or as a result of New Year's Resolutions. In short, cross-sectional designs only alert us to patterns of behavior that may vary by age (age differences). They cannot explain age changes.

Longitudinal designs (Chappell, 1983) can provide a more complete explanation of age changes over time (i.e., a panel study). However, this type of study is expensive, time-consuming, and susceptible to the loss of subjects, especially when older subjects are included. Moreover, longitudinal designs are often highly dependent on volunteers, and thus sources of potential intracohort bias (e.g., higher than average levels of health, physical activity, intelligence, or mobility) must be controlled if valid conclusions are to be drawn. An additional weakness of longitudinal designs is that generalizations about the aging process or about the behavior of the elderly may reflect a situation that is unique to only one cohort. This is known as "cohort-centrism." Thus, to account for intercohort variation, longitudinal studies of aging phenomena should include at least two birth cohorts, preferably separated by 5 to 10 years. In this way, period (historical) effects and variations in socialization experiences (cohort effects) may be identified and controlled.

In order to eliminate some of the inherent weaknesses of the above designs, researchers in gerontology are increasingly employing the technique of cohort analysis (Schaie, 1965; Glenn, 1977, 1981). In this design, similar information is collected at different time periods, but different individuals within the same age cohort are sampled each time. This is a common method in national surveys that are repeated at regular intervals. This design accounts for age changes due to maturation, to cohort differences, and to period or historical effects. In many instances this design is used in retrospective secondary analyses of data stored in archives. However, it is essential to determine whether the meaning and wording of questions are similar from survey to survey; otherwise, changes over time could be due to changes in the instruments rather than to changes with age (i.e., aging effects).

Another concern related to experimental designs in gerontology is that one control group may not be sufficient. This is especially true because of potential intracohort variations among elderly subjects on key variables such as health, past experience in physical activity, economic status, or degree of physical mobility. More specifically, in studies using "well-being" or other psychological constructs, one sedentary control group used in conjunction with an experimental exercise group may not be sufficient. Rather, as Morgan (1984) notes, other forms of therapy or diversion that may distract the individual from stress or boredom should be accounted for by the use of additional control groups. In short, more than one control group should be utilized in exercise and activity studies to control for intra- and intercohort variations among elderly subjects.

A final design consideration is the extent to which aging-related research should be unidisciplinary, interdisciplinary, or multidisciplinary. With respect to the sport sciences, while the nature of the problem or topic should dictate the approach, there could very well be greater levels of explanation achieved concerning aging phenomena and the elderly if sport scientists from different disciplines were to pool their expertise. Specifically, greater attention needs to be directed to possible interactions among social, psychological, biological, and physiological variables. As members of multidisciplinary departments and professional associations, we have a unique opportunity to demonstrate leadership in the integration of various disciplines to enhance the study of aging phenomena.

The Population and Sampling

Investigators working in this area must be aware of the increasing heterogeneous composition of the adult population with age, and the decreasing sex ratio (fewer males than females) with age, especially after age 65. The elderly are perhaps the most heterogeneous age cohort in society because of great variation in lifelong experiences; because of varying degrees of health status, marital status, employment status, degree of independent living, mobility, and income; and because of higher death rates among males. At present the sex ratio in Canada and the United States is 86 and 68 males per 100 females, respectively, for the population 65 years of age and older. It is projected that this ratio will decline to about 78 in Canada and to about 65 in the United States by the year 2000. Not surprisingly, for increasingly older cohorts beyond age 65 the sex ratio decreases even more dramatically. To illustrate, in Canada the decline at present is as follows: .83 (70 to 74), .71 (75 to 79), .63 (80 to 84), .59 (85 to 89), and .54 (90+).

As a result of this decreasing sex ratio and the potential of extreme intracohort individual differences on important demographic and lifestyle characteristics, those 65 years of age and over should not be grouped into a single age category, as occurs in many studies. Rather, at least two or three categories of older subjects should be utilized to account for cohort differences, as well as age-related individual differences. Furthermore, females should be proportionately sampled for each age cohort in order to accurately represent the composition of older age groups.

As with any population with unique characteristics, there are difficulties in identifying the elderly population and drawing a truly representative sample. Hence, many studies have utilized volunteers from readily visible and available groups of senior citizens, namely, church members or attendees at senior citizen centers. Members of these volunteer, handy groups are not representative of the general population of older adults, and, indeed, to use these subjects may introduce biases that favor the more active, healthy, mobile, and independent older adult. This has serious ramifications for the generalizability of findings that pertain to sport or physical activity domains. Moreover, males may be underrepresented when samples are drawn from church or senior citizen center groups.

One approach to selecting a more representative sample of older adults is to employ a two-stage sampling design (Lee & Finney, 1977). The first stage identifies and describes the elderly who reside within a large probability sample of residences (institutionalized and/or noninstitutionalized) within a community, region, or country. In the second stage a representative sample is drawn—one that accounts for the sex ratio, intracohort sociocultural variations (e.g., class, ethnicity, education), and other important factors in the specific study—and the consent of those selected is obtained. In short, when studying the elderly population, do not ignore or underrepresent females, and ensure that the heterogeneity of the elderly population on potentially important variables is considered when defining the criteria for sampling. Otherwise, interpretations may be misleading or invalid, and the generalizability of the findings will be seriously restricted.

Measurement and the Elderly Population

Collecting data from the elderly, especially the very old, can create special problems for an investigator. While many of these concerns are unique to particular research methods (e.g., fear about using treadmills or bicycles, apprehension concerning blood samples and biopsies), some general concerns are prevalent. For example, older subjects may be skeptical or misinformed about the research process, in general, and may feel insecure and apprehensive in the presence of scientists and their staffs. This applies especially to social scientists, who are unlikely to wear white lab coats, and who are likely to ask for "personal" information. Thus, it is essential that rapport and open communication be established early to obtain their cooperation and thereby enhance the quality of the data collection process. It may also take more time to collect information from older subjects, and this must be considered when designing the budget and scheduling staff and subjects for test sessions.

With respect to the social sciences, there are a number of specific concerns that must be addressed when studying the older population. First, at least for the immediate future, many older people have not been "raised" on questionnaires, multiple-choice questions, and inquisitions about "personal" matters. Second, older respondents, like young children, may be more likely to respond in socially approved directions and thereby report a situation that is better or higher than reality would warrant, especially as it relates to personal matters such as income, well-being, quality of housing, or degree of independence. They may also be more likely to respond with "no opinion" or "don't know," or be unwilling or unable to reveal true feelings or facts. Third, they may be suspicious of interviewers who appear unannounced at the door, they may be unable to recall information, or they may misinterpret questions because of hearing deficiencies, fatigue, or a short attention span. Finally, questionnaires must be carefully pretested for meaning, readability (e.g., size of type), and clarity of instructions for completing and returning the instrument. Fortunately, all of the above concerns can be resolved, but they must be specifically considered when designing studies that involve older subjects (McPherson, 1983).

A final measurement concern relates to the use of behavioral, cognitive, and social indicators during the middle and later years of adulthood. Some specific questions that must be addressed include: Are the measures appropriate and sufficiently sensitive to tap variation among older respondents? Does the wording of the question(s) account for cultural and educational variations among the elderly? Do attitude and behavioral questions tap daily fluctuations or long-term permanent characteristics or patterns? Are single-question indicators adequate or should multidimensional indicators be used to enhance reliability and conceptual completeness? Are the theoretical and operational definitions for the major independent and dependent variables similar (e.g., the wording of questions) from survey to survey so that aging and cohort effects can be identified across time? For example, what does "degree of physical activity" or "amount of sport involvement" mean to respondents of varying ages? Is walking, which is frequently reported as a major activity by the elderly, conceptualized as a low, moderate, or high intensity activity? In short, employing common theoretical and operational definitions across studies is essential.[2]

Physical Activity, Sport, Exercise, and Aging

This section provides an overview of patterns of physical activity involvement across the life cycle. While it is beyond the scope of this paper to review or debate the meaning of concepts (e.g., Is swimming a sport, exercise, or both?), scholars in the sport sciences must derive and employ common theoretical and operational definitions for such concepts as sport, exercise, and physical activity. In general, at least in North America, physical activity is used as a more global rubric that encompasses sport and exercise, whereas sport and exercise are more specific concepts that should be operationalized consistently from study to study. As a starting point, "sport" usually refers to watching or participating in some form of organized competitive game that requires varying degrees of skill, conditioning, and knowledge (e.g., tennis, golf, baseball). In contrast, "exercise" is less institutionalized, is not normally bound by rules, does not involve competition with others, requires less skill and knowledge of rules, and demands varying degrees of physical capacity and training (e.g., walking, jogging, cycling, calisthenics, aerobics, aquatics).

These concepts may also have different meanings to specific respondents. Hence, the definition must be stated in each study so as to establish a common response set. Furthermore, the meaning of a concept to a given individual may vary from one stage in the life cycle to another, among varying age cohorts, or within cohorts. To illustrate, it has been found that females are generally more interested and involved in "exercise" activities, whereas males are generally more involved in "sport" activities (Canada Fitness Survey, 1982). Thus, both concepts need to be measured to account for sex differences in physical activity involvement at varying points in the life cycle and for possible changes in the type of participation across the life cycle.

Based on a large number of cross-sectional studies in a variety of countries (Anderson et al., 1956; McPherson, 1978, 1982, 1984; McPherson & Kozlik, 1980; Boothby et al., 1981; Unkel, 1981; Stones & Kozma, 1982; d'Epinay, 1983; Curtis & White, 1984; Snyder & Spreitzer, 1984), there appears to be an almost universal pattern of declining involvement in physical activity with age, especially after adolescence. This pattern of less involvement by successively older cohorts is more significant among specific subgroups: the less educated, those who dwell in rural areas or smaller communities, women (especially if married and with preschool children), and those employed in manual or blue-collar occupations. Furthermore, only a small minority of older adults, primarily males, report being regularly involved in any type of physical activity (Cunningham et al., 1968; Harootyan, 1982; d'Epinay, 1983; Curtis

---

[2]A valuable source concerning the use, reliability, and validity of research instruments in social gerontology is the three volume series edited by Mangen and Peterson (1982).

& White, 1984), while in a recent Canadian study, only 7% of those 65 to 69 years of age were found to have reached a recommended level of cardio-vascular fitness on the Canada Home Fitness Test (Canada Fitness Survey, 1982). Clearly, the need and capacity for physical activity continues with chronological aging (Shephard, 1978; Smith & Serfass, 1981). Moreover, physiological and medical evidence suggest that most older adults have the ability to engage in some type of physical activity to some degree (McPherson, 1983). Yet, why do so few participate regularly and consistently during middle and later adulthood, and is this trend likely to continue?

Before reporting some of the many alternative explanations for this universal pattern of declining involvement by age, recent data collected for five age cohorts (15-19, 20-34, 35-54, 55-64, 65+), at two points in time (1976 and 1981), are reported to illustrate that cohort effects as well as aging effects must be identified (*Highlights*, 1983).[3] In this Canadian study, all age groups reported greater participation in both sport and exercise in 1981 than in 1976. Particularly large increases were reported by the oldest (65 and over) age cohort (an increase from 13% to 38% for sport; from 50% to 68% for exercise). In fact, those 65 and over were as likely to be active as much younger Canadians.

To date, a number of alternative explanations have been proposed for the generalized pattern of declining involvement by age and for the low levels of fitness and involvement found in those over 60 years of age (Spreitzer & Snyder, 1974, 1983; Wohl & Szwarc, 1981). Some of these sociological and psychological explanations include: inadequate early life socialization experiences; lack of opportunity (programs and facilities) during adulthood because of discrimination (ageism); learned helplessness in the later years; normative beliefs leading to a self-fulfilling prophecy that middle-aged and older adults should not participate in this type of leisure activity; a lack of role models; a lack of time due to competing family, work, or leisure responsibilities or interests; the presence of myths that physical activity is unnecessary or harmful in the middle or later years; and, as a remnant of disengagement theory, there is an inevitable and universal process of social and psychological disengagement that begins at retirement or widowhood. Thus, while chronological age per se does not appear to be a barrier to participation in physical activity, we have yet to derive a complete explanation as to why participation rates decrease by age, and why some elderly persons are active, while most are not. Herein lies a challenge to sport scientists so that policies and programs might be developed and initiated to change existing patterns.

In addition to the pursuit of a more complete explanation for existing patterns of involvement across the life cycle, there are a number of unanswered research questions that merit immediate inquiry. A number of these, primarily from a sociological perspective, have been raised in a recent paper by McPherson (1984). However, there are also more general questions that remain unaddressed or only partially answered with respect to the relationship between physical activity, health, and well-being across the life cycle. The following shopping list may serve as a stimulus for further research:

---

[3]The necessity of temporal and cohort analysis is further reinforced by the findings of Stones and Kozma (1982) that cross-sectional data reveal a pattern of decline in athletic performance with age that is approximately twice as steep as that suggested by a longitudinal design.

1. While regular physical activity at all stages in the life cycle may not increase longevity, to what extent, and how, can it enhance the quality of life and well-being in the middle and later years?
2. What impact does a life of physical labor at work have on health status and well-being following retirement?
3. Does the degree and type of physical activity involvement throughout the life cycle influence age at death or the health status of older persons?
4. To what extent is involvement at work in fitness programs related to absenteeism, job efficiency, productivity, rate of staff turnover, and morale? Some recent studies suggest that fitness and activity programs are important. But, might the provision of free video games or movies similarly reduce absenteeism and turnover and increase productivity and morale? That is, competing leisure activities have not been used as possible explanatory factors in controlled studies in corporate settings. Moreover, during periods of high unemployment, such as those that exist today, absenteeism declines since employees are more concerned about being positively evaluated to insure being retained. Many of the studies concerning corporate fitness programs for employees have been conducted during recent years when high levels of employment have been a factor in the labor force market.
5. Does the influence of physical activity on well-being during the middle and later years vary by whether the activity is competitive sport, recreational sport, or an informal exercise program? Does it vary by early-life activity patterns, sex, marital status, ethnic background, geographical region or place, and type of residence?

Health, Physical Activity, and Aging

Health and Aging

The relationship between health and aging has been a long-standing interest of some specialties within the medical profession. It is only in recent years that gerontologists with a social science, behavioral medicine, or health perspective have sought to examine health-related research questions (Hickey, 1980; Wantz & Gay, 1981; Kart & Metress, 1984). As a result there has been a shift within the field of gerontology from a "medical model" (with a focus on the incidence, cause, treatment, and medical response to illness or disease among the elderly) to a "functional model" of health and aging. This latter model seeks to describe and explain how individuals cope with age-related chronic disabilities; how acute and chronic illnesses influence social behavior within such domains as the family, work, and leisure; and how older persons adapt socially and psychologically when faced with increasing dependency because of age-related physical or mental illness. This functional model is also concerned with the economic and social costs of health care for the elderly; the relationship between the quantity and quality of life; and with the impact on physical and mental health of such potentially stressful events as later-life divorce, widowhood, forced loss of employment in midlife, or retirement.

As a result of increased research concerning the relationship between health and lifestyles, valid evidence is available to refute the myth of the frail, sick-ly, and socially isolated, elderly person. That is, among the elderly there is a range of individual differences in the onset and severity of acute and chronic conditions; in the availability of access to and use of health care facilities and services and in the physical, social, emotional, and cognitive reactions to varying degrees of changing health status. Some of these individual differences in reactions reflect former and present lifestyles (e.g., attitudes toward physical activity, use of alcohol or tobacco, nutritional habits); some are related to environmental factors (e.g., type of housing, urban vs. rural living, geographical region); some are related to achieved or ascribed social characteristics (e.g., sex, race, ethnicity, education, socioeconomic status, marital status); and some are related to the availability and use of informal (e.g., family, friends) and formal (e.g., social services, institutions) support systems. In short, the presence of varying levels of health status is not just a biological or medical problem but rather a significant personal and social concern that can influence adaptation and the degree of independence and mobility in the middle and later years. Thus, personal health status is an important independent and intervening variable in the study of age-related processes, especially because a change in health status is accompanied by changes in mood, attitudes, and type and degree of social participation, including physical activity.

Unfortunately, health status and health-related concepts are difficult to measure, and many objective and subjective measures have been utilized. For example, while both physical and mental health need to be assessed, seldom are both measures included in a given study. In fact, mental health is seldom measured. Moreover, a single objective or subjective measure of health status, regardless of age, is usually inadequate (Hickey, 1980; Mangen & Peterson, 1982). Thus, composite indicators are needed to determine the relationship between present level of health status and a variety of dependent variables, including level, type, and frequency of exercise or sport involvement.

Ideally, assessment of health status should involve some combination of a physician's rating of acute and chronic physical health, based on observations over a period of time; the subjective evaluations, perceptions, and expectations of the individual; the subjective evaluation of significant others (e.g., spouse, children); and objective and subjective assessments of functional health status. As a minimum, at least one measure should be obtained from a global health status dimension (e.g., perceived health status, degree of nutritional risk, perceived level of sensory and motor ability, level of mental health) and one from a functional dimension (e.g., ability to perform varying types of daily activities, level of cognitive functioning). More specifically, Wolinsky et al. (1984) recommend that perceived health status and number of activities of daily living be used because both are brief, reliable, and valid.

Despite the recognized need to use multiple indicators, valid, reliable, and conceptually clear measures of health status are unavailable. For example, many measures have been constructed to assess functional capacity or functional health[4] (Shanas et al., 1968; Lawton, 1971; Hickey, 1980;

---

[4]For example, the Canada Health Survey of 1978 used the following classification scheme to note the presence or absence of, and the severity of, long-term disability. In order of decreasing severity the categories were: cannot do major activity; restricted in the kind or amount of major activity performed; not restricted in major activity, but otherwise restricted; no long-term activity limitation. (cf. Wilkins and Adams, 1983).

Mangen & Peterson, 1982; Wilkins & Adams, 1983). This type of measure is important to physical activity scientists as it could be used to select and assign subjects to experimental groups, or it could serve as an independent, intervening, or dependent variable. However, most of the existing measures are of limited use because they tend to be too simplistic and conceptually incomplete; they lack the precision to discriminate in a meaningful and useful way; they are unclear as to the appropriate normative or reference group to which an individual is being compared; and they may be designed for use in a clinical setting with geriatric patients (i.e., the frail elderly). Similarly, subjective indicators that assess the "personal and social meanings of symptoms" (Hickey, 1980) seldom are administered over a period of time to identify consistency or change (i.e., control for mood or physical changes), and seldom, if ever, is an appropriate and consistent frame of reference provided to the respondent for comparison. Hence, an individual's self-perception may vary hourly, daily, or weekly and may vary according to whether the perceived standard is one's age peers, oneself last year or earlier in life, or one's ideal level. Moreover, it has not been determined that an individual can accurately and consistently rate his or her own health without exaggerating or underrepresenting the objective or desired level.

In order to overcome some of the above concerns, scholars interested in the relationship between health and physical activity should seek and use measures that not only monitor health status but that categorize the degree and type of activity limitation. This information is also important when planning physical activity programs for senior citizens with varying levels of activity restriction. These measures would enable an investigator to consider the behavioral consequences of chronic health impairment, rather than the mere presence of health problems, and to identify the number of years of expected disability-free life. This distinction is important because most middle-aged and elderly persons will report at least one health problem. But the problem is not usually perceived to be serious enough to limit them in their preferred activities. Some specific measures worth considering are the Index of Health Expectancy and the Quality-Adjusted Life Expectancy Index used by Wilkins and Adams (1983). For example, they found that 49% of those 65 and over reported conditions serious enough to limit their activities. More specifically, for all age groups they found lower levels of reported activity restriction for males, for those who live in large metropolitan regions, and for those in the highest income groups.

Because of increased longevity and the aging of the baby-boom generation, the amount of activity restriction can be expected to increase substantially in the future unless individually designed programs can be implemented to delay the onset and to increase the individual's ability to remain active, mobile, and independent. It is important for practitioners to recognize that until the year 2011 this increase can be expected in those who are 45 to 64 years of age, as well as those over 65. After 2011 almost all of the reported increase in activity restriction will be due to the increased number of persons over 65 years of age.

Physical Activity, Health, and Aging

With increasing age the need for physical activity as an important component of one's lifestyle does not decrease. Yet, as we have often seen, participation in physical activity decreases with age. Moreover, a physical health problem is frequently given as a major reason for the lack of involvement in sport or physical activity during middle and later adulthood. Yet, older persons may actually benefit more than younger persons from an appropriate exercise or physical activity program. Similarly, older persons often report more interest in their health than younger persons and often report being more interested in their health if they exercise (Yamaguchi, 1984). While a causal linkage has not been supported, although one is often assumed, participation in physical activity is generally highly correlated with subjective and objective ratings of physical health status at all ages. However, it may be that level of physical activity has a more profound influence on health status in the earlier years. In contrast, health status may have an increasingly greater effect on the type and degree of physical activity in the middle and later years.

With respect to the relationship between mental health and physical activity, little valid research evidence is available (Ostrow, 1980; Morgan, 1984). Again, many studies have found a correlation between activity and some hypothesized measure of mental health, but these studies have generally used volunteers (e.g., those who are already moderately or highly active), and many have used personality inventories that measure single components of mental health that are strictly psychological in nature (e.g., tension, anxiety, well-being, or personality traits). That is, psychological parameters rather than degree of mental health have been assessed. As Morgan (1984) succinctly states:

> The view that physical fitness training leads to improved mental health should be considered as hypothetical rather than factual. The correlational, cross-sectional and epidemiological data upon which this hypothesis is based reflects *necessary* rather than *sufficient* evidence. . . . While exercise may have caused the observed changes, there are many alternative hypotheses.

While this quote does not specifically address the issue of alternative hypotheses being used at varying stages in the life cycle, it is quite likely that alternative explanations for the observed relationship may vary by cohort or by stage in the life cycle. Indeed, observed relationships between activity and mental health across the life cycle may be represented by a linear, curvilinear, or inverted-U pattern. These theoretical and conceptual matters need to be addressed before further research is initiated on this topic.

The following are some possible questions and issues that need to be considered with respect to the relationship between physical activity and mental or physical health at various stages in middle and later life:

1. To what degree is physical fitness a component of physical and mental health at various stages in the life cycle?
2. Does physical activity enhance the quality of life at one stage more than at another?
3. To what extent, and how, can physical activity maintain or enhance functional independence in the later years (Canadian Public Health Association, 1983)?
4. What is the relationship between functional independence in later life and mental health?
5. Can physical activity retard, prevent, or assist in the rehabilitation of some acute and many chronic health conditions?

6. If the ability to cope with stressful events significantly influences mental health in the later years (McPherson, 1983), what is the influence of reduced physical health and reduced levels on the ability to cope with stress?
7. What are the dietary and nutritional needs of older persons who engage in varying levels of physical activity? Do these needs vary by sex and activity?
8. What is the impact of poverty on the dietary practices of older persons with varying levels of activity?
9. What role can various forms of exercise or sport play in maintaining health and productivity through the middle years and into old age?
10. How can persons be encouraged to adopt physical activity and health-promoting behaviors in the later years?
11. To what extent, and how, can exercise or sport compensate for age-related deficits and impairments so as to maintain levels of independence that will enable the individual to remain in the community rather than enter an institution?

Well-Being, Physical Activity, and Aging

Physical Activity and Well-Being

As noted earlier, a positive relationship is often reported between the type, degree, or level of physical activity, and subjective reports of well-being. But what is not known is to what extent this relationship varies across the life cycle, and if it varies, when and why it does so. Unfortunately, a major limitation of research on this subtopic is that, regardless of age, subjects are often volunteers who are more active, more educated, and in better physical and mental health. Thus, more attention needs to be directed to selecting samples that adequately represent the population of the age cohort being studied and to the use of valid and reliable indicators of well-being.

Well-Being and Aging

For much of its history, the field of gerontology has been concerned with the "problem" of the elderly and how to improve the lifestyle or quality of life of older persons. One outcome of this early orientation was a preoccupation with "successful" aging, especially the factors that might be related to some ideal way of aging. Hence, much of the research in social gerontology has involved correlational studies which examine the relationship between a variety of independent variables and a dependent variable that has variously been operationalized as life satisfaction, well-being, adjustment, happiness, morale, or quality of life (Lawton, 1975; Larson, 1978; George & Bearon, 1980; Lohmann, 1980; Sauer & Warland, 1982; Horley, 1984). In effect, all of these concepts are likely a subset of mental health and therefore highly intercorrelated.

Not surprisingly, sport scientists have also become interested in the relationship between the degree and type of physical activity involvement in the later years and the various measures of well-being, life satisfaction, or quality of life.[5] Moreover, because an increasing number of companies in the private sector are now offering employees mental health and lifestyle assistance programs, including fitness and sport programs, the number of sport scientists conducting research on well-being and aging is likely to increase. Therefore, this section introduces a number of methodological concerns that must be addressed when using such concepts as well-being, life satisfaction, morale, and quality of life.

To date, some of the predictors or correlates of life-satisfaction, well-being, or morale that have frequently been used include: health, number and type of personal resources, economic status, social class, education, satisfaction with housing, availability of transportation, marital status, widowhood, degree of social participation, social support from others, sex, and race. Of these, "research shows reported well-being to be most strongly related to health, followed by socioeconomic factors and degree of social interaction, for the general population of Americans over 60" (Larson, 1978). In most cases, subjective measures of these dependent variables have been used, especially those related to well-being. Unfortunately, these diverse measures of the various components of "successful" aging are frought with conceptual and methodological weaknesses. Some of these include:

• Varying degrees of conceptual overlap among the constructs of well-being, morale, happiness, life satisfaction, and adjustment. The constructs are frequently used interchangeably with little regard for conceptual or operational uniqueness. In fact, high intercorrelations between the scales are frequently observed.

• The measures are often too global. They lack a specific frame of reference for the respondent, and they fail to tap specific elements of well-being (e.g., symptoms of stress, quality of support from significant others, feelings of deprivation).

• The measures are not sensitive to temporal or seasonal variations in mood states, which, in fact, can influence one's score on most of these constructs. Indeed, few longitudinal studies have used the various measures of well-being.

• The same construct has been theoretically and operationally defined in so many ways that researchers cannot agree on what a particular construct means or how it should be measured. There is a need for greater concern with construct validity.

• The constructs have been measured mostly by unidimensional scales and seldom by multidimensional scales. There has been little attempt to determine whether a uni- or multidimensional approach is more reliable or valid.

• Little attention has been directed to developing or understanding the theory concerning the structure and meaning of the concept or their relationship to the various independent variables with which they have been correlated.

---

[5]For example, sport sociologists have been interested in the degree of adjustment (i.e., well-being, morale, life satisfaction) to retirement from sport by age-group swimmers (Brown, 1983), college athletes (Snyder & Baber, 1979), professional athletes (Arviko, 1976; McPherson, 1980; Lerch, 1981; Reynolds, 1981; Rosenberg, 1981b; Brandmeyer & Alexander, 1982; Lerch, 1982), and in the general process of retirement from a sport career (Rosenberg, 1981a; Coakley, 1983; Lerch, 1984; Rosenberg, 1984).

To illustrate, measures of economic, social, psychological, or environmental well-being could be included as a discrete item, or various combinations of these elements could be combined to form a composite indicator of well-being.

- There has been an overemphasis on the psychological or individual level of analysis, with little concern for environmental, cultural, or societal factors that may also be related to these various concepts.
- Seldom are controls for health status, marital status, ethnicity, education, age, economic status, or gender introduced into the analysis.
- Most studies have involved bivariate correlational analyses rather than multivariate analyses or causal models.
- Some of the instruments have been used with inappropriate populations. That is, an instrument designed for use with institutionalized geriatric patients should not, in most situations, be used with the noninstitutionalized population of the well elderly.
- Where both objective and subjective indicators are used, seldom are tests conducted for possible interactions between the two types of measures.
- Where age differences in the dependent measure are observed, they may reflect cohort differences in the response to some item(s), or they may reflect subcohort variation because of biased sample selection (e.g., the well-educated, those with the highest levels of health).
- Finally, seldom is the possibility of feedback or reciprocal influence considered for the independent and dependent variables.

In summary, despite the proliferation of studies employing the various concepts concerning well-being or successful aging, the many conceptual and methodological difficulties summarized above should alert sport scientists to the problems of research in this area. In fact, as Larson (1978) noted, only a small percentage (0-16%) of the variance has been explained by any one correlate of well-being. Thus, prior to initiating research concerning physical activity and well-being, sport scientists should diligently evaluate the use and limitations of existing measures (George, 1981) and develop a valid and logical theoretical rationale for the specific relationships to be studied.

Conclusion

As a result of the increasing interest by sport scientists and practitioners in age-related phenomena, it is essential from the outset of this new thrust of inquiry and practice that unique theoretical, conceptual, and methodological issues, already identified and addressed by gerontologists, be understood and incorporated into research designs and program development. This paper has attempted to raise and review some of these issues. Moreover, if valid and reliable research, policies, and programs are to be initiated, scholars and practitioners in the sport sciences must first acquire substantive knowledge concerning aging processes and the aged, from both a unidisciplinary and an interdisciplinary perspective. In addition, they must understand the conceptual and methodological issues unique to the study of an aging individual or population. More specifically, we must not, as we have with other topics at earlier stages in the development of our disciplines, ignore the existing experience and knowledge accumulated by other disciplines and professions. Nor can we ignore the many social, historical, cultural, environmental, political, and economic factors that can influence physical activity involvement patterns or potential in the middle and later years of life. Hence, to enhance the amount of explanation concerning physical activity and age-related phenomena, interdisciplinary cooperation and designs are desirable, if not essential. As will be noted throughout this volume, most research papers are unidisciplinary in orientation. Hopefully, by the next Olympic Scientific Congress the level of conceptual and methodological sophistication will have increased and more interdisciplinary or multidisciplinary studies will have contributed to our level of understanding concerning physical activity and sport at various stages in the life cycle.

References

Anderson, H., Bo-Jensen, A., Elkaer-Hansen, H., & Sonne, A. (1956). Sports and games in Denmark in the light of sociology. *Acta Sociologica, 2*, 1-28.

Arviko, I. (1976). *Factors influencing the job and life satisfaction of retired baseball players*. Unpublished master's thesis, Department of Kinesiology, University of Waterloo, Ontario, Canada.

Boothby, J. et al. (1981). Ceasing participation in sports activity: Reported reasons and their implications. *Journal of Leisure Research, 13*, 1-14.

Brandmeyer, G., & Alexander, L. (1982). Dealing with tempered dreams: Reflections of aging ballplayers on careers that used to be. In A. Ingham & E. Broom (Eds.), *Proceedings of the Conference on Career Patterns and Career Contingencies in Sport* (pp. 454-461). Vancouver, British Columbia, Canada: University of British Columbia.

Brown, B. (1983). *Factors influencing the process of withdrawal by female adolescents from the role of competitive age group swimmers*. Unpublished doctoral dissertation, Department of Kinesiology, University of Waterloo, Ontario, Canada.

Canada Fitness Survey. (1982). *Fitness and Aging*. Ottawa: Fitness Canada.

Canadian Public Health Association. (1983). *National Conference on Fitness in the Third Age*. Ottawa: Canadian Public Health Association.

Chappell, N. (Ed.). (1983). *Longitudinal design and data analysis in aging*. Winnipeg: University of Manitoba Center on Aging.

Coakley, J. (1983). Leaving competitive sport: Retirement or rebirth. *Quest, 35*(1), 1-11.

Costa, P., & McCrae, R. (1982). An approach to the attribution of aging, period and cohort effects. *Psychological Bulletin, 92*(1), 238-250.

Cunningham, D., Montoye, H., Metzner, H., & Keller, J. (1968). Active leisure time activities as related to age among males in a total population. *Journal of Gerontology, 23*, 551-556.

Curtis, J.E., & White, P.G. (1984). Age and sport participation: Decline in participation with age or increased specialization with age? In N. Theberge & P. Donnelly (Eds.), *Sport and the sociological imagination* (pp. 273-293). Fort Worth, TX: Texas Christian University Press.

d'Epinay, C. (1983). *Vieillesses*. Geneva, Switzerland: Editions Georgi.

George, L. (1981). Subjective well-being: Conceptual and methodological issues. In C. Eisdorfer (Ed.), *Annual Review of Gerontology and Geriatrics* (Vol. 2) (pp. 345-384). New York: Springer.

George, L., & Bearon, L. (1980). *Quality of life in older persons: Meaning and measurement*. New York: Human Sciences.

Glenn, N. (1977). *Cohort analysis*. Beverly Hills: Sage.

Glenn, N. (1981). Age, birth cohorts and drinking: An illustration of the hazards of inferring effects from cohort data. *Journal of Gerontology, 36*(3), 362-369.

Grupe, O., Kurz, D., & Teipel, J.M. (1973). *Sport in the modern world—Chances and problems*. New York: Springer-Verlag.

Harootyan, R. (1982). The participation of older people in sports. In R. Pankin (Ed.), *Social approaches to sport* (pp. 122-147). East Brunswick, NJ: Associated University Presses.

Hickey T. (1980). *Health and aging*. Monterey, CA: Brooks/Cole.

Highlights (No. 14). (1983). Ottawa: Canada Fitness Survey.

Hobart, C. (1975). Active sports participation among the young, the middle-aged and the elderly. *International Review of Sport Sociology, 10*(3-4), 27-44.

Horley, J. (1984). Life satisfaction, happiness and morale: Two problems with the use of subjective well-being indicators. *The Gerontologist, 24*(2), 124-127.

Kart, C., & Metress, S. (1984). *Nutrition, the aged, and society*. Englewood Cliffs, NJ: Prentice-Hall.

Landry, F., & Orban, W. (Eds.). (1978). *Physical activity and human well-being*. Miami: Symposia Specialists.

Larson, R. (1978). Thirty years of research on the subjective well-being of older Americans. *Journal of Gerontology, 33*(1), 109-125.

Lawton, M.P. (1971). The functional assessment of elderly people. *Journal of the American Geriatrics Society, 19*, 465-481.

Lawton, M.P. (1975). The Philadelphia Geriatric Center Morale Scale: A revision. *Journal of Gerontology, 30*, 85-89.

Lawton, M.P. (1980). *Environment and aging*. Monterey, CA: Brooks/Cole.

Lee, G., & Finney, J. (1977). Sampling in social gerontology: A method of locating specialized populations. *Journal of Gerontology, 32*(6), 689-693.

Lerch, S. (1981). The adjustment to retirement of professional baseball players. In S. Greendorfer & A. Yiannakis (Eds.), *Sociology of sport: Diverse perspectives* (pp. 138-148). West Point, NY: Leisure Press.

Lerch, S. (1982). The life satisfaction of retired ballplayers. *Baseball Research Journal, 11*, 39-43.

Lerch, S. (1984). Athletic retirement as social death: The applicability of two thanatological models. In N. Theberge & P. Donnelly (Eds.), *Sport and the sociological imagination* (pp. 259-272). Fort Worth, TX: Texas Christian University Press.

Lohmann, N. (1980). Life satisfaction research in aging: Implications for policy development. In N. Datan & N. Lohmann (Eds.), *Transitions of aging* (pp. 27-40). New York: Academic Press.

Mangen, D., & Peterson, W. (Eds.). (1982). *Research instruments in social gerontology* (Vols. 1-3). Minneapolis: University of Minnesota.

McPherson, B. (1978). Aging and involvement in physical activity: A sociological perspective. In F. Landry & W. Orban (Eds.), *Physical activity and human well-being* (Vol. 1) (pp. 111-128). Miami: Symposia Specialists.

McPherson, B. (1980). Retirement from professional sport: The process and problems of occupational and psychological adjustment. *Sociological Symposium, 30*, 126-143.

McPherson, B. (1982). Leisure life-styles and physical activity in the later years of the life-cycle. *Recreation Research Review, 9*(4), 5-14.

McPherson, B. (1983). *Aging as a social process: An introduction to individual and population aging*. Toronto: Butterworths.

McPherson, B. (1984). Sport participation across the life-cycle: A review of the literature and suggestions for future research. *Sociology of Sport Journal, 1*(3), 213-230.

McPherson, B., & Kozlik, C. (1980). Canadian leisure patterns by age: Disengagement, continuity or ageism? In V. Marshall (Ed.), *Aging in Canada: Social perspectives* (pp. 113-122). Don Mills, Ontario: Fitzhenry & Whiteside.

Ministry of Tourism and Recreation. (1983). *Physical activity patterns in Ontario* (Vol. II). Toronto: Government of Ontario Bookstore.

Morgan, P., Shephard, R.J. Finucane, R., Schimmelfing, L., & Jazmaji, V. (1984). Health beliefs and exercise habits in an employee fitness programme. *Canadian Journal of Applied Sport Sciences,* 9(2), 87-93.

Morgan, W.P. (1984). Physical activity and mental health. In H. Eckert & H. Montoye (Eds.), *Exercise and health* (pp. 132-145). Champaign, IL: Human Kinetics.

Ostrow, A. (1980). Physical activity as it relates to the health of the aged. In N. Datan & N. Lohmann (Eds.), *Transitions of aging* (pp. 41-56). New York: Academic Press.

Reynolds, M. (1981). The effects of sport retirement on the job satisfaction of the former football player. In S. Greendorfer & A. Yiannakis (Eds.), *Sociology of sport: Diverse perspectives* (pp. 127-137). West Point, NY: Leisure Press.

Rosenberg, E. (1981a). Gerontological theory and athletic retirement. In S. Greendorfer & A. Yiannakis (Eds.), *Sociology of sport: Diverse perspectives* (pp. 118-126). West Point, NY: Leisure Press.

Rosenberg, E. (1984). Athletic retirement as social death: Concepts and perspectives. In N. Theberge & P. Donnelly (Eds.), *Sport and the sociological imagination* (pp. 245-258). Fort Worth, TX: Texas Christian University Press.

Sauer, W., & Warland, R. (1982). Morale and life satisfaction. In D. Mangen & W. Peterson (Eds.), *Research instruments in social gerontology* (Vol. 1). Minneapolis: University of Minnesota Press.

Schaie, K.W. (1965). A general model for the study of developmental problems. *Psychological Bulletin,* 64(2), 92-107.

Shanas, E., Townsend, P., Wedderbum, D., Friis, H., Milhoj, P., & Stehouwer, J. (1968). *Old people in three industrial societies.* New York: Atherton Press.

Shephard, R. (1978). *Physical activity and aging.* London: Croom Helm.

Sinnott, J., Harris, C., Block, M., Collesano, S., & Jacobson, S. (1983). *Applied research in aging: A guide to methods and resources.* Boston: Little, Brown.

Smith, E., & Serfass, R. (Eds.). (1981). *Exercise and aging: The scientific process.* Hillside, NJ: Enslow.

Smith, T. (1979). Happiness: Time trends, seasonal variations, intersurvey differences, and other mysteries. *Social Psychology Quarterly,* 42(1), 18-30.

Snyder, E., & Baber, L. (1979). A profile of former collegiate athletes and nonathletes: Leisure activities, attitudes toward work and aspects of satisfaction with life. *Journal of Sport Behavior,* 2, 211-219.

Snyder, E., & Spreitzer, E. (1984). Patterns of adherence to a physical conditioning program. *Sociology of Sport Journal,* 1(2), 103-116.

Spreitzer, E., & Snyder, E. (1974). Correlates of life satisfaction among the aged. *Journal of Gerontology,* 29(4), 454-458.

Spreitzer, E., & Snyder, E. (1983). Correlates of participation in adult recreational sports. *Journal of Leisure Research,* 15(1), 28-38.

Stones, M., & Kozma, A. (1982). Cross-sectional, longitudinal and secular age trends in athletic performances. *Experimental Aging Research,* 8(4), 185-188.

Unkel, M. (1981). Physical recreation participation of females and males during the adult life cycle. *Leisure Sciences,* 4(1), 1-27.

Wantz, M., & Gay, J. (1981). The aging process: A health perspective. Cambridge, MA: Winthrop.

Wilkins, R., & Adams, O. (1983). *Healthfulness of life.* Montreal: The Institute for Research on Public Policy.

Wohl, A., & Szwarc, H. (1981). The humanistic content and values of sport for elderly people. *International Review of Sport Sociology, 16*(4), 5-13.

Wolinsky, F., Coe, R., Miller, D., & Prendergast, J. (1984). Measurement of the global and functional dimensions of health status in the elderly. *Journal of Gerontology, 39*(1), 88-92.

Yamaguchi, Y. (1984). *Socialization into physical activity in corporate settings: A comparison of Japan and Canada*. Unpublished doctoral dissertation, Department of Kinesiology, University of Waterloo.

2

Life Course Socioeconomic Transitions and Sport Involvement: A Theory of Restricted Opportunity

William J. Rudman
UNIVERSITY OF ILLINOIS AT URBANA-CHAMPAIGN
URBANA, ILLINOIS, USA

For millions of Americans sport activities are an important part of life. Current findings suggest the social and economic implications of increased sport participation go far beyond participation in the sport itself. As a social force, sport serves as an acceptable method of teaching social norms, reinforcing cultural values, and facilitating social integration (Kenyon & McPherson, 1974; Guttman, 1978; McPherson, 1983; Snyder & Spreitzer, 1983). Economic aspects focus on sports as a forum to display economic and status disparity, as an escape from the drudgery of work, and as a means of upward social and economic mobility (Dunning & Sheard, 1976; Ingham, 1978; Rigauer, 1981).

The purpose of this paper is to explore variations in sport participation at various stages in the adult socioeconomic life course of the individual. Unlike much of the previous research where age-related determinants are operationalized to have a constant effect on sport behavior at different ages (DeGrazia, 1962; Kenyon, 1966; Wohl, 1979; McPherson, 1983); this study looks at differential effects of sport determinants within specific age categories. This allows for a direct examination of social and economic factors over the life course of the individual. Implicit assumptions made about aging and social processes are: (a) transitions through socioeconomic periods are the underlying determinants of sport participation; (b) factors affecting sport involvement vary across age categories; (c) there is a common standard of acceptable behaviors centered around a shared value system where sports are viewed as positive social activities.

In addition to traditional resource explanations of sport behavior, the interpretation of the current findings will center around various types of the social opportunity dimensions. Many of the hypothesized results are speculative in nature and are presented in the form of alternative explanations. An effort will be made to integrate different facets of opportunity theory found primarily in the criminology literature (Hirschi, 1969; Cohen & Felson, 1979), along with resource-based explanations (Yiannakis, 1975; Ingham, 1978; Lueschen, 1983). Opportunity processes are broadly conceptualized as age-dependent socioeconomic transitions related to: (a) attachment to significant others—interpersonal bonds; (b) commitment—beliefs in desirability of sports; (c) geography—environmental factors; and (d) economic opportunity—social class, education, income. These measures are intended to designate varying degrees of exposure and access to sport activities. Sport participation is expected to be limited when exposure is limited. For example, past research suggests that married couples are more likely to be involved in home-centered activities (Cohen & Felson, 1979). Because access and exposure to sport activities are limited for married couples, sport participation should decrease. A summary of expected effects in propositional form is presented in Table 1.

Data and Methods

Data for this study were collected from a national survey on Americans' beliefs, interests, and participation in sport conducted by the Miller Lite Beer Company. Data came from a simple random phone survey of 1,319 adults, over the age of 13, October 1-October 30, 1983. After deleting missing data and restricting the analysis to those 18 and older, results are based on a sample of 970.

Ordinary least squares regression analysis using pairwise deletion as a method of dealing with missing data was the statistical technique used in this study. Use of regression analysis allows for simultaneous control over the effects of each independent variable and provides adequate tests of statistical significance for expected patterns of sport participation. Separate regression analyses were performed for three different age groups of 18-34, 35-54, and over 55 in order to test for interactions between age and various dimensions of opportunity.

Variations in sport participation are the dependent variables in this study. Both type and degree of sport involvement were examined. The following sports were used as dependent variables: tennis, golf, bike riding, ice skating, basketball, and football. These sports were chosen because they seemed to represent a broad range of individual and team sports. Specific demographic and opportunistic dimensions are the independent variables in this study. Attachment is operationalized on the basis of family commitments. First, marital status is coded as 1 = married and 0 = not married; second, the effect of having children is coded as number of children living in the household. Using factor analysis as a method of grouping variables, commitment was scaled according to the following questions measuring the social desirability of sport:

1. "Competition is good for kids because it teaches them to do their best?"

Table 1. Summary table of hypotheses related to sport participation

	Main effects	Type of sport	Age
Age	As age increases—participation decreases	Age effect strongest for team sports	
Sex	Males more likely to have higher rates of participation	Sex effect strongest for team sports	Age effect strongest for males
Race	Whites more likely to have higher rates of participation	Whites more likely to participate in individual sports	Age effect strongest for blacks
Marriage	Married individuals less likely to participate in sport	Marriage effect strongest for team sports	Marriage effect strongest among younger age groups
Children	Number of children increases— participation level decreases	Child effect weakest for team sports	Child effect strongest for the middle age groups
Region	Participation decreases where environmental and spatial factors are prevalent		
Population	As size of population increases— participation level increases	Population size effect strongest for team sports	
Skill	As skill level increases— participation increases	Upper social class more likely to participate in individual sports	Age effect increases as social class decreases
Education	As education increases— participation increases	As education increases—the more likely participation in individual sports	Age effect increases as education decreases
Income	As income increases— participation increases	As income increases—the more likely participation in individual sports	Age effect increases as income decreases
Commitment	The greater the belief in the desirability of sport the higher the level of participation		

2. "There are more opportunities in sport than any other field for the social advancement of blacks and other minorities?"
3. "Athletes are often the best role models children can have?"
4. "Increased participation in sport by youth would greatly reduce crime?"
5. "The US should use the same procedure as East Germany and Russia to identify and train potentially outstanding young athletes so we can achieve sport superiority?"

Income and education measures of economic opportunity were operationalized using traditional definitions from past stratification research. Education is categorized as less than eighth grade, some high school, high school, some college, college, and postgraduate work. Income is coded into five categories ranging from less than $10,000 to over $50,000 a year for household income. Social class is a dummy variable based on current neo-Marxist conceptions of the workplace (Braverman, 1974; Edwards, 1979) where 1 represents professionals and upper-level management, sales, clerical, transportation, skilled and unskilled blue-collar workers, and laborers. The other variables were coded as follows: age into the numerical age of the respondent; race, 1 = white and 0 = nonwhite; sex, 1 = male and 0 = female.

Results

Findings reported in this study suggest that a strong consistent relationship exists between sport involvement and various social and economic processes. Analysis of the entire sample before disaggregating by age provides support for much of the previous work. First, as age increased, participation levels in sport decreased. Age was the primary determinant of sport participation in most cases. Second, the effect of age was stronger for team sports. The slopes of the regression lines are steeper and the effect of age within the different models is stronger. Respondents are more likely to participate in individual sports at older ages.

Regression results disaggregated by age are presented in Tables 2 and 3. By focusing on different age groupings, several behavioral patterns not found in previous research are apparent. Results clearly show how sport involvement is related to social processes that integrate society and to economic processes that distinguish stratified segments of society. Attachment and economic opportunity dimensions have important effects that vary in terms of type and level of involvement by age of the individual. As expected, the negative effect of getting married is strongest in the 18-34 age category. Surprisingly, the difference does not seem to be based on type of sport but on levels of male and female participation. Where sex was not a determinant of participation (tennis, bike riding, ice skating) sport involvement seems to be an important meeting place where single individuals are able to interact. Participation may serve as a way of initiating prospective dating relationships.

Unlike the negative effect of being married on sport participation, having children had a strong positive effect on certain types of sport involvement within the 35-54 age group. Family-oriented sports (football, basketball) enabled

Table 2. Participation level in sport disaggregated by age of respondent: Controlling for the effects of sex, race, attachment, geographic variations, commitment, and economic opportunity

	Tennis			Golf			Bike Riding		
	18-34	35-54	55+	18-34	35-54	55+	18-34	35-54	55+
Sex	.1547 (.0528)	-.0463 (-.0211)	-.0638 (-.0397)	.3626 (.1659)**	.2362 (.1071)*	.2467 (.1287)	-.2427 (-.0618)	-.0653 (-.0181)	.0549 (.0196)
Race	.1425 (.0389)	-.0908 (-.0330)	.3494 (.0929)	.2419 (.0884)	.0119 (.0041)	-.1017 (-.0227)	-.4819 (-.0981)*	-.2151 (-.0449)	.2963 (.0542)
N. England	.4853 (.0913)	.0378 (.0096)	1.0070 (.2356)**	-.1199 (-.0280)	-.1619 (-.0449)	.7384 (.1536)	-.0685 (-.0096)	-.0461 (-.0075)	1.7635 (.2835)**
East	.1147 (.0173)	.0197 (.0064)	.2375 (.0964)	.0565 (.0180)	-.1874 (-.0608)	-.1964 (-.0669)	-.2896 (-.0519)	.0354 (.0068)	-.3290 (-.0918)
South	-.0019 (-.0006)	-.0059 (-.0026)	.3153 (.1859)*	-.2340 (-.0999)	-.1645 (-.0730)	-.0243 (-.0121)	-.3855 (-.0917)	-.2707 (-.0732)	.1340 (.0547)
West	.2090 (.0483)	-.2121 (-.0597)	.0515 (.0222)	.1217 (.0397)	.2415 (.0674)	.0217 (.0098)	-.3197 (-.0551)	-.2359 (-.0401)	-.4697 (-.1394)*
City	-.0519 (-.0463)	-.0668 (-.0768)	.0186 (.0294)	.0071 (.0085)	.0033 (.0037)	-.0034 (-.0046)	.1127 (.0756)	-.0204 (-.0142)	-.1249 (-.1364)*

(cont.)

Table 2. (Cont.)

Married	−.4451 (−.1522)**	.0993 (.0402)	.2339 (.1466)	.0981 (.0450)	.2219 (.0892)	.0053 (.0027)	−.5030 (−.1284)**	−.0464 (−.0114)	−.1472 (−.0634)
Child	−.0805 (−.0519)	.0901 (.0891)	.2640 (.1288)	−.0320 (−.0261)	−.0608 (−.0597)	.3506 (.1435)*	.0131 (.0063)	.3466 (.2073)**	.2296 (.0769)
S. Class	−.1584 (−.0464)	.0272 (.0116)	.4158 (.2433)**	.1395 (.0547)	.2989 (.1264)*	.0533 (.0271)	−.1865 (−.0408)	.0444 (.0114)	−.1102 (−.0634)
Education	.1880 (.1400)**	.1374 (.1892)**	.1291 (.2508)**	.0621 (.0637)	.0156 (.0214)	.1522 (.2481)**	.1551 (.0885)	.1206 (.1005)*	.1037 (.1385)*
Income	.0069 (.0094)	.0537 (.1075)	.0113 (.0275)	.0308 (.0561)	.0706 (.1403)**	.0903 (.1897)**	.0208 (.0210)	.0095 (.0116)	−.0562 (−.0940)
Commitment	−.1158 (−.0913)	.0210 (.0290)	−.0024 (−.0055)	.0124 (.0130)	.0160 (.0219)	.0610 (.0309)	.0103 (.0061)	−.0566 (−.0473)	−.1068 (−.1695)*
R squared	.08134	.09720	.2733	.07670	.11283	.22263	.03980 (ns)	.07467	.17282
N of cases	390	412	150	390	412	150	390	412	150

p value one-tailed test ** .001, * .05
( ) Standardized regression co-efficients

Table 3. Participation level in sport disaggregated by age of respondent: Controlling for the effects of sex, race, attachment, geographic variations, commitment, and economic opportunity

	Ice Skating			Basketball			Football		
	18-34	35-54	55+	18-34	35-54	55+	18-34	35-54	55+
Sex	-.2573 (-.1069)*	.0082 (.0049)	-.0180 (-.0982)	.9891 (.2973)**	.3156 (.1507)**	.0881 (.1875)*	.8148 (.2780)**	.3396 (.2903)**	.0876 (.1879)*
Race	-.2182 (-.0724)	.0414 (.0186)	.0093 (.0298)	-1.0010 (-.2403)**	-.1471 (-.0530)	.0643 (.0581)	.2211 (-.0602)	.0412 (.0168)	.0636 (.0583)
N. England	-.1834 (-.0420)	-.0523 (-.0183)	.1742 (.4939)**	-.1343 (-.0222)	-.1344 (-.0377)	.0188 (.0151)	.2744 (-.0522)	.1533 (.0486)	.0190 (.0154)
East	.0441 (.0128)	-.0605 (-.0258)	.0168 (.0819)	-.0732 (-.0153)	-.1115 (-.0391)	-.0236 (-.0328)	-.0054 (-.0013)	.0181 (.0070)	-.0235 (-.0329)
South	-.2169 (-.0841)	-.2719 (-.1583)**	.0085 (.0604)	-.2042 (-.0530)	-.1504 (-.0702)	.0551 (.1111)	-.0972 (-.0310)	.1009 (.0534)	.0550 (.1117)
West	-.3714 (-.1044)	-.2376 (-.0870)	.0095 (.0492)	-.0772 (-.0157)	-.0904 (-.0014)	-.0060 (-.0089)	-.2778 (-.0641)	-.0562 (-.0187)	-.0057 (-.0084)
City	-.0598 (-.0649)	-.0531 (-.0795)	.0002 (.0038)	-.0200 (-.0157)	-.0019 (-.0014)	.0200 (.0200)	-.0050 (-.0044)	-.0402 (-.0547)	.0196 (.1075)

(cont.)

Table 3. (Cont.)

Married	-.3698 (-.1615)**	.0228 (.0120)	.0146 (.1109)	-.3146 (-.0947)	.0937 (.0897)	.0694 (-.1488)*	-.0961 (-.0329)	-.0510 (-.0245)	-.0698 (-.1490)*
Child	.0683 (-.0029)	.1416 (.2362)**	-.0022 (.0333)	-.0258 (-.0146)	.1871 (-.1932)**	.0087 (.0146)	.1429 (-.0921)	.2952 (.3458)**	.0087 (.0147)
S. Class	.0765 (.0277)	.0949 (.0527)	.0146 (.2111)**	-.0340 (-.0088)	-.0750 (-.0377)*	-.0727 (-.1457)*	-.3574 (-.1046)*	.0809 (.0408)	-.0716 (-.1444)**
Education	.0155 (.0144)	.0777 (.1392)**	-.0004 (-.0103)	-.0895 (-.0596)	-.0344 (-.0721)	.0198 (.1316)*	-.11501 (-.1140)*	-.0403 (-.0706)	.0196 (.1314)*
Income	.0251 (.0416)	-.0266 (-.0694)	-.0018 (-.0527)	-.0228 (-.0273)	.1275 (.1835)**	-.0012 (-.0098)	-.0084 (-.0113)	-.0347 (-.0822)	-.0013 (-.0111)
Commitment	-.0697 (.1169)	.0140 (.0189)	-.0063 (-.0013)	.0152 (.0106)	.0638 (.0921)	.0076 (.0597)	-.0148 (-.0117)	.0319 (.0521)	.0074 (.0052)*
R squared	.05580	.08949	.27984	.18279	.11513	.07229	.14039	.16623	.07209
N of cases	390	412	150	390	412	150	390	412	150

p value one-tailed test **.001, *.05
( ) Standardized regression co-efficients

family members to simultaneously participate. Skill level did not seem to be a deterrent of group participation. These were sports where access was easy and where cost of additional participants was minimal. Sport seems to be used by parents to provide relatively inexpensive entertainment, exercise, and training of valuable social skills that aid communication and cooperation techniques in other nonsport activities.

In addition to the varying effects of the attachment dimension of opportunity, strength, and direction of the effect of economic opportunity, indicators varied across type of sport and age of the individual. The importance of social class, education, and income determinants increased as age increased. In the older age groups, sport seems to serve as an important social activity distinguishing upper from lower socioeconomic groups. The effects of the economic factors were especially strong in the two traditional upper social class sports: tennis and golf. For both football and basketball, economic restraints were the most important underlying determinants of sport participation in the older age groups.

Although the effects of economic opportunity in traditional blue-collar team sports were not as strong as expected, there was a remarkable shift in the type of individual participating in team sports as age increased. Both basketball and football are predominantly male dominated and involve those from the lower social class. As age increases the effect of sex decreases, and participation shifts from the lower social classes to middle-class college-educated individuals. This pattern of sport behavior suggests that easy access to facilities and scheduling freedom to participate at various hours in the day where competition for facilities is at a minimum is an important determinant in participation. Those individuals in the lower social classes may still want to participate, as the data show (Miller Lite Study, 1983), but opportunity to participate is restricted.

Implications and Discussion

Implications of these results have far-reaching consequences in both future research on the aging effect on sport involvement and in the interpretation of the importance of sport in society. Studies where consideration is not given to the interaction between age and various dimensions of socioeconomic opportunity will be unsuccessful in accurately assessing the pattern of sport participation over the lifetime of the individual. Further, to better understand the importance of sport in society, it is necessary to examine participation patterns within various age groupings. These results clearly show that sport as a social and economic factor serves as means of social integration and of maintaining the existing social structure.

Depending on the age of the individual, sport serves either as an important setting where single individuals participate in socially accepted dating and courting activities, or as a source of family integration. Sports where both males and females participate together on an equal basis seem to facilitate the courting and marriage process. Sports where family members participate together serve as socially acceptable forms of behavior and provide further support of the traditional family structure. Further, these are sports that emphasize traditional societal norms and values associated with teamwork, cooperation, and the interdependence of the social system on each individual. Sport in this sense serves as an important place where the child can learn how to interact within society.

Economic opportunity dimensions relate directly to the social class base of sport within society. These findings are consistent with the literature on various forms of voluntary activity, which shows that as age increases, differences in the level of participation in voluntary activities between upper and lower social class individuals significantly increase. Upper social class individuals are much more likely to be involved in social activities at older ages. Consequently, these individuals directly control social processes related to the consumption and production of societal goods and services. Indirectly, control is over economic and political processes where power positions are traditionally associated with seniority in the system.

Additional support of the social class and economic base of sport in society are found in the patterns of the type of lower social class participation in sport. Generally, those in the lower social classes tend to participate in highly visible and professionally oriented team sports. This pattern of participation raises two serious questions related to the use of sport as a method of social control. First, there is a trend of individuals to enter sport as a means of upward mobility instead of a redirection of lower social class individuals into other professional areas where competition is reduced and success over the lifetime of the individual is less problematic. Second, because lifetime participation in team sports is limited by time and space restrictions, questions concerning the health of an entire segment of a population are important social and political concerns where sport has a direct relationship. Although these results are preliminary, they do suggest that further research on the aging process and an expanded conceptualization of the importance of sport in society needs further consideration.

References

Braverman, H. (1974). *Labor and monopoly capital*. New York: Monthly Review Press.

Cohen, L.E., & Felson, M. (1979). Social change and crime rate trends: A routine activity approach. *American Sociological Review,* **44**, 588-607.

DeGrazia, S. (1962). *Of time, work, and leisure*. New York: 20th Century Fund.

Dunning, E., & Sheard, K. (1976). The bifurcation of Rugby Union and Rugby League: A case study of organized conflict and change. *International Review of Sport Sociology,* **11**(2), 31-71.

Edwards, R. (1979). *Contested terrain: The transformation of the workplace in the twentieth century*. New York: Basic Books.

Guttman, J. (1978). *From ritual to record: The nature of modern sport*. New York: Columbia University Press.

Hirschi, T. (1969). *Causes of delinquency*. University of California Press.

Ingham, A.G. (1978). *American sport in transaction: The maturation of industrial capitalism and its impact upon sport*. Doctoral dissertation, University of Massachusetts, Amherst.

Kenyon, G.S. (1966). The significance of physical activity as a function of age, sex, education, and socio-economic status of northern United States adults. *International Review of Sport Sociology*, **9**(1), 70-96.

Kenyon, G.S., & McPherson, B.D. (1974). An approach to the study of sport socialization. *International Review of Sport Sociology*, **9**(1), 127-139.

Lueschen, G.R.F. (1983). The system of sport: Problems of methodology, conflict, and social stratification. In G.R.F. Lueschen & G.H. Sage (Eds.), *Handbook of social science of sport* (pp. 197-213). Champaign, IL: Stipes Publishing Co.

McPherson, B.D. (1983). *Aging as a social process*. Toronto, Canada: Butterworth.

Rigauer, B. (1981). *Sport and work*. New York: Columbia University Press.

Snyder, E.E., & Spreitzer, E. (1983). Sport, education and schools. In G.R.F. Lueschen & G.H. Sage (Eds.), *Handbook of social science of sport* (pp. 119-143). Champaign, IL: Stipes Publishing Co.

Wohl, A. (1979). Sport and social development. *International Review of Sport Sociology*, **14**, 5-20.

Yiannakis, A. (1975). A theory of sport stratification. *Sport Sociology Bulletin*, pp. 22-33.

3

Physical Activity and Aging in a Post-Industrial Society

Roy J. Shephard
UNIVERSITY OF TORONTO
TORONTO, ONTARIO, CANADA

Developed nations currently face the twin problems of an aging society and the rapid introduction of high technology. The present paper examines interactions between physical activity and aging in the context of this cultural change, drawing upon the recent experience of populations at "primitive," intermediate, and advanced stages of development.

Primitive Technology

The Setting

Studies of the Eskimo or Inuit people (Rode & Shephard, 1971; 1984) allow us to follow adjustments on a vastly accelerated time scale. Our observations have been centered on Igloolik (69° 40′N). This particular community of 700 people was selected for study in the early 1960s because many of the population were still following a traditional nomadic hunting lifestyle. Over the past 2 decades, the villagers have moved from a neolithic to a technological culture. The energy demands of daily living have dropped dramatically, and there have been associated alterations in the aging curve for fitness-related functions.

The Neolithic State

In 1969/70, the energy cost of eight different types of hunt was 15.4 MJ•day^{-1} (Godin & Shephard, 1973), comparable with traditional mining (15.3 MJ•day^{-1}) and forestry (15.4 MJ•day^{-1}). The Inuit woman of this epoch also faced a scarcity of household equipment, skins to chew and scrape, and a baby to carry on her back. Within the settlement her energy expenditure averaged about 10 MJ•day$-^{1}$—at field camps, costs were undoubtedly higher.

Physiological consequences of the vigorous lifestyle included a virtual absence of subcutaneous fat, strong leg muscles, and a large maximum oxygen intake (Rode & Shephard, 1971). Oxygen transport of the Inuit was better preserved until middle age, but the loss of function beyond 45 years was more rapid than in "white" society. This can probably be explained in cultural terms. As a grandparent, the traditional Inuit no longer went hunting but was nevertheless accorded first pick from the chase. A dramatic drop of daily energy expenditures was then associated with a rapid deterioration of fitness. It was also socially acceptable for the grandmother to accumulate quite a large amount of subcutaneous fat.

Early Acculturation

By 1970, many of the Inuit had accepted an intermediate level of technology, working at "blue-collar" jobs within the settlement—tasks such as ice-delivery and sewage bag collection. The average cost of 25 governmental and commercial activities for a 4- or 5-day week was about 13.7 MJ•day^{-1} (Godin & Shephard, 1973).

A simple job classification (hunter, intermediate status, or settlement worker) showed higher aerobic power and lesser body fat in traditional Inuit (Shephard, 1980). A more formal index of acculturation considered education level, housing type, geographic mobility, wage income, and household equipment stock. In both sexes, the move from primitive to intermediate technology was associated with an increase of subcutaneous fat; in men it was also negatively correlated with leg extension force and maximum oxygen intake.

Longitudinal Observations

Over the past decade, Igloolik has seen the rapid introduction of mechanical equipment including: motor launches, seaplanes, 180 powerful snowmobiles, and snow-clearing graders. Homes enjoy video and satellite television plus high-fi sets. A new runway allows 5-hour journeys to the night life of Montreal.

Repetition of our physiological observations (Rode & Shephard, 1984) has shown a marked decrease of maximum oxygen intake, an increase of subcutaneous fat, and a loss of muscle strength by all groups except young boys (see Figure 1). The longitudinal change is far greater than would be expected from normal aging, and much of the functional loss must be attributed to a decrease of habitual activity over the decade. Cross-sectional data now show much of the deterioration occurring during the late teens and early adult life, at ages when snowmobile ownership has become the community norm.

One unexpected finding was that all adult Inuit had become 1-2 cm shorter over the decade of observation (Rode & Shephard, 1984). The change far exceeded that expected from kyphosis and compression of intervertebral discs, particularly in the younger subjects. The intervertebral distance was decreased, and the change was largest in frequent snowmobile users. We thus suspect that spinal injury had been caused by driving snowmobiles long distances at high speeds over rough packed ice.

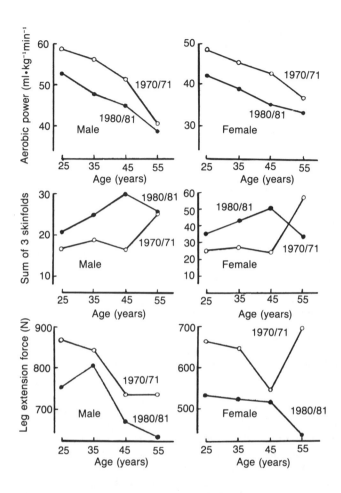

Figure 1. Cross-sectional aging data for an Inuit community examined in 1970/71, and again in 1980/81 after 10 years of rapid technological change. Based on data of Rode & Shephard (1984) for predicted maximum oxygen intake (ml·kg⁻¹min⁻¹ STPD), body fat (sum of 3 skinfolds, mm) and knee extension force (N).

Intermediate Technologies

Some studies of people using intermediate technologies have reported improbably small daily energy expenditures, possibly because of the difficulties inherent in determining food intake. On the other hand, indirect calorimetry has indicated quite high rates of energy expenditures. Thus Viteri, Torun, Galicia, and Herrera (1971) reported values of 13.2-17.9 MJ•day⁻¹ for Guatemalean highlanders, whereas on the technically more advanced farms of Israel (Edholm, Humphrey, Lourie, Tredre, & Brotherhood, 1973), many tasks demanded 25-32 kJ•min⁻¹, with a daily load of 12 MJ.

Post-Industrial Societies

Energy Cost of Daily Living

Edholm (1970) made the provocative suggestion that mechanization would cause people to work faster, without reducing their daily energy expenditures. This may be true at the intermediate level of technology. For example, a peasant maneuvering a rotary cultivator in heavy soil finds little opportunity to rest or to vary the pace of work. However, there is already data to disprove Edholm's view for more advanced societies (see Table 1), and the need for human power will decline further as robots begin to control production lines.

Physical Limitations and Mandatory Retirement

Until recently, mandatory retirement was justified in physically demanding jobs because of deteriorating physical ability. The maximum energy expenditure tolerated over an 8-hour workday was 40% of maximum oxygen intake, corresponding at age 65 to a loading of 15.7 kJ•min⁻¹ in a man, and 11.1 kJ•min⁻¹ in a woman. Allowing also for a 20% interindividual variation of aerobic power, 1 man in 40 would have an upper working limit of 9.4 kJ•min⁻¹, while 1 woman in 40 would have an upper limit of 6.7 kJ•min⁻¹.

Many tasks in a traditional intermediate technology appear too strenuous for 65-year-old workers. However, complaints of physical fatigue are infrequent. Possible explanations include: promotion from physically demanding jobs, fitness preservation by regular job activity, delegation of strenuous tasks, slowing of pace, and efficiency enhancement by long experience.

Impact of Technological Change

Has technological change abolished the need for mandatory retirement? Certainly, there has been extensive mechanization of traditional, heavy industries such as forestry, coal-mining, farming, steel work, and building trades. However, a compressed work week has increased the daily energy expenditure in some occupations. Heavy work tasks that remain involve walking, carrying, and climbing stairs (e.g., mail carrying and marine surveying). The walking speed of mail carriers is frequently discussed in contract negotiations, and the retirement age of marine surveyors is also hotly debated. Marine surveying is relatively resistant to automation, although as cargo holds become larger, a power-operated inspection chair may become a possibility. Mail carrying is plainly threatened by the development of electronic mail systems.

Table 1. The decrease in energy cost of some common tasks on changing from traditional to intermediate or advanced technology

Task	Type of technology and energy cost (kJ·min⁻¹) Traditional		Intermediate or Advanced	
Mowing	Scythe	(23-43)	Tractor	(7-19)
Grain harvest	Binding & Stacking	(21-36)	Combined harvester	(8-13)
Milking	Hand	(9-21)	Machine	(6)
Tree planting	Hand	(27)	Machine	(12)
Horizontal sawing	Hand	(30)	Power saw	(23)
Digging	Pick & shovel	(20-42)	Mechanical digger	(15-31)

Note. Based on data collected by Durning and Passmore (1967).

It is unlikely that technical progress will extend the work span of the present generation, because the oldest employees tend to remain in traditional crafts (Sachuk, 1971). Whether future generations will continue working beyond the age of 65 depends in part upon employment availability and extent of voluntary efforts to maintain personal health and fitness, thus compensating for lack of physical activity at work.

Implications for Health

Epidemiological studies suggest that low-energy expenditure at work can double the risk of death from ischaemic heart disease, even after allowance for such covariables as cigarette smoking and high systemic blood pressure. The risk of physical injury is also great if physical demand is normally low, but high on rare occasions (Guthrie, 1963). Automation can further lead to job dissatisfaction and worker alienation. The usual problem is that task demand is too low so that work seems repetitive and boring. But on occasion, the required speed of operation or the degree of responsibility are beyond the individual's tolerance (Coburn, 1981). Younger employees often express work dissatisfaction by absenteeism, alcohol and drug abuse, poor work quality, and strikes. The need to maintain a family and concern about possible difficulty in finding alternative employment reduce such outward manifestations of dissatisfaction in the older worker. However, covert problems lead to perceived poor health.

Benefits From Leisure Activity

Physical gains from a compensatory increase of leisure activity are of special importance to an older person. A well-designed training program not only increases life satisfaction, but also augments maximum oxygen intake by at least 20%, with associated increases of muscle strength and joint flexibility, dispersal of accumulated fat, and halting of bone mineral loss. The subsequent rate of aging is unchanged, but it takes many more years to reach the situation where working capacity is insufficient to meet the demand of either occupation or personal care.

Implication for Society

In the short-term, aging of the population may require adoption of an older retirement age. However, many economists predict that technological advances will eliminate 10-14% of present jobs by the year 2025. Rapidly changing skill requirements will also place the elderly at a serious disadvantage in the post-industrial job-market, and they will need to accept leisure not as a weekend luxury or an interjob episode, but rather as a permanent way of life. Unfortunately, this is a difficult adjustment for an older person to make. Early socialization has favored the protestant "work ethic," with expectations of a long work week and little play. Such attitudes are often reinforced by age-stratification of behavioral norms. A 50-year-old executive expects to be overworked just because he or she has reached the age of 50. Much reeducation is thus needed to assure self-fulfillment rather than disgrace in any enforced leisure. Recreational programs specifically designed for the older individual make an important contribution in this situation, reversing the self-fulfilling expectation that activity declines with age.

Recreation programs for the elderly are by nature labor intensive, so that they offer the further dividend of providing employment for those displaced by industrial automation.

Conclusions

Modern technology has reduced energy expenditures in both industry and the home, thereby causing a decrease of physical fitness. However, leisure activity can counter the adverse health effects, generating new employment while providing self-fulfillment for those with boring jobs or excessive free time. Voluntary activity cannot slow biological aging, but it can give meaning to life, setting back the time when the citizen of our post-industrial society is unable to care for himself or herself.

References

Coburn, D. (1981). Work alienation and well-being. In D. Coburn, C. D'Arcy, P. New, & G. Torrence (Eds.), *Health and Canadian Society* (pp. 420-437). Toronto: Fitzhenry & Whiteside.

Durnin, J.V.G.A., & Passmore, R. (Eds.). (1967). *Energy, work and leisure*. London: Heinemann Educational Books Ltd.

Edholm, O.G. (1970). The changing pattern of human activity. *Ergonomics, 13*, 625-643.

Edholm, O.G., Humphrey, S., Lourie, J.A., Tredre, B.E., & Brotherhood, J. (1973). Energy expenditure and climatic exposure of Yemenite and Kurdish Jews in Israel. *Philosophical Transactions of the Royal Society of London*, Series B, *266*, 127-140.

Godin, G., & Shephard, R.J. (1973). Activity patterns of the Canadian Eskimo. In O.G. Edholm & E.K.E. Gunderson (Eds.), *Polar human biology* (pp. 193-215). London: William Heinemann.

Guthrie, D.I. (1963). A new approach to handling in industry. A rational approach to the prevention of low back pain. *South African Medical Journal, 37*, 651-656.

Rode, A., & Shephard, R.J. (1971). Cardiorespiratory fitness of the Canadian Eskimo. *Journal of Applied Physiology, 31*, 519-526.

Rode, A., & Shephard, R.J. (1984). Ten years of "civilization"—fitness of the Canadian Inuit. *Journal of Applied Physiology, Environmental Exercise Physiology, 56*, 1472-1477.

Sachuk, N.N. (1971). The aging worker's abilities and disabilities in relation to industrial production. In J. Huet (Ed.), *Work and aging* (pp. 147-162). Paris: Int. Centre of Social Gerontol.

Shephard, R.J. (1980). Work physiology and activity patterns. In F.A. Milan (Ed.), *The human biology of circumpolar populations*. London: Cambridge University Press.

Viteri, F.E., Torun, B., Galicia, J.C., & Herrera, E. (1971). Determining energy costs of agricultural activities by respirometer and energy balance techniques. *American Journal of Clinical Nutrition, 24*, 1418-1430.

4

Sport Voluntary Association Involvement and Happiness Among Middle-Aged and Elderly Americans

Edwin Rosenberg
UNIVERSITY OF PITTSBURGH AT BRADFORD
BRADFORD, PENNSYLVANIA, USA

Introduction and Review of Literature

Over the years numerous gerontological studies have theorized about and attempted to measure the relationship between social activity level and happiness, life satisfaction, or social adjustment. Much social activity occurs within voluntary associations: groups or organizations that vary in form and function with optional membership. Voluntary associations play a functional role in American society, and there is a substantial body of research examining the relationship between such organizations and the older population. The pattern of voluntary association membership by age tends to be curvilinear across the life cycle, peaking in the 20-year range that brackets the act of retirement, and declining thereafter.

In recent years there has been an apparent increase both in the number of voluntary associations for older persons and elderly participation in these organizations (McPherson, 1983). This enhances the relevance of various gerontological investigations of such topics as the age profiles of members of different types of voluntary associations (Cutler, 1976), the impact of aging on voluntary association participation (Cutler, 1977), and the importance the aged place on voluntary association participation (Ward, 1979).

One type of voluntary association is the sport organization. Few studies exist of the link between sport voluntary association membership and life satisfaction, and their findings are inconsistent. While the effects of exercise on physiological well-being are extensively documented and irrefutable, the psychological and/or social benefits of exercise are more difficult to assess accurately. Researchers who have attempted to do just that (McPherson, 1965; Ostrow, 1980) report that exercise seems to enhance well-being, self-confidence, and emotional stability while decreasing tension, anxiety, and depression. In a metropolitan area sample Snyder and Spreitzer (1974) reported a positive relationship between sport involvement and feelings of psychological well-being, especially for women. Rosenberg and Chelte (1980), however, using a national data base, found that self-reported happiness was not higher for members of sport (as opposed to nonsport) voluntary associations and, in fact, was lower for women.

These mixed results—especially those not showing a positive relationship between sport participation and socioemotional well-being—may be due in large part to a combination of physiological decrements and societal age norms. For instance, a 1975 National Council on the Aging report showed that public perception of the problems and concerns of the aged often differed significantly from the personal experiences reported by senior citizens. The data showed that "the essentially negative stereotype of the sedentary, isolated, and unstimulated old person that is held by the total public does not correspond with old people's actual experiences" (Harootyan, 1982).

Nonetheless there was fairly close agreement between public perception of and elderly participation in sports. Only 5% of those surveyed felt that most people over 65 spend a lot of time in such sports as swimming, golf, or tennis; however, this is close to the 3% of the elderly surveyed who reported frequent participation in such sports (National Council on the Aging, 1975). The findings mean that there is little public expectation that the aged will be active in sports, and even less actual activity on the part of the elderly. Thus age norms guide, reflect, and reinforce elderly nonparticipation in active sports, effecting a cycle detrimental to both physiological health and self-esteem.

Some might argue that disassociating from sport groups and physical activity is in line with disengagement theory and thus functional for the elderly. However, the bulk of the evidence suggests that successful adjusters to old age are more likely to be regular participants in physical activity (Palmore, 1979; Teague, 1980). Still, "in spite of the well-documented and publicized benefits of remaining physically active, there is increasing evidence of a decline in physical activity participation with advancing age" (Ostrow, 1984; for factors specifying the magnitude of this decline, see McPherson, 1983). This pattern has been observed in such nations as Canada, Czechoslovakia, Denmark, Finland, France, Great Britain, and Norway, as well as in America. (For a substantial citation list, see McPherson, 1983.)

A 1982 study by Harootyan shed light not only on age-related activity decline but also on activity type. Dividing his sample into under-60 and 60-and-over groups, he concluded that as people age they apparently decrease their physical activity level and the intensity of their physical activity by substituting or continuing to participate only in less strenuous pursuits. The physical activities of old age are also more likely to be of a solitary rather than group-oriented nature, a finding with obvious consequences for sport voluntary associations for the middle-aged and elderly.

There are, of course, biological changes which necessitate a scaled-down level of physical activity as people age. But there are many nonphysiological reasons for declining physical activity in middle and old age. Among those reported by various researchers are cohort differences in awareness of the benefits of exercise, educational attainment, and previous opportunity for physical activities; negative attitudes toward participation based on childhood or adolescent experiences in sport or exercise; other activities (e.g., hobby, family) competing for a limited amount of leisure time; different role commitments according to sex, race, socioeconomic status, family life cycle stage, or nationality; a lack of sport/exercise role models who are elderly; limited access to facilities; a breakdown of relevant social contacts and networks; lack of encouragement from the medical establishment; stereotypes of the aged as frail and noncompetitive; and the belief that the need for exercise diminishes and disappears with advancing age (Boothby, Tungatt, & Townsend, 1981; McPherson, 1983; Pardini, 1984).

Other current data hint that, perhaps due to cohort and/or period effects, the aged are becoming more aware of the activity-health link and are acting on this awareness. A recent insurance company survey (TIAA/CREF, 1983), admittedly unrepresentative of all retirees, found that 34% of its annuitants participate in sport or physical fitness programs.

The current situation, then, is one in which the benefits of exercise are indisputable; yet the middle-aged and older populations are not significantly responding to this knowledge. What does sport participation, both per se and as a form of exercise, mean for these people? What role do or can voluntary associations play in facilitating physical activity and thus improved health for the middle-aged and older populations?

Few studies exist on the meaning of sport involvement for the elderly and the process by which aged involvement is initiated, maintained, and discontinued (Curtis & White, 1984; Ostrow, 1982). Thus, the literature on the relationship between sport voluntary association participation and life satisfaction is inconclusive. Despite signs of increasing retiree participation in sport and physical fitness programs, the relationship of such participation to life satisfaction among the aged remains uncertain. This paper explores that issue by examining a sample of middle-aged and elderly Americans. The research question centers on a comparison of self-reported life satisfaction levels of late middle-aged (55-64) and elderly (65-74 and 75+) Americans whose voluntary association memberships range from 0 to 2 or more and may or may not include a sport voluntary association.

Methodology

The 1980 National Opinion Research Center's General Social Survey provided a sample of 1,527 Americans, of whom 468 were age 55 and over. There were 238 respondents age 55-64, 163 age 65-74, and 67 age 75 and over. Crosstabulations and regression analyses were conducted using SPSS.

The dependent variable was avowed happiness (coded high, medium, or low). Independent variables were sex, age (in the above-mentioned groupings), number of voluntary association memberships (ranked 0, 1, or 2 or more), and membership in a sport voluntary association (ranked yes or no). The last two variables were also combined to form Voluntary Association Status, categorized as 0 voluntary association memberships, 1 nonsport membership, 1 sport membership, 2 or more nonsport memberships, and 2 or more memberships including at least 1 sport association.

Two hypotheses were tested:

1. There is a positive relationship between the number of voluntary association memberships and avowed happiness.
2. The avowed happiness of members of sport voluntary associations will be greater than the avowed happiness of members of nonsport voluntary associations.

Gender and age differences were examined where relevant and where sample size was sufficiently large to permit meaningful analysis and interpretation.

Results

Overall there were no significant differences between males and females in terms of avowed happiness. The same can be said when happiness was cross-tabulated with the three age groups on which this study focuses. Thus subsequent differences in happiness levels might in fact be attributed to voluntary association membership patterns.

Hypothesis 1

For the entire NORC sample, there was indeed a positive relationship between the number of voluntary association memberships and avowed happiness. Respondents who rated themselves "very happy" increased from 25.8% of those in 0 voluntary associations to 39.5% of those in 2 or more voluntary associations, with a highly significant chi-square ($p < .0001$).

When controlling for age, only the 65-74 age group data conformed to the hypothesis ($X^2 = 11.16$, df $= 4$, $p < .03$). In the 55-64 group and especially in the 75+ group (which was hampered by small cell frequencies), the happiest respondents were those in 1 voluntary association.

When controlling for sex, the percentage of males rating themselves as "very happy" increased significantly ($p < .001$) as the number of voluntary association memberships increased. Females in voluntary associations were significantly ($p < .01$) happier than those not in voluntary associations, but there was no difference in happiness between women in 1 and women in 2 or more voluntary associations.

Further analysis included a comparison of avowed happiness of members of no voluntary associations to that of members of various voluntary association statuses for the entire NORC sample. Respondents who were members of 1 nonsport, 1 sport, 2 or more nonsport, and 2 or more including at least 1 sport voluntary association were all more likely to be "very happy" and less likely to be "unhappy" than were members of no voluntary associations.

A breakdown by age group continued to support the hypothesis. This conclusion is weakened, however, by small numbers of 55- to 64-year-olds in 1 sport association, 65- to 74-year-olds in 1 sport or 2 or more with at least 1 sport association, and respondents age 75+.

Hypothesis 2

In examining whether sport voluntary association members express greater happiness than nonsport voluntary association members, the data were recoded so that the happiness of members of no sport associations could be compared to that of members of sport associations. For each of the 3 age groups under consideration, no differences of statistical or substantive significance were discerned. Small cell frequencies again created an obstacle for analyzing data for the 65-74 and 75+ groups in the sport voluntary association category. Further, both on total sample and age-group levels, no significant differences in expressed happiness were found between members of equivalent numbers of sport versus nonsport voluntary associations. This analysis, too, was hampered by small cell frequencies.

Men in one voluntary association tended to be happier if they were in a sport voluntary association; men in 2 or more groups were happiest when none was sport-oriented. Women in 1 nonsport voluntary association were twice as likely to rate themselves "very happy" as women in 1 sport-oriented group; however, women in 2 or more voluntary associations were slightly happier if one of those groups involved sports.

Regression analysis to assess the predictive power of voluntary association status (as well as other variables in this study) on avowed happiness was unproductive. The explained variation was less than 5% in all runs.

Discussion and Conclusions

There are several problems with the data in this study. First, they are no longer the most recent available. More recent General Social Surveys can and should be examined, especially considering the cohort and period effects that constantly change the complexion of the middle-aged and elderly populations. Second, to the extent that these populations find satisfaction through exercise and sport outside voluntary associations, this study does not measure the relationship of exercise and sport to the life satisfaction of the late middle-aged and elderly. Third, the data set characteristics preclude examination of participation variables (active versus passive participation; frequency, intensity, and duration of participation) of interest to gerontologists and sport sociologists.

Finally, in interpreting the data presented, one should keep in mind potential problems of reliability and validity when using subjective well-being indicators (life satisfaction, happiness, morale). For instance, Horley (1984) has noted that these indicators lack both conceptual clarity and a common scale of assessment (e.g., overall life satisfacton, happiness in the past month, week, or day). Horley (1984) recommends that, as a minimum, researchers specify their measures and underlying constructs, and that "a new methodology permitting multi-level assessment" be developed.

Keeping in mind the above-mentioned limitations, the main findings from this analysis of a national sample are:

1. the number of voluntary association memberships is positively related to avowed happiness (reinforcing prior research); (a) this is true for both males and females; (b) among the middle-aged and elderly, the relationship is strongest for the 65-74 age group;
2. introducing membership in a sport voluntary association as a specification variable does not alter the original relationship;
3. in general, membership in a sport (versus nonsport) voluntary association does not result in higher levels of avowed happiness;
4. men who are members of only one voluntary association are more happy if it is a sport organization, whereas women are less happy by a factor of 2.

The preliminary conclusion must be that despite growing literature on the benefits of physical activity for the aged, increases in life expectancy and health status, and general growth of "fitness consciousness" in the United States, late middle-aged and elderly Americans who are members of sport voluntary associations generally do not report higher life satisfaction levels than their age peers who are members of nonsport voluntary associations. This does not mean that the elderly do not enjoy or participate in exercise and sport activities—it merely implies that recent cohorts of the elderly do not tend to derive great happiness from such activities in formal group settings. This is consistent with previous research (Harootyan, 1982) that suggests as people enter the later years there is a tendency to scale down physical activity and to move from group-oriented activities to solitary pursuits. Thus, the data are not an indictment per se of America's unfit elderly, but rather an indication that voluntary associations serve a limited function at best in terms of promoting exercise, sport, and physical fitness among the aged.

Can the aged be more active? The answer is yes. A National Center for Health Statistics survey (described in Harootyan, 1982) reported that 55.9% of elderly Americans (53.7% of males and 57.4% of females) suffer no activity limitations. The gap between potential participation in sports (55.9%) and actual participation (3%) is a crude yet startling indicator of the extent to which nonphysiological factors influence the aged's sport participation.

It would be hard to deny that age grading and age stratification affect the athletic self-image and perceived opportunity structure of middle-aged and elderly Americans. For instance, McPherson (1978) has argued that physical activity participation is subject to age grading and that the norms, values, and sanctions for athletic participation and exercise may vary from one social age category to the next. If we find from middle age into old age that sport and exercise participation is increasingly devalued, we are well along the way to a social explanation for observed age-based declines in physical activity.

It is often noted that the elderly are among the staunchest believers in and supporters of negative stereotypes about themselves. To have to cope with social pressures to disengage from physical activity is a serious burden when added to the reality of declining physical abilities. Sport and exercise skills, like all others, must be practiced regularly to be improved or maintained. When discontinued, they tend to atrophy. As the social breakdown theory (Kuypers & Bengston, 1973) would predict, this produces a vicious cycle where role loss can lead to negative labelling, withdrawal from activity, skill atrophy, and subsequent failure at attempted re-engagement, completing the self-fulfilling prophecy of lost competence and perhaps leading to further role relinquishing.

To some extent the effects of age grading, age stratification, and negative stereotyping of the elderly are generational and will be ameliorated naturally in the future. Accompanying this trend, general societal attitudes linking age with sport and exercise participation should be altered for the better. Alternative performance standards and goals, such as those currently found in senior or master competitions, must be publicized and legitimized. The difference between physical ability decline with age and decline due to societally induced withdrawal and consequent skill atrophy must be made clear, as must the potential for re-engagement and skill recovery with appropriate support. The physical, psychological, and social benefits of continued participation in exercise and sport must be emphasized. If voluntary associations are to play a role, exercise and sport organizations for the aging and aged, which can provide positive role supports and social as well as physical activity, must increase in number, variety, accessibility, and responsiveness to the needs of America's current and future elderly.

References

Boothby, J., Tungatt, M.F., & Townsend, A.R. (1981). Ceasing participation in sports activity: Reported reasons and their implications. *Journal of Leisure Research,* **13**, 1-14.

Curtis, J., & White, P. (1984). Age and sport participation: Decline in participation with age or increased specialization with age? In N. Theberge and P. Donnelly (Eds.), *Sport and the sociological imagination* (pp. 273-293). Fort Worth, TX: Texas Christian University Press.

Cutler, S. (1976). Age profiles of membership in sixteen types of voluntary associations. *Journal of Gerontology,* **31**, 462-470.

Cutler, S. (1977). Aging and voluntary association participation. *Journal of Gerontology,* **32**, 470-479.

Harootyan, R.A. (1982). The participation of older people in sports. In R.M. Pankin (Ed.), *Social approaches to sport* (pp. 122-147). East Brunswick, NJ: Associated University Presses.

Horley, J. (1984). Life satisfaction, happiness, and morale: Two problems with the use of subjective well-being indicators. *The Gerontologist,* **24**, 124-127.

Kuypers, J.A., & Bengston, V.L. (1973). Competence and social breakdown: A social-psychological view of aging. *Human Development,* **16**, 37-49.

McPherson, B.D. (1965). *Psychological effects of an exercise program for postcardiac and normal adult men.* Masters thesis, University of Western Ontario, London, Ontario.

McPherson, B.D. (1978). Aging and involvement in physical activity: A sociological perspective. In F. Landry & W. Orban (Eds.), *Physical activity and human wellbeing* (pp. 111-125). Miami, FL: Symposia Specialists.

McPherson, B.D. (1983). *Aging as a social process*. Toronto: Butterworths.

National Council on the Aging. (1975). *The myth and reality of aging in America*. Washington, DC: The National Council on the Aging.

Ostrow, A.C. (1980). Physical activity as it relates to the health of the aged. In N. Datan & N. Lohmann (Eds.), *Transitions of aging* (pp. 41-56). New York: Academic Press.

Ostrow, A.C. (1982). Age role stereotyping: Implications for physical activity participation. In G. Rowles & R. Ohta (Eds.), *Aging and mileau: Environmental perspectives on growing old*. New York: Academic Press.

Ostrow, A.C. (1984). *Physical activity and the older adult*. Princeton, NJ: Princeton Book Company.

Palmore, E. (1979). Predictors of successful aging. *The Gerontologist, 19*, 427-431.

Pardini, A. (1984). Exercise, vitality, and aging. *Aging*, April-May, 19-29.

Rosenberg, E., & Chelte, A. Avowed happiness of members of sport and nonsport voluntary associations. *International Journal of Sport Psychology, 11*, 263-275.

Snyder, E., & Spreitzer, E. (1974). Involvement in sports and psychological well-being. *International Journal of Sport Psychology, 5*, 28-39.

Teague, M.L. (1980). Aging and leisure: A social psychological perspective. In S.E. Iso-Ahola (Ed.), *Social psychological perspectives on leisure and recreation* (pp. 219-257). Springfield, IL: Thomas.

TIAA/CREF. (1983).A new look at retired participants. *The Participant*, August, pp. 1-5.

Ward, R. (1979). The meaning of voluntary association participation to older people. *Journal of Gerontology, 34*, 438-445.

5

The Effect of Recreational Sports on the Quality of Life of the Unemployed

Kari Fasting
NORWEGIAN COLLEGE OF PHYSICAL EDUCATION AND SPORT
KRINGSJAA, OSLO, NORWAY

In recent years unemployment has increased all over the world. Even if unemployment now touches people in all kinds of occupations, it seems to affect young and old, men and women, skilled and unskilled very unevenly. Rapoport (1982) characterizes the unemployed in the following way: "The unemployed is disproportionately composed of the unskilled, the less fit, the low paid, employees of small firms, and the oldest age groups." In this connection it is relevant to focus on the fact that the participation rate in recreational sport varies according to socioeconomic and educational status (Rodgers, 1977). The same disparities that exist between people who are active and passive in sport seem to exist between the employed and unemployed. The strongest barriers toward sport participation can perhaps be found in those groups which are hardest stricken by unemployment.

How then does unemployment affect people? People who become unemployed seem to undergo different experiences. Based on other studies Smith and Simpkins (1980) describe these as follows:

1. Euphoria—the experience of being liberated from work.
2. Shock—which among other things contains the realization of the economic implication of being unemployed.
3. Optimism—where one tries to get a new job.
4. Pessimism—where one experiences depression and defeat. This phase can lead to major personality disorganization.
5. Fatalism—this phase may also result in personal disorganization, but more generally involves the acceptance of the stigma of being unemployed.

According to Heinemann (1979), leisure time interests seem to undergo changes when a person becomes unemployed. In a West German study the interest for sport diminished with the length of unemployment. At the same time there came an increasing interest in receptive sedentary activities such as reading, listening to the radio, watching TV, and so forth. The same has been found in a study in England (Bunker, Dewbarry, & Kelvin, 1983). Other studies have found that unemployed people spend a longer time in bed than before, and lose interest in previous hobbies (Smith & Simpkins, 1980). In a newly published study in England, Pahl (1983), however, summarized the results as follows:

> Contrary to popular opinion, typical daily activity is centered around the house. The mornings are spent shopping, doing housework, gardening and job hunting, whereas the afternoon's activities are more diversified, with television viewing and preparing the evening meal being more important. (p. 27)

The conclusions that can be drawn from these studies are that unemployed people tend to be more physically inactive than before they became unemployed.

The unemployed describe themselves as "financially disadvantaged, aimless, useless, and boring" (Vink, 1980). The major material experiences of unemployment, therefore, seem to be humiliation, poverty, isolation, and feelings of uselessness (Corrigan, 1982). The psychological effects of unemployment, however, are loss of personal identity, feelings of degradation, boredom, loneliness, inadequacy, loss of drive, anxiety, and depression (Stokes, 1983). Quite often these reactions manifest themselves in health and social problems. The correlation between unemployment and higher rates of physical and mental illness, for example, has already been established (Ravnmark, 1976).

On the other hand, studies have shown that physical training can have a positive effect on some of these psychological consequences of unemployment and on related variables, for example, depression, self-concept, nervousness, anxiety, and emotional instability (Greist et al., 1978; Brown, Ramirez, & Taub, 1978; Michevic, 1982). This seems first of all to apply to persons who initially are in poor physical and mental condition (Fasting, 1982).

Based on these results, and the results from the effect-studies of unemployment, a research project among the unemployed was set up at the University of Odense in Denmark.[1] The purpose of the project was to study the effect of physical training on health and quality of life.

Methods

Based on different theories the positive effect of physical training on indicators of mental health such as depression, emotional instability, and so forth is explained differently. Folkins and Sime (1981) divide the explanations into four groups: somatopsychic theory, physiological viewpoints, psychological viewpoints, and a cognitive oriented model.

---

[1]The study was done in 1982 at the Institute of Physical Education, University of Odense, in collaboration with Preben K Pedersen, Karsten Froberg, Bjarne Andersen, Ole Lammert, and Jens A Rokkedal.

On the whole the explanations can be divided into two main groups—physiological theories and psychological theories. Physiological theories claim that the changes are due to neurophysical and biochemical alterations as a result of physical activity. Psychological explanations assume that physical fitness improvements give people a sense of mastery, which then can be associated with an experience of well-being and/or that exercise provides a distraction or diversion from, for example, anxiety-provoking cognitions (Solomon & Bumpus, 1978; Morgan, 1979).

These explanations could mean that other types of activities would have the same effect on mental health and quality of life as physical training. To test this assumption, the design of the study was set up with 3 different groups: 64 men and women, age 25-45, were divided into an exercise group, a study group, and a control group. The participants were, prior to the study, physically inactive, in the sense that none did regular physical training. They had all been unemployed from 4 to 27 months.

Before and after the research period, which lasted 3 months, the subjects went through physiological tests as well as an interview where medical, psychological, and sociological data were gathered. Altogether 17 persons dropped out of the project. The reasons for this were sickness, employment, or educational courses.

The exercise group trained 2 hours, twice a week. The training was led by a female and a male physical education teacher. The activities were calisthenics, volleyball, or badminton. Every training session ended with swimming.

The training was organized so that the participants had some influence on the content and the form of the training. This was necessary to create a "we-feeling" in the group in order to have a meaningful, motivating exercise period.

The study group met twice a week at the same time as the exercising group. A social worker with experience from different areas led the group. His objectives were to create positive social relations in the group and to teach different subjects. In this group, too, the participants could partly choose the subjects. The following topics were presented by speeches, discussions, and excursions: social conditions, working environments, narcotics and alcohol problems, ways of living, art, and culture.

The concept of health and quality of life was operationalized and measured in different ways. In this paper only results from the scales measuring the participants' quality of life are presented.

Researchers in this area use different approaches. Moum (1984) mentions four alternatives in measuring people's quality of life:

1. the use of a third person (friend, neighbor, or a professional psychologist);
2. medical symptoms as indicators (headache, etc.);
3. the person's own behavior (demonstrations, etc.); and
4. asking people directly about their feelings and well-being.

It was this last approach that was used in our study. The different alternatives all have weaknesses. Concerning number 4, quality of life scales, three types of systematic errors can occur: yeasaying, social desirability, and trait desirability. According to Moum (1984), however, these biases seem to have relatively little influence on the scales.

On one scale we asked the participants how satisfied they were with different areas in their lives. On the other scale, the participants were asked to describe their lives at that moment on an adjective scale.

Each scale consists of either 14 different domains (for example, friends, neighborhood, etc.), or 14 adjective pairs (for example, good . . . bad). The participants were asked to mark on a 7-point scale either how satisfied they were with their friends, neighborhood, and so on, or how their lives were at that moment. The sum score then on both scales could vary from 14 to 98 points. Low scores indicate low quality of life, and high scores indicate high quality of life. A difference score was constructed by subtracting the post- from the prescore. This difference was tested separately for each group with a two-tailed t-test.

Results

The results presented in Tables 1 and 2 show that all groups have a higher score on the post- than on the pretest. The increase in difference score was greatest for the exercise group. Only the exercise group has shown significant statistical improvement on both scales. However, the improvement for the study group was significant on the domain scale, but the difference here was stronger for the exercising than the study group. The changes in the control group on both scales were not statistically significant.

Two conclusions must be drawn from these results. Physical exercise can have a positive effect on the unemployed's quality of life. Participation in an exercise group seems to be more effective in producing a better quality of life than participation in a study group.

Discussion

Because the exercise group improved more than the study group, and improved significantly on both scales, we may conclude that the improvement was not only caused by psychological factors. The effect of physical activity per se (e.g., the physiological and biochemical changes that take place in the body as a result of training) seems to be of importance. The explanation is probably multifactorial. Ismail and Young (1977) claim that there is a connection between certain chemical substances and behavior, and that the concentration of these substances is affected by physical activity.

The results were also confirmed by a personal qualitative interview after the research period. Almost all the participants in the exercise group claimed that they "felt better," they were looking forward to the two days they should exercise, and they had more energy, which for some had led to greater activity concerning job seeking. It is also worth mentioning that after the project was finished, the participants in the exercise group founded their own sport club, which today has more than 400 members. Contrary to most sport clubs, physical training is offered during daytime, for both sexes of all ages. Dif-

Table 1. The mean score on "quality of life scale (domain)" for the three groups

Group	N	Pre-score M	Pre-score SD	Post-score M	Post-score SD	Diff-score M	Diff-score SD	Significance level
Exercise	20	36	8	44	10	8	8	$p < 0.001$
Study	14	32	9	36	7	4	6	$p < 0.05$
Control	13	36	13	38	9	2	7	ns

Table 2. The mean score on "quality of life scale (adjective pair)" for the three groups

Group	N	Pre-score M	Pre-score SD	Post-score M	Post-score SD	Diff-score M	Diff-score SD	Significance level
Exercise	20	39	13	48	12	9	12	$p < 0.01$
Study	14	36	11	39	13	3	14	ns
Control	13	37	15	40	12	3	11	ns

ferent sports are offered in the same training session, which is not competitive in orientation. All who have the possibility to exercise during daytime are welcome, for example, housewives, shift workers, and so forth.

This sport club organized by the unemployed themselves has had greater success in activating unemployed than both the trade unions and the traditional voluntary sport clubs. In planning for a future society, with less work and more leisure time, this may be important to take into account.

In discussing the results of this research project a comparison of work and sport could be useful. Can participation in recreational sport give people some experiences they normally get through their work which directly or indirectly influence their quality of life?

The following three factors are mentioned by Glyptis (1983):

1. Work involves going out. Participation in recreational sport can provide this opportunity.
2. Work provides social contacts. Through participation in sport one can maintain friendships and make new friends.
3. Participation in recreational sport may play a significant role in alleviating the monotonous isolation and anomie of unemployment.

In addition, it should be mentioned that having a job structures the day. Time disturbances are therefore not unusual among the unemployed. In a study by Hepworth (1980), for example, the best single predictor of mental health during unemployment was whether or not a man *felt* his time was occupied. Through sport participation the day can be better structured (Heinemann, 1979).

Leisure is usually defined as free time, which in this connection means time free from work. Defined in this way one may argue that unemployed people don't have leisure time at all, or at least, that it is meaningless to discuss the concept in this way. Many people do have a job that is meaningless and problematic. As Robert, Noble, and Duggan (1982) express it, this has had the effect that leisure has become "the deferred reward for working (r 178)." The individual difference may of course vary to a great extent. This is illustrated clearly by Stokes (1983) when he stated that : "For certain people meaning in life may be derived from non-working activities, for others their occupation may provide them with only limited access to the latent consequences of work in employment (r 276)."

There is no doubt that the first group is the biggest group. In spite of this, Kelvin (1982) states that being "unemployed carries a stigma in a world of work, not so much because it is *bad*, but because it is being *different* (r 43)." Stokes (1983) focuses on the fact that retirement research gives support to the view that separation from the work role itself may have little negative effect on quality of life and health. The important difference between an unemployed and a retired person is, however, the fact that retirement may incur less social stigma and be less unexpected.

Thinking about the future, Smith and Simpkins (1980) state that "education for non-work is as important as education for work." This implies that we must learn how to live and fill our time with meaningful activities that probably give no income. One factor that could facilitate such a process is a change in people's values toward the relationship between work and leisure. If this attitude could change, it probably would be easier to get unemployed people more involved in sport. This may be of great importance because the results from the research project presented in this paper suggest that sport may have some advantages over other more sedentary recreational activities.

References

Brown, R.S., Ramirez, D.E., & Taub, J.M. (1978). The prescription of exercise for depression. *The Physician and Sportsmedicine, 6*, 35-45.

Bunker, N., Dewberry, C., & Kelvin, P. (1983). Unemployment and use of time; methods and preliminary results of a research enquiry. In S. Glyptis (Ed.), *Newsletter Supplement*, No. 1, Leisure Studies Association, 6-8.

Corrigan, P. (1982). "The trouble with being unemployed is that you never get a day off." In T. Veal, S. Parker, & F. Coalter (Eds.), *Work and leisure, unemployment, technology and life-styles in the 1980s*. Leisure Studies Association, Conference Paper No. 21., 50-56.

Fasting, K. (1982). Leisure time, physical activities and some indices of mental health. *Scandinavian Journal of Social Medicine* (Suppl. 29), 113-119.

Folkins, C.H., & Sime, W.E. (1981). Physical Fitness Training and Mental Health. *American Psychologist, 36*, 373-389.

Glyptis, S. (1983). Business as usual? Leisure provision for the unemployed. *Leisure Studies, 2*, 287-300.

Greist, J.H., Klein, M.H., Eischens, R.R., & Faris, J.T. (1978). Running out of depression. *The Physician and Sportsmedicine, 6*, 49-56.

Heinemann, K. (1979). Arbeitslosigkeit und sportsoziale Lage und psychische Verfassung der Arbeitslosen. *Arbeitslosigkeit und sport*. Deutscher Sportbund, 15-35.

Hepworth, S. (1980). Moderating factors of the psychological impact of unemployment. *Journal of Occupational Psychology, 53*, 139-146.

Ismail, A.H., & Young, R.J. (1977). Effect of chronic exercise on the personality of adults. Part XI. Psychological considerations of long distance running. *Annals of the New York Academy of Science, 301*, 958-969.

Kelvin, P. (1982). Work, unemployment and leisure: Myths, hopes and realities. In S. Glyptis (Ed.), *Prospects for leisure and work*. Proceedings of Regional Seminars. Leisure Studies Association, Conference Papers No. 12, 35-49.

Michevic, P.M. (1982). Anxiety, depression and exercise. *Quest,* **33**, 140-153.

Morgan, W.P. (1979). Anxiety reduction following acute physical activity. *Psychiatrics Annals,* **9**, 34.

Moum, T. (1984). Idrett og livskvalitet. Måle-og modelleringsproblemer. *Proceedings of the 1st Annual Conference of the Norwegian Association for Sport Research*. Sanner Turist Hotell 31.10-1.11, 1983, Universitets-forlaget, Oslo, 199-215.

Pahl, R.E. (1983). *The Thatcher Crisis*. (Review of economist intelligence unit, coping with unemployment: The effects on the unemployed themselves). *New Society*, Jan. 6.

Rapoport, R. (1982). *Unemployment and the family Loch memorial lecture*. London: Family Welfare Association.

Ravnmark, H. (1976). *Arbejdsløshed og sygelighed, en litteraturgjennomgang socialmed*. Inst. Univ. Århus, Denmark.

Robert, K., Noble, M., & Duggan, J. (1982). Youth unemployment: An old problem or a new life-style? *Leisure Studies,* **1**, 171-181.

Rodgers, B. (1977). *Rationalising sport politics. Sport in its social context. International comparisons*. Strasbourg: Council of Europe. Committee on Sport.

Smith, M.A., & Simpkins, B.S. (1980). *Unemployment and leisure: A review and some proposals for research*. U.K.: The Centre for Leisure Studies, University of Salford.

Solomon, E.G., & Bumpus, A.K. (1978). The running meditation response: An adjunct to psychotherapy. *American Journal of Psychotherapy,* **32**, 583-592.

Stokes, G. (1983). Work, unemployment and leisure. *Leisure Studies,* **2**, 269-286.

Vink, G. de. (1982). Unemployment and leisure—An ignored dimension. In T. Veal, S. Parker, & F. Coalter (Eds.), *Work and leisure, unemployment, technology and lifestyles in the 1980s*. Leisure Studies Association, Conference Paper No. 15, 41-48.

6

Sport and the Unemployed: An Evaluation of Experimental Provision in England and Wales

Susan A. Glyptis
LOUGHBOROUGH UNIVERSITY OF TECHNOLOGY
LOUGHBOROUGH, LEICESTERSHIRE, UNITED KINGDOM

The Unemployed as a Target Group in the United Kingdom

Since the late 1970s public sector sport providers in the United Kingdom have shown a progressive shift from a facility to a community orientation, and toward increasing market segmentation. Hitherto "Sport for All" was (and still remains) a prime objective, but it lacked both focus and direction. Participation data (e.g., Office of Population Censuses and Surveys, 1976, 1979, 1980) continue to show sport as socially selective, with several sectors of society conspicuously absent through lack of interest or lack of opportunity. National agencies, with the Sports Council and its 10 Year Strategy (1983) at the forefront, have increasingly adopted a strategic approach to future priorities, including, within the development of participation, special attention to the needs (or assumed needs) of particular target groups whose access to sport opportunities may be limited for personal, physical, social, or financial reasons. Prominent among these target groups are the unemployed.

Registered unemployment in the United Kingdom as of March 1984 was 3.14 million (Department of Employment, 1984). To these must be added a

---

The research projects on which this paper is based were funded by the Sports Council and carried out with the assistance of Ms. T. Kay and Mr. A.C. Riddington. The views expressed in the paper are those of the author alone.

substantial number (probably well in excess of one million) who are out of work but not registered as such or not eligible to register because they are temporarily engaged on government-sponsored work experience schemes. In common with other West European countries the most dramatic increases have occurred since 1980 (see Table 1). The problem is not merely short term. Forecasters are in broad agreement that, whatever the future economic scenario, employment prospects are bleak: Continuing economic decline means continuing shrinkage of the labor force; yet economic recovery too will require the shedding of labor to make way for machine and microprocessor production. Individuals remain unemployed for long periods. Over a third of the U.K. unemployed, and almost half of those aged 55 and over, have been out of work for over a year (see Table 2). For leisure providers—and for service provision generally—the unemployed are a client group comprising more people, with more time on their hands, for longer periods.

There are certain complications in treating the unemployed as a target group. The first is their heterogeneity. Unemployment is socially and geographically concentrated but touches all sectors of society: young and old, men and women, all social classes, and all ethnic backgrounds. The unemployed vary in their characteristics, circumstances, needs, and constraints. The second complication is their individuality: They have no group identity or corporate existence; they are in no sense a pressure group. The effects of unemployment (charted fully in social science literature)—loss of income, loss of routine, lack of purpose, isolation—are borne almost entirely by individuals and families, not groups or communities. The third complication is their fluidity. The unemployed do not have a fixed membership over time. People drift into and out of unemployment, and so the composition of the target group is continually changing. Recent years have seen a steady net inflow into unemployment, though this was reversed in March 1984 in the UK when a net monthly outflow of 47,000 resulted from 319,000 people entering unemployment and 366,000 leaving. Two months earlier there had been a net inflow of 104,000 new entrants (Department of Employment, 1984). Providing for the unemployed means providing for a moving target.

The Role of Leisure

Public sector providers have been quick to recognize high levels of unemployment as a major challenge to leisure provision. In the academic sphere there is much debate and substantial dissent about the ability of leisure to replace work by providing the same personal satisfactions. Neulinger (1982), for example, recognized that ''people may be incapable of turning newly gained free time or economic freedom into perceived freedom, as long as their values are rooted in a character structure that would see such freedom as inappropriate.'' For most people free time is not easily instilled with structure and purpose. The work ethic runs deep, its effects powerfully portrayed by Hughes (1951): ''A man's work is one of the things by which he is judged, and . . . by which he judges himself . . . one of the more important parts of his social identity,

Table 1. Unemployment rates: Selected West European countries

Country	1973	Registered unemployed as % of civilian working population 1980	1983
United Kingdom	2.4	6.3	11.7
West Germany	1.0	3.3	8.4
France	1.8	6.4	8.9
Italy	4.9	8.0	11.9
Netherlands	2.9	6.2	14.3
Belgium	2.8	9.1	14.4
Eire	5.6	8.3	15.2
Denmark	0.7	6.1	9.7

Note. From Eurostat, 1984, Table 1V/3.

Table 2. Duration of unemployment in the United Kingdom

	% of unemployed out of work for more than one year (as of January 1984)
Men	41.4
Women	27.1
Age (years)	
Under 25	27.6
26-54	42.6
55 +	46.5
All	37.1

Note. From Department of Employment, 1984, Table 2.5.

of his self.'' Jahoda (1978), reporting on empirical enquiries, writes in similar vein: ''Being unemployed is very different from having leisure time . . . their (i.e., the unemployed) sense of time disintegrated.'' Very few empirical studies have examined the time use or leisure life styles of the unemployed, although a substantial enquiry in England by Kelvin and Morley-Bunker is nearing completion.

Practitioners, meanwhile, have been concerned or coerced to act. The Sports Council, as the national agency responsible for the promotion of sport, has identified the unemployed as one of the most disadvantaged and deserving causes in its implementation of ''Sport for All.'' Local authorities, too, have responded in large number by identifying the unemployed as worthy of special provision. Alongside a genuine desire to promote sport or alleviate some of the hardship of unemployment have been objectives of a more instrumental or political nature. The early 1980s heralded not only dramatically higher rates of unemployment but also a spate of inner-city unrest and violence. It would be hard to dissociate these events entirely from high levels of unemployment, as the Scarman enquiry (1981) argued, although cause and effect have probably been oversimplified. The evidence is tenuous at best, but leisure provision has been seen by some—central government included—as a vital preventive or cure for antisocial behavior; unemployment, crime, and leisure provision have thus become locked into a policy triangle.

Whatever the objectives directing it, there has been very little evidence about the likely response of the unemployed to sport and recreation provision, and, because of the rapidity of growth of unemployment, no guidance on the design, establishment, and operation of appropriate schemes. Within the sphere of sport a number of experimental provisions have been started. This paper, based on two research studies, presents a review and evaluation of schemes currently or recently operated by public sector providers, draws conclusions about the role of sport in the lives of the unemployed, and highlights some issues pertinent to future provision.

England and Wales:
The National Context of Provision

Concerned to promote suitable schemes itself and to give appropriate advice to local authorities and other providers, the Sports Council recently commissioned a review of local authority policies and provision in England and Wales, with the aim of distilling successful (and unsuccessful) practice and identifying the factors contributing to success. The methodology and results are reported in full elsewhere (Glyptis & Riddington, 1983). Given the exploratory nature of the enquiry and the complete absence of information on the extent of current provision it was decided to attempt a complete census of the 399 local authorities. The bulk of the information was gathered by correspondence and postal questionnaire. An initial letter to the departments responsible for recreation asked whether any specific policies or provision had been formulated with regard to sport and the unemployed. Authorities making such provision were then asked to complete a brief postal questionnaire comprising a series of open questions regarding the details of policies and provisions currently operating, the objectives behind them, methods of management, staffing, financing and marketing, and the response from the target group. Once a broad categorization of types of provision could be established, visits were made to a small number of each type to observe them in action and discuss their operation more fully with the managers and staff involved. It should be noted that leisure provision other than sport, and sports schemes offered by providers other than local authorities (e.g., voluntary groups) were beyond the purpose of this study. This review is not, therefore, a comprehensive compilation of all leisure provision for the unemployed.

Responses were obtained from 316 (79%) of the authorities contacted. Their constituent areas vary considerably in geographical extent, population size and structure, economic base, and political complexion, but their responses, in terms of leisure provision, to the issue of unemployment fell into four basic types:

1. Forty-seven percent were making no special provision for the unemployed. Included within these are 7% of authorities who operated off-peak price reductions at existing facilities for all sectors of the community, including

the unemployed. The remaining 40% were operating no concessions or provisions at all from which the unemployed could benefit. Many of these authorities were in areas of relatively low unemployment, notably the southern and southeast regions, and did not recognize unemployment as a problem. Some hoped or intended to respond but had been unable to decide upon the most appropriate action to take within the resources available; many authorities in rural areas, for example, were acutely aware of "need" but unable to design or fund provision that could effectively serve a dispersed population. Others had explicitly decided not to act, on the grounds that special concessions for the unemployed might stigmatize them or imply discrimination against other groups in need.

Provision by the other 53% of authorities comprised three basic types. A small number (1%) were offering an amalgam of two or more of them.

2. Forty-two percent offered price concessions specifically for the unemployed, comprising junior rates, special rates, or entry free of charge. Such concessions applied to existing provisions and were usually confined to off-peak hours; most required that the unemployed identify themselves as such on each admission by showing a UB40 registration card.
3. Five percent offered a slightly more sophisticated version of a price concession, in the form of a "leisure pass" or "concession card" scheme. In these schemes, after showing proof of unemployment once, users were issued a concession card in the form of a season ticket, whereby reduced price or free entry could be gained over a defined period at specified facilities. In some cases concession card holders could also purchase sport equipment at discount prices at local shops.
4. Five percent operated sport leadership schemes, involving paid or volunteer staff as leaders, motivators, or support workers, and with a program of activities designed and aimed specifically to attract the unemployed.

Few schemes have been monitored closely, but from the evidence submitted by those involved in running them some initial generalizations can be made. Price concessions have mostly attracted a rather low response. Some authorities attribute this to lack of interest by the unemployed or to the stigma that may be generated by having to show proof of unemployment on each admission. The evidence points to other reasons too: Many schemes have been given minimal publicity, and several are confined to a very narrow range of activities at unpopular times of day. Nonparticipants are hardly likely to respond in great number to publicity located only at leisure centers or other sport venues or to be motivated purely by the written message that something they have never been inclined or able to take part in is now available at reduced cost. Sensitive promotion and sensitive pricing have, however, generated a response; in Telford, for example, Wrekin District Council has experimented over some 3 years with different pricing schemes and concluded that free access attracts substantially higher usage rates than even minimal entry costs. Leisure pass schemes have had rather greater success. Authorities involved in operating them find that the unemployed tend to make frequent use of their concession cards, and this enables the development of friendship and a sense of belonging among the cardholders, which further enhances their enjoyment and their participation in sport. Most successful, however, are sport leadership schemes.

Sport leadership schemes are distinguished from pricing schemes by the appointment of workers or motivators whose specific task is to work with the unemployed, organizing events, activities and courses, generally free of charge or at a nominal fee. Many such schemes have been set up on the initiative of the Sports Council working in partnership with local authorities and often making a substantial input of funds. Three schemes, in particular, were launched by the Council in 1981 for a 3-year period as national pilot projects (see Table 3). All three bring together a team of sport leaders at new or existing facilities, with transport and equipment provided to operate a variety of sporting activities. All have involved the Manpower Services Commission as a provider of additional staff (unemployed people allocated to the projects on work experience schemes and paid at standard MSC rates), and the back-up resources of a host authority—local authorities in Leicester and Derwentside and a voluntary group in Birmingham. All three aim to provide sport opportunities for the jobless and their families. In addition to funding the schemes the Sports Council has also funded an extensive monitoring program designed to evaluate the effectiveness of the schemes and to obtain guidance for future provision. Monitoring is still in progress, but some selected issues and interim data are considered here for two of the schemes.

The Leicester and Birmingham Pilot Schemes

The schemes are similar in objectives, in the fact that neither requires proof of unemployment to be given by users, and neither makes a charge for activities except in special cases (e.g., residential trips) where a nominal contribution may be charged. Both concentrate on what they term the "unattached" unemployed, casual users who come of their own accord, rather than "attached" users who are brought to the scheme by other organizations like community colleges or drop-in centers. Some important contrasts exist. STARS is a city-wide scheme using existing facilities, whereas Hockley Port is site-based, including some new facility provision. STARS has been provided in conjunction with a local authority leisure department, whereas Hockley Port is run by a voluntary group, the Cut Boat Folk. Although set up initially for 3 years, both schemes will be continued beyond the experimental period, STARS having been incorporated into Leicester City Council's main program

Table 3. Three sport leadership schemes

Scheme	Partner authority	Location
1. Sports Training and Recreation Scheme (STARS)	Leicester City Council	Leicester
2. Derwentside Recreation Scheme	Derwentside District Council	Consett & Stanley, Co. Durham
3. Hockley Port	Cut Boat Folk	Handsworth, Birmingham

provision, and the sport for the unemployed element of Hockley Port being continued as fully as possible with the resources of the Cut Boat Folk and other sponsors to be obtained.

Continuation of the schemes beyond the initial pump-priming by the Sports Council is, in itself, a major achievement. At a more specific level, the achievements and failures of the schemes are subject to detailed scrutiny in the monitoring and evaluation program. Research approaches employed to date comprise:

Leicester "STARS" Scheme

1. Attendance records have been designed by the researchers and maintained by the sport leaders for all sessions, sites, and facilities involved in the schemes since their inception. Records for "STARS" comprise a complete register of usage from the outset of the scheme, showing names (or nicknames) of users, their age, sex, and employment status, and whether present or absent on each occasion when sessions take place. These records are the most detailed ever compiled for any sport provision in the United Kingdom and allow many types of analysis, including the following: total usage levels, totals per activity or venue, breakdown of usage by employed and unemployed people, breakdown of usage by age and sex, and—uniquely—the facility, through being able to identify individual users, to examine the participation "career" of *each user*, the rates of turnover and wastage of participants in different sessions, and multiple attendance at different sessions by the same participant.
2. Interview with scheme participants to obtain information regarding: (a) user characteristics—age, sex, employment history, ethnic origin, and household circumstances; (b) sporting interests and sporting history; other recreation interests, especially activities newly started or abandoned since becoming unemployed; (c) reactions to the STARS scheme; motivations for attending, and satisfactions or frustrations derived from doing so.
3. Interviews with other unemployed people in the city to ascertain: (a) their awareness of STARS and (if nonusers) reasons of nonuse, (b) the interests of specific sectors of the target groups (e.g., the older unemployed), and (c) their interest and involvement in sport and other recreation activities (which might perhaps be incorporated into STARS if demand appears to exist).
4. Participant observation and user interviews on residential trips.
5. Monitoring the effectiveness of a publicity campaign.
6. Survey of lapsed participants to investigate reasons for dropping out of the schemes.
7. Interviews and discussions with sports leaders and scheme managers regarding their perceptions of their job, the scheme, and the target group.
8. Facilities survey, examining the range of facilities being used by STARS, and their suitability for purpose as judged by the sport leaders.

Hockley Port

1. Attendance records for Hockley Port are less detailed than those for Leicester because the site has open access, and operates a wide range of

community activities (including youth clubs, playschemes, a city farm, canal boat cruises) over and above its sport provisions for the unemployed. Attendance records here comprise site counts built up over a substantial period of time, comprising 3 daily counts of users divided into male and female and by 3 areas of the site.

2. Participant observation and informal interviews and discussions with Hockley Port users, to obtain information equivalent to that in the STARS user survey.
3. Interviews with other unemployed people in Handsworth.
4. Sport interest survey among unemployed people engaged in life and social skills programs at a local Job Preparation Unit, one of six centers for post-school teenagers run by the City of Birmingham Education Department.

A detailed account of all aspects of the monitoring is beyond the compass of this present paper. Attention here is focused on a number of key results, concentrating especially on the extent of participation generated and the importance of social factors in facilitating the involvement of the unemployed and influencing the satisfaction or frustration they derive from taking part.

Participation Levels

In its first year of operation STARS attracted 1,600 users. The second year saw a virtual doubling of response to 2,993 users, who between them generated some 10,778 attendances (an average of 3.6 attendances per person). This amounts to attendance on at least one occasion by approximately 1 in 7 of the city's registered unemployed people, although as noted earlier there are substantial numbers of unregistered unemployed too. All but a few users (2%) are unemployed, the vast majority (92%) are "unattached" unemployed who come along as casual participants. There is some evidence too that the scheme is reaching the longer term unemployed: half of users have been out of work for over a year, and one third for over 2 years.

Response to the scheme has not come uniformly from throughout the target group, as Table 4 indicates. To date men outnumber women 3 to 1, and the age profile is highly skewed toward the younger unemployed. These variations are scarcely surprising given the imbalance in sport participation across society as a whole, as indicated for example by data from recent General Household Surveys (Office of Population Censuses and Surveys, op cit). From the organizers' viewpoint, however, there is concern to spread opportunities as equitably as possible throughout the target group and conscious efforts to diversify the activity program in year 2 have resulted in some stretching of the age range, with nearly one quarter of users now aged over 25.

As might be expected, a large proportion of users (60%) had previously taken part in the activity undertaken at STARS. But 40% had never previously taken part, and even among the 60%, half had long since given up. STARS is, therefore, attracting newcomers into sport for the first time, and retrieving a number of lapsed participants. In terms of promoting "Sport for All" these are encouraging results.

Success, however, tends to be short-lived. A small core of users (approximately 6%) attend very frequently, becoming strongly committed to the activity or some other aspect of the scheme (e.g., its social elements). But large

Table 4. User profile, Leicester "STARS" scheme

	Year 1 (base = 1,600 users) %	Year 2 (base = 2,993 users) %
Sex		
Male	71	76
Female	29	24
Total	100	100
Age (years)		
Under 15	0.5	0.5
15-19	64.0	43.0
20-24	21.0	33.0
25-29	7.6	12.0
30 +	6.9	11.5
Total	100.0	100.0

proportions attend only once (42%) or between 2 and 5 times (41%) and then drop out; there is high recruitment, but high drop-out, and the latter, being of considerable concern to the organizers, is the subject of a particular research exercise at present.

Usage of Hockley Port (including community projects as well as the sport for the unemployed initiative) currently averages 550 attendances per week, excluding special events. Attendance levels have varied markedly during the first 2 years, largely as a result of staff changes and the consequent need to rebuild community contacts and trust when new staff take over. Most users are young unemployed members of the local community, the majority from the ethnic minority groups, most of whom have been unemployed for over a year. As in Leicester, most are in the age range 17-30 years, and women are relatively underrepresented (69% of users are men, 31% women). Sport facilities contribute substantially to the Port's attractions, the sports hall and kick-about area together accounting for almost two-thirds of all usage.

Social Incentives and Barriers

In addition to the quantitative data summarized above, the interviews and follow-up surveys of lapsed users have been concerned with participants' qualitative assessments of the schemes. Users have been asked how they first heard about the schemes, what made them come along, and what they like or dislike about the schemes. Lapsed users have been asked what, if anything, put them off attending. Social reasons have proved important in motivating people to take part with social benefits prominent among the satisfactions gained and social barriers significant in causing them to drop out. The following results relate to the Leicester scheme.

People heard about the scheme mostly from friends, and all but a few came along with friends. The stigma of joblessness may prevail, but unemployed people live within a culture of unemployment: 54% of STARS users had other members of the immediate family unemployed, and 73% had best friends unemployed. Word of mouth *within* the target group can thus be a very powerful method of promotion.

Scheme users have been asked what, if anything, they enjoy about the scheme. Mixing with other people, gaining confidence, and being able to relate to sport leaders were important benefits, as the following verbatim extracts indicate:

> I have become more confident with people since starting these sports.
>
> Before I went I hated myself because I wasn't putting anything into society but now I feel fit and more sure of myself.
>
> Our leader was very helpful.
>
> All the staff were extremely friendly and helpful. Tony was exceptional. He organized, coached and encouraged every one of the players both with their game and with their efforts to find work, and was good at using people to help others.

At the same time, social barriers and deterrents feature strongly in wastage from the scheme. Follow-up surveys among 145 users who dropped out of STARS in November-December 1982 revealed various problems, including dislike of the activities provided, prohibitive travel costs or distances, and lack of information or understanding about the scheme. Social reasons, though, were much more widespread. Typical of comments made in response to the question, "Why did you stop attending (a named session)?" were the following:

> I haven't got anyone to go with me and I'm not very good at sport anyway.
>
> Meeting different people.
>
> I would not have any friends to keep me company.
>
> I am white and my boyfriend is black. If we go together . . . the skinheads would probably cause trouble.

Some of the reasons cited by female respondents are worth special mention:

> The other girls were very unfriendly. We felt like intruders because we started later than them and they all knew each other.
>
> I was the only female and the men didn't like being beaten by a woman.

The social stigma attached to unemployment has complex effects. For some the idea of special provision is a form of stigma in itself:

> I feel that the STARS scheme is an insult to a person's identity . . . a bit like going on an outing for underprivileged kids and everyone feeling sorry for you because you've never seen the sea before. Being unemployed is bad enough without new stigmas being created (for which someone is getting paid to organize them).

For others, the idea of special provision is not in itself abhorrent, but guilt and stigma already firmly rooted are barriers to becoming involved:

> At first I felt like a sponger. I felt guilty at not having to pay.

Conclusions

The review and monitoring studies reported here provide a number of detailed operating guidelines to assist in the design and management of future schemes.

For present purposes attention is confined to the major issues and problems arising.

The overall success of schemes owes much to the employment of leaders or motivators and the empathy they develop with the target group. Continuity of key staff is therefore crucially important. At Hockley Port changes in key personnel at intervals throughout the scheme have badly disrupted the program; attendances plummeted, and the loss of momentum was such that new staff virtually had to start afresh in establishing links with the local community. A long-term objective is to generate sufficient voluntary involvement of local people for the scheme to be run much more by the community itself, but the experiment to date indicates that the establishment phase is quite long, and schemes need as much continuity and stability as possible if achievements are to be consolidated.

If staffing is important, so too are other elements of recurrent funding, notably transport and equipment. There is some evidence from the national review that a number of schemes experience difficulty in financing over a period of time because revenue implications have not been fully appreciated at the planning stage.

Objectives can become confused and complicated. There is some reluctance in leisure provision generally to promote sport or recreation for its own sake, and a tendency has evolved to attempt to solve an amalgam of society's problems (e.g., unemployment and crime) in a single scheme, and to assume policy burdens which arguably lie more centrally within the remit of other policy concerns (e.g., industry, housing). In many schemes sport is being used as a means to other ends, notably group development and community development. There are implications here both for coordination with other policy agencies, and for the training of sport leaders who are called upon increasingly to fulfill the roles of community worker, support worker, and counselor, in addition to coaching.

Experiments need to be given a fair trial. Schemes for the unemployed need the freedom and the time to experiment and, indeed, the freedom to fail. They need time to consolidate, adapt, and review. The national pilot schemes have had sufficient timescale and flexibility to do this, but several other initiatives have been tried for only very short periods of 3-4 months.

Most schemes are launched and operated with short-term objectives only. But unemployment has long-term implications, both for the individuals concerned and as a societal problem. The STARS scheme is beginning to feed its participants into established clubs and to assist participants in setting up their own clubs where opportunities do not already exist within established community sport provision.

Catering for the unemployed has become a competitive market, with several agencies involved, often operating in isolation from each other in jealously guarded areas. There is risk of considerable duplication of effort and resources in a policy field where total resources are severely limited.

Except for a minority of users, the main attractions of schemes to date appear to lie as much in the social benefits of being involved as in the activities per se. Publicity and marketing need, therefore, to stress the potential social benefits of involvement, and sport leaders need to be particularly sensitive to the need to integrate newcomers into established groups and to ensure that participants are not isolated either through lack of integration encouraged by the group or lack of self-confidence.

Sport is still a minority activity within society as a whole. Unemployment strikes disproportionately at the young, the manual and unskilled sectors, and ethnic minorities; long-term unemployment mainly afflicts older people. These are precisely the missing sectors in sport participation generally even among the employed, and any assessment of sport schemes for the unemployed needs to be set in this perspective. Schemes such as those in Leicester and Birmingham are beginning to fulfill some needs for some of the unemployed and beginning to reach sectors of society that have remained largely untouched by conventional sports provision.

References

Department of Employment. (1984, April). *Employment Gazette, 92*(4).

Eurostat. (1984). *Employment and unemployment.* Luxembourg: Statistical Office of the European Communities.

Glyptis, S., & Riddington, A.C. (1983). *Sport for the unemployed: A review of local authority projects.* Sports Council Research Working Paper 21.

Hughes, E. (1951). Work and the self. In J.H. Rohrer & M. Sherif (Eds.), *Social Psychology at the Crossroads.* Harper & Row.

Jahoda, M. (1979, September 6). The psychological meanings of unemployment. *New Society.*

Kelvin, P., & Morley-Bunker, N. (research in progress). *Leisure and the unemployed.* Project funded by the Joint SSRC/Sports Council Panel on Recreation and Leisure Research.

Neulinger, J. (1982). Leisure lack and the quality of life. *Leisure Studies, 1,* 53-64.

Office of Population Censuses and Surveys. (1976, 1979, unpublished). *General Household Surveys 1973, 1977, and 1980.* London HMSO.

Scarman, Right Hon. Lord. (1981, April). The Brixton Disorders. *Report of Inquiry,* pp. 10-12. CMND. 8427, London, HMSO.

Sports Council. (1983). *Sport in the community. The next ten years.* London: Sports Council.

7

Participation in Physical Activity and Male Adult Development

Michael J. Dixon
UNIVERSITY OF ALBERTA
EDMONTON, ALBERTA, CANADA

Investigations concerned with involvement in regular physical activity have, in general, focused on the phenomenon of attrition from easily monitored exercise programs. Despite an awareness of the potential physiological and psychological benefits of regular exercise, attrition rates of between 30 and 70% have been commonly reported (Dishman, Ickes, & Morgan, 1980). Evidence supports the widespread belief that the number of people involved in physical activity has increased dramatically in recent years. However, the rates of attrition associated with exercise programs have not changed during the last decade (Dishman, 1982). Researchers have compiled various characterizations of the "adherent" and the "drop-out," based on a number of demographic, physiological, and psychological characteristics (Shephard, 1983). Although these characterizations may have some practical value, they have contributed very little to an understanding of the factors underlying the predominance of the sedentary lifestyle in modern society. More importantly, by focusing on these characterizations, researchers investigating involvement in physical activity have paid little attention to the reasons why large numbers of individuals choose to lead an active life. As a direct result of the lack of progress in this field, increased attention is now being directed toward different perspectives, particularly those concerned with the sociopsychological determinants of involvement in regular exercise (Shephard, 1983). Despite this apparent shift in the focus of attention, the research paradigm traditionally used in this field does not appear to have been critically reviewed.

As a result of a review of the literature related to involvement in physical activity, it was apparent that the superficial approach typically adopted in this field had not provided an appropriate perspective to interpret the processes underlying an extremely complex situation. Consequently, the aim of this study was to examine the role and importance of involvement in physical activity in the lives of a number of men, from a phenomenological perspective.

The study included 40 men between 23 and 67 years of age. In order to obtain a group in which the subjects differed widely in their origins and their styles of living, it was decided to choose four occupations as diverse as possible. Those chosen were "Academics," "Accountants," "Garbage Collectors," and "Managers." In order that the study fulfill its aims, it was decided to select the sample from groups more likely to contain individuals for whom physical activity occupied an important place in everyday life.

Biographical interviewing is not a research technique widely used in this field. However, it was particularly striking that in a number of studies where biographical interviewing had been used, the authors noted the influence of physical activity in peoples' lives (Rapoport & Rapoport, 1975; Levinson, Darrow, Klein, Levinson, & McKee, 1978; Davitz & Davitz, 1979). In view of the phenomenological nature of the study, it was decided to conduct a series of loosely structured biographical interviews. A rigorous interview schedule was not used. However, a number of subject areas were used to shape the interview. These included: family of origin, school, occupational history, marriage and the family, friendships, leisure, and physical activity. Each man was interviewed privately, and the duration of the interviews ranged between 2 and 7 hours.

The use of biographical interviewing in this study provided access to important information that could not have been measured quantitatively. The biographies obtained from the subjects provided a number of examples of individuals whose lives illustrated the complex fashion in which participation in physical activity was interwoven with patterns of daily living.

It was evident that physical activity functioned in different ways for different men—and perhaps more importantly—functioned in different ways for the same man, at different times in his life. In view of this finding, the concept of male adult development became central to the study.

Although the lifecycle concept was first enunciated by Erikson in 1960, more recent researchers have developed various conceptualizations of the adult lifecycle; and the subject has received a great deal of attention in the popular press (Vaillant, 1977; Gould, 1978; Davitz & Davitz, 1979; Nicholson; 1980). One conceptualization of the male adult life course has proved to be particularly influential. Levinson, Darrow, Klein, Levinson, and McKee (1978) argued that the male life structure evolves through a relatively orderly sequence of periods during the adult years. The sequence was argued to consist of an alternating series of structure-building and structure-changing periods. The primary task of a structure-building period was identified as trying to form a life structure where certain key choices must be made and certain values and goals can be pursued. A transitional period terminates a life structure and begins with the advent of a period of life structure evaluation. The primary tasks of every transitional period are to reappraise the existing life structure, explore the various possibilities for change, and make choices to form the basis of the ensuing period (Levinson et al., 1978). Throughout life, one or two components are said to have a central place in the life structure. These components receive the largest share of time and energy and have a profound influence on the self and the evolving life course (Levinson et al., 1978).

For a number of the men in this study, regular physical activity could certainly be regarded as a central component throughout life. These individuals made many unsolicited references to physical activity and clearly illustrated several different ways involvement in physical activity influenced their lives. Above all else, it was regarded as a way of life. Consider the following statements made by one of these men.

> Physical activity enabled me to be accepted by the system . . . and by the people around me. . . . I was a very nervous and apprehensive person and whenever any changes took place in my life I became very anxious. . . . physical activity and the friends it helped me make and all this type of thing enabled me to settle in. . . . physical activity was the only continuous thread among changing scenes, changing skills and changing friends and it enabled my life to be linked in some kind of way.

> (Academic, Aged 52)

The recurring expression of thoughts and sentiments such as those clearly articulated by the Academic make it tempting to speculate that physical activity, in some way, functions as a means of coping in many different situations. In view of this finding, it is appropriate to examine possible explanations of the processes underlying this phenomenon.

Although the areas of coping, adaptation, and competence are relatively new areas of psychological research, Antonovsky (1979) developed an insightful theory to explain the relative success of certain people, and certain social groups, in coping with stress. Antonovsky (1979) argued that Generalized Resistance Resources (GRR) were important characteristics influencing the global orientation of an individual, leading to the development and maintenance of an individual's sense of coherence. GRRs, it was argued, may be considered to be physical, biochemical, artifactual-material, cognitive, emotional, valuative-attitudinal, interpersonal-relational, or macrosociocultural. The implications of this theory, and the multidimensional nature of physical activity, appeared to provide a unique perspective from which to consider involvement in physical activity throughout the life course.

During a stable life structure, physical activity could be seen to contribute, in a number of important ways, to the lives of many of the men who participated in the study. Physical activity was repeatedly seen to act as an important means of social experience and a facilitator of social interaction. Not surprisingly, involvement in physical activity was regarded as an important influence on health and fitness. The cathartic nature of physical activity was also described frequently. A number of men clearly articulated modifications in self-concept, which had occurred as a result of changing involvement in physical activity. It was also evident that physical activity appeared to blend harmoniously with the stable lifestyles typically associated with the "Entering the Adult World" and, particularly, "Settling Down" life structures (Levinson et al., 1978).

In contrast, circumstances reported by men in relation to life around the age of 30 were less harmonious. The "Age Thirty Transition" is said to extend, roughly, between 28 and 33 years (Levinson et al., 1978). The period is characterized by an opportunity to work on the flaws and limitations evident from decisions made since entering adulthood. During an "Age Thirty

Transition" a man is said to strive to create the basis for a more satisfactory life structure. This is achieved by making conscious decisions to include or exclude or modify in some other way, major aspects of life. Although some men remain relatively untroubled by the experience, it can also produce a great deal of anxiety. Several men provided graphic descriptions of this period in their lives.

> I questioned the whole concept of working a regular job, settling down, getting a house, paying it off, having a wife, all that sort of stuff. . . . I thought "What's it all about?"

> (Accountant, Aged 35)

This man, and three others who took part in the study, subsequently made a number of decisions, which affected several important areas of their lives. In each case, these changes resulted in an increased participation in physical activity. Although other factors were undoubtedly important in the lives of these men at this time, exercise appeared to assume an important place in day-to-day life. In particular, valuative-attitudinal and interpersonal-relational aspects of regular involvement in physical activity were greatly emphasized. These findings provided some support for the argument that physical activity may function as a basis for GRRs and facilitate effective coping.

The "Age Forty Transition" can also be a traumatic period in a man's life. Rather than the emphasis being on possible modifications to an evolving life structure, the focus is on the past. A man is said to consider his achievements in life and to reflect upon his relationships with family, occupation, and community. The answers to these questions may cause deep concern and may result in lifestyle changes so that certain desires, values, talents, and aspirations may be expressed. A number of authors have written about the importance of physical concerns to men of this age (Davitz & Davitz, 1980; Nicholson, 1980). The typical 40-year-old has not fallen significantly below the levels of maximal body functioning. However, the common cosmetic changes that may occur (baldness, wrinkles, excess fat) appear to dramatically increase the salience of physical characteristics (Levinson et al., 1978). Although it was difficult in this study, with such small numbers, to provide support for the argument that physical activity can be important to a man in his forties, consider the following statements made by one of the men who participated in the study.

> Last June, last birthday, I was 42 and I started to have a serious think about myself and how I fit in the world and what my responsibilities are and everything and I started to get a bit worried because I was fat, unfit, smoking heaps, drinking too much, and I could see myself getting into an early grave. So I said "There are three things you're going to do in the next 12 months: lose weight, get fit, and stop smoking" . . . and I've done it.

> (Manager, Aged 42)

Once again, in view of the comments made by the subjects about this period in their lives, it was tempting to speculate that physical activity played an important role as a means of coping with the difficulties associated with day-to-day life and with adult development. In contrast to the functions of physical activity that appeared to predominate in relation to the "Age Thirty Transition," the "Age Forty Transition" appeared to be associated with the physical, cognitive, and emotional functions of involvement in regular exercise. In particular, the effect of involvement in regular exercise. In particular, the effect of physical activity in relation to body shape and appearance and self-concept, in general, was certainly important.

> I didn't use to care, but now it means a lot to me to look O.K. I don't want to be big and fat . . . people think garbos just sit around drinking . . . big fat drunks. . . . I like people to think that I look after myself. . . . I like to think I set an example.

(Garbage Collector, Aged 42)

Once again, although other factors were certainly influential in the lives of these men around the age of 40, exercise appeared to assume an important place in their day-to-day lives. These findings provided further support for the belief that physical activity is a useful means of providing the GRRs necessary to facilitate effective tension management.

Although tentative, the results of this exploratory study strongly suggest that involvement in physical activity plays an important part in the process of adult development. In particular, it appears that physical activity is in some way related to the way some of the men in the study coped with periods of stress in their lives. It was beyond the scope of this study to examine the possible mechanisms underlying this process in detail. Consequently, further research should be directed toward the relationship between involvement in physical activity and adult development and the possible influence of this relationship on coping processes.

References

Antonovsky, A. (1979). *Health, stress and coping.* San Francisco: Jossey-Bass.

Davitz, J., & Davitz, L. (1979). *Making it: 40 and beyond.* New York: Dutton.

Dishman, R.K. (1982). Compliance/adherence in health related exercise. *Health Psychology, 1*, 237-267.

Dishman, R.K., Ickes, W., & Morgan, W.P. (1980). Self-motivation and adherence to habitual physical activity. *Journal of Applied Social Psychology, 10*, 115-132.

Erikson, E.H. (1960). The problem of ego identity. In M.R. Stein, A.J. Vidich, & D.M. White (Eds.), *Identity and anxiety.* Illinois: Free Press.

Gould, R.L. (1978). *Transformations: Growth and change in adult life.* New York: Simon & Schuster.

Levinson, D.J., Darrow, C.N., Klein, E.B., Levinson, M.H., & McKee, B. (1978). *The seasons of a man's life.* New York: Alfred Knopf.

Nicholson, J. (1980). *Seven ages.* London: Fontana.

Rapoport, P., & Rapoport, R. (1975). *Leisure and the family life cycle.* London: Routledge & Kegan Paul.

Shephard, R.J. (1983). Physical activity and the healthy mind. *Canadian Medical Association, 128*, 525-530.

Vaillant, G.E. (1977). *Adaptation to life.* Boston: Brown.

8

The Effects of "Being Housebound," of Receiving a Meal Program Supplement, and Use of Dietary Aids on the Dietary Behavior of Senior Adults

David R. Stirling and Stephen Meehan
SIMON FRASER UNIVERSITY
BURNABY, BRITISH COLUMBIA, CANADA

Melvin G. Ralston
WHITE ROCK BAPTIST CHURCH
WHITE ROCK, BRITISH COLUMBIA, CANADA

The nutritional status of older adults in North American communities has become an area of growing concern to many health care professionals (Axelson & Penfield, 1983; Bowman & Rosenberg, 1982; Exton-Smith, Santon, & Windsor, 1972; Grandjean, Korth, Kara, Smith, & Schaefer, 1981). One portion of this population where limited information in all areas of health care appears available is on housebound seniors. A recent review of the literature identified only two nutritional studies in this area (Exton-Smith et al., 1972; Johnson & Feniak, 1965). Of the two studies, one was completed using a North American sample (Johnson & Feniak, 1965). This study reported the food practices and nutrient intake of elderly "housebound" individuals. The dietary analysis of these housebound seniors was not reported.

This study was supported by grant funds from Employment and Immigration Canada. The authors would like to acknowledge the assistance of Mr. and Mrs. A. Graham, Mrs. J. Poelvoorde, Mr. and Mrs. D. Sherwin, Mr. and Mrs. F. Griggs, and Mrs. R. Ralston in completing this project.

Although being housebound is a factor uncommonly reported in the literature, its effect on behavior and nutritional habits can be significant (Kirschmann, 1975). The effect of being housebound on the dietary intake of adult seniors has not been reported. The purpose of this study was to investigate the effect of being housebound, of participating in a subsidized 3-day per week meal program, and of using dietary supplements on the dietary intake of senior citizens.

Methods

Selection of Subjects

Twenty-eight subjects age 74 ± 8 years were drawn from a referral list provided by community contacts (friends, social services, and church people) of persons interested in a community service program called "Active Health for Seniors." This program was initiated and supported by a local church group, the White Rock Baptist Church, and the Department of Kinesiology, Simon Fraser University. Apart from this survey, "Active Health for Seniors" was attempting to provide quality contact and programs for each senior participating in the Active Health project. This survey was a part of a seniors visitation program.

Collection of Data

Over the duration of the study six personal contacts were made with each participant. Two contacts were made to establish rapport with each subject and explain the purposes of the study. Three contacts were used to collect the dietary intake data. A final contact was used to explain the results for each individual.

Having explained the purpose of the study and the procedures to be followed, a 3-day 24-hour recall method was used to document dietary intake. Portion size was established with the aid of measuring cups, glasses, bowls, and food models. By carefully interviewing each participant, accuracy and completeness of the data collected were maintained. The quantities of foods cited by each subject were converted to grams using the food tables of the nutrition almanac. Nutrient composition was calculated using an SFU dietary analysis computer program (Drinkwater, 1980).

Subjects participating in the study were grouped and regrouped into three categories according to their state of being housebound, their use of dietary supplements, and their receiving a 3-day per week meal supplement program. The matched control groups were created out of the original sample of 28 and identified accordingly for the particular characteristic being studied. For example, the housebound group was matched with a control group of nonhousebound individuals. For the purpose of this study, a housebound person was defined as any individual who only left his or her home or apartment on the average of two occasions or less each week in the previous 6-month period. This information was obtained during the initial interview with each individual.

Statistical analyses of the data were carried out using analysis of variance (ANOVA) and t-tests to show mean differences. Values of $p < .05$ were considered significant.

Follow-Up From the Study

In this study, most of the observed dietary information was within the recommended limits for seniors (Read & Graney, 1982). These results were communicated to each individual through personal follow-up interviews. However, of the 28 seniors, dietary information on 13 subjects suggested poor eating habits, and advice was given to improve their dietary intake. In one case, the dietary data was referred to the individual's physician for further follow-up.

Results

The response by the seniors to participate in this study was relatively low. Of those seniors invited to take part in the study, 54% responded. These data according to sex and marital status are given in Table 1.

Using 66% of the recommended daily intake as a critical or minimum level to determine the adequacy of the diet (Read & Graney, 1982), all groups of seniors in this study were found to be eating an adequate diet. Table 2 shows the results of the dietary intake for the 28 seniors studied, grouped according to being housebound, taking dietary supplements, and receiving a 3-day per week hot meal program. Table 3 shows the data for each of the control groups. Figures 1, 2, and 3 show the percent RDIs for total calories consumed and mean total nutrient intake for housebound seniors, seniors taking dietary aids, and seniors receiving a 3-day per week meal supplement program. The mean percent RDIs were 384%, 438%, and 327% for the housebound group, the dietary supplement group, and the meal supplement group, respectively. With respect to energy consumption, no differences were observed between any of

Table 1. Participation of senior shut-ins in the White Rock Area Nutrition Survey

| | Single | | Married | |
	Men	Women	Men	Women
Number approached	11	29	11	14
Number completing 3-day recall survey	3	8	7	10
Number rejecting	8	21	4	4

Table 2. Dietary intake for housebound, meal supplement, and dietary supplement groups

Variable	Housebound n = 15 age = 75.2 ± 8 yrs			Meal supplement n = 10 age = 72.7 ± 8 yrs			Dietary supplement n = 14 age = 73.7 ± 8 yrs		
	M	SD	% of RDI	M	SD	% of RDI	M	SD	% of RDI
Energy (Kcal)	1522.1	424.5	80	1592.6	378.6	78	1664.1	532.0	84
Protein (gm)	67.2	21.2	153	71.5	25.0	147	66.7	26.2	145
Thiamine (mg)	11.5	5.0	1040	8.2	4.9	646	13.0	5.1	1157*
Niacin (mg)	25.3	20.2	176	33.7	23.6	222	32.9	20.3	220*
Riboflavin (mg)	10.3	4.6	757	8.6	4.9	550	11.5	4.8	832*
Ascorbic acid (mg)	295.4	84.6	974	294.0	97.5	984	367.4	306.1	1213*
Vitamin A (IU)	7523.5	2451.2	88	9873.6	3260.5	105	8372.4	2400.4	92
Calcium (mg)	723.5	342.4	100	773.7	352.1	103	674.2	142.9	92
Iron (mg)	12.2	3.8	94*	13.0	4.8	115	13.2	4.3	111
	mean % of RDI = 384 ± 75*			mean % of RDI = 327 ± 69			mean % of RDI = 438 ± 81*		

*Significant values $p < .05$; comparisons were made between each group and the respective control.

Table 3. Dietary intake of the controls used for Group I, Group II, and Group III

Variable	Housebound $n = 13$ age $= 73.3 \pm 9$ yrs			Meal supplement $n = 18$ age $= 72.7 \pm 8$ yrs			Dietary supplement $n = 14$ age $= 73.7 \pm 8$ yrs		
	M	SD	% of RDI	M	SD	% of RDI	M	SD	% of RDI
Energy (Kcal)	2068.4	850.4	94	1877.6	821.3	91	1664.1	532.0	84
Protein (gm)	80.9	36.3	156	75.1	32.1	157	66.7	26.2	145
Thiamine (mg)	3.0	3.5	199	7.1	3.4	653	1.0	0.5	89*
Niacin (mg)	31.9	10.9	176	25.4	7.9	151	15.4	7.4	105*
Riboflavin (mg)	3.4	4.2	199	6.4	3.0	469	1.4	0.7	103*
Ascorbic acid (mg)	200.4	109.2	657	227.6	221.0	740	92.6	74.7	309*
Vitamin A (IU)	9843.6	5678.3	100	7983.5	6436.0	87	4265.2	668.7	49
Calcium (mg)	882.1	587.1	11	810.1	533.0	106	611.8	518.1	84
Iron (mg)	16.4	7.5	141*	14.8	6.8	117	11.4	3.9	95
	mean % of RDI = 204 ± 21*			mean % of RDI = 286 ± 53			mean % of RDI = 118 ± 11*		

*Significant values $p < .05$; comparisons were made between each group and the respective control.

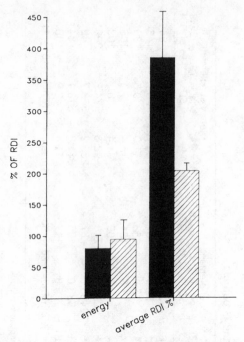

Figure 1. Effect of "being housebound" on dietary intake of 15 individuals; solid bar = housebound, hatched bar = controls

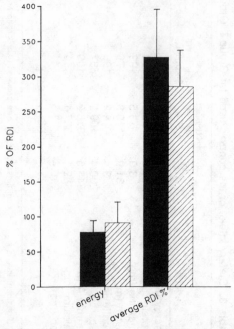

Figure 2. Effect of meals program on dietary intake of 10 individuals; solid bar = 3-day/week hot meal program, hatched bar = controls

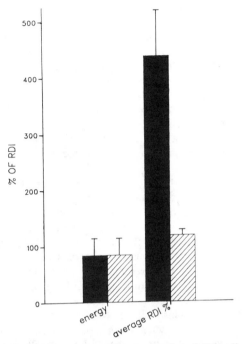

Figure 3. Effect of dietary aids on dietary intake of 15 individuals; solid bar = dietary supplement, hatched bar = control groups

the three study groups and the matched controls. The mean percent RDI, however, was significantly higher in the case of the housebound group (housebound mean % of RDI = 384 ± 75; controls mean % of RDI = 204 ± 21; $p < .01$). The energy consumption for the shut-in group, the dietary supplement group, and the meal supplement group was 80%, 78%, and 84% of RDI, respectively. The 8 nutrients for which RDIs were available are also reported in Tables 2 and 3.

Although some of the nutrient intakes were below percent RDI in some of the groups, none of these values were below the minimum level, 66% of RDI. Vitamin A intake was 88% of RDI for the housebound group; iron intake was 95% of RDI for the group without meal supplements and 94% of RDI for the housebound group. When comparisons were made between each of the three study groups and their respective control groups, using analysis of variance, the following F values were obtained: housebound and nonhousebound group $F = 14.68$ (mean % of RDI) and $F = 2.08$ (% of RDI for energy); dietary supplements and control group $F = 58.18$ (mean % of RDI) and $F = 1.00$ (% of RDI for energy); and meal supplement group and the control group $F = 1.08$ (mean % of RDI) and $F = 3.18$ (% of RDI for energy).

Comparing caloric and nutrient intake for men and women, no differences were found. Caloric intake for men was 2154.2 ± 847 KAL, 86% of RDI, and for women was 1565.6 ± 520 KAL 88% of RDI. The mean percent of RDI for men was 291.1 ± 54.4 and for women was 310.1 ± 64.7 (not significantly different).

Discussion

One fact often referred to and reported in the literature is the low response rate for seniors participating in various nutritional studies (Leitcher, Angel, & Lee, 1978). It was felt that this low participation was a result of lack of time spent in contacting and explaining the purposes of the proposed research and in establishing rapport with each individual. This study was conducted with this in mind. An emphasis was placed on making personal contact and establishing rapport with each senior. However, our results are similar to others reported in the literature. Seniors contacted during this study were reluctant to participate in the survey due to a general disinterest and mistrust of research in general.

The nutritional status of the three groups of seniors (Tables 2 and 3) participating in this study was adequate, even though the caloric intake was below the recommended daily intake. These data are in agreement with work published by Reid and Niles (1972) and Johnson and Leitcher (1978). In a study of 50 noninstitutionalized senior citizens Reid reported 36% of the cases with caloric intakes below the recommended standard. Johnson's study of 74 "housebound" individuals reported 67% of the sample had mean caloric values below the standard. Leitcher et al. (1978), studying a similar group to the one reported here with respect to age and geographical location, reported energy intakes well below the dietary standard. There are several possibilities to explain the reduced caloric intake values when compared to the recommended standard. Some evidence suggests that using the 24-hour recall method for dietary analyses can significantly underestimate the actual caloric intake. Research (Madden, Goodman, & Guthrie, 1976) would suggest that this may not be true in studies of the type reported here. More importantly, these results may be due to the inappropriate use of the dietary standards suggested by Nutrition Canada National Survey (1970-1972). The standards suggested for an older population may not take into account those factors that best reflect the energy requirements of the elderly. For example, it is difficult to predict and therefore control the effect that various geriatric disease processes could have on actual energy requirements. Research (Williamson et al., 1964) shows that men and women over the age of 65 on the average suffer from over three different disease processes. As a result the recommended standards may overestimate the true energy requirements of the seniors.

The deficiencies observed for three of the nutrients (vitamin A, calcium, and iron) were not below the minimum level (i.e., 66% of RDI). We suggest considering the potential difficulties in using recommended standards, that the intake of these three nutrients was adequate for the subjects studied.

Dietary Supplements

Fifty percent of the subjects participating in this study used dietary supplements. These supplements included vitamin C, multivitamins, iron, multiminerals, and calcium.

As shown in Tables 2 and 3 the dietary intake for those individuals was sufficient without the use of the dietary supplements. These supplements appeared to provide no specific nutritional benefit, yet they do increase the intake of certain nutrients to excessive levels.

Although some work has been reported on the use of food supplements by the elderly (Read & Graney, 1982; Rae & Burke, 1978), there appear to be no previous reports in the literature on the nutrient intakes of the elderly with and without diet supplements. The data reported here would support earlier suggestions that the nutrient supplements provide little if any unique health benefit (Rae & Burke, 1978).

Meal Supplement Program

There was no difference found between the group supplementing their diet with the hot meal program and those who prepared their own meals. This would suggest that the hot meal program has become an integral part of the diet of seniors on the program. From data collected through personal interviews the persons using the hot meal supplement program depended heavily on the meal. The shopping habits of this group were less particular and regular compared to the matched control group. On the days when the hot meal was provided the two other meals were light in content, often consisting of toast, cheese, and/or salad. In some cases portions of the hot meal provided would be saved for the days when the meal was not provided.

The findings reported in this study are limited and as a result no conclusions drawn. These limitations are due to sample size, biased nature of the sample, and the fact that no data were collected on the income backgrounds of the subjects.

Summary

Although the caloric intake of the subjects in this study was below the recommended standards, in almost all cases the seniors tended to overeat many of the essential nutrients. Fifty percent of the subjects participating in the study were taking dietary supplements. These supplements provided no unique health benefit and tended to provide quantities of essential nutrients in excess of the daily requirements. There was no observed difference between males and females in any aspect of their dietary intakes. The hot meal supplement program was an integral part of the diet of those seniors who participated in the meal supplement program. The seniors participating in a hot meal program tended to avoid purchasing essential grocery items. Some seniors would try to spread the meal supplement provided over a 2-day period. The difference between the mean total percent RDI for each pair of study and control groups appeared significant just for the housebound/nonhousebound pair. The housebound seniors in this study consumed amounts of protein, thiamine, niacin, riboflavin, ascorbic acid, vitamin A, calcium, and iron in excess of the recommended standards. Further study is needed, particularly in isolating the effect of "being housebound" on dietary intake.

References

Axelson, M.L., & Penfield, M.P. (1983). Food and nutrition-related attitudes of elderly persons living alone. *Journal of Nutrition Education*, **15**(1), 23.

Bowman, B.B., & Rosenberg, I.H. (1982). Assessment of the nutritional status of the elderly. *The American Journal of Clinical Nutrition*, **35**, 1142.

Davies, L., Purves, R., & Haldsworth, M.D. (1983). Longitudinal study on elderly recipients of meals on wheels. *Journal of Human Nutrition*, **35**, 442.

Drinkwater, D. (1980). *Dietary analysis computer program*. Department of Kinesiology, Simon Fraser University, B.C.

Exton-Smith, A.N., Santon, B.R., & Windsor, A.C.M. (1972). *Nutrition of housebound old people*. London: King Edwards Hospital Fund.

Grandjean, A.C., Korth, L.L., Kara, G.C., Smith, J.L., & Schaefer, A.E. (1981). Nutritional status of elderly participants in a congregate meals program. *Journal of Dietetic Association*, **78**, 324.

Habson, E.L. (1983). Meals delivery systems. *The American Journal of Clinical Nutrition*, **26**, 1150.

Johnson, B., & Feniak, E. (1965). Food practices and nutrient intake of elderly homebound individuals. *Canadian Nutrition Notes*, **21**(6), 61.

Kirschmann, J.D. (1975). *Nutrition almanac*. Nutrition Search Inc. New York: McGraw-Hill.

Kohrs, M.B., Norstrom, J., Plowman, E.L., O'Hanlon, P., Movre, C., Davis, C., Abrahams, B., & Eckland, D. (1980). Association of participation in a nutritional program for the elderly with nutritional status. *American Journal of Clinical Nutrition*, **33**, 2643.

Leichter, J., Angel, J.F., & Lee, M. (1978). Nutritional status of selected group of free-living elderly people in Vancouver. *Journal of Canadian Medical Association*, **118**, 40.

Luhrs, C.E. (1973). Feeding the elderly. *The American Journal of Clinical Nutrition*, **26**, 1150.

Madden, J.P., Goodman, S.J., & Guthrie, H.A. (1976). Validity of the 24-hour recall. *Journal of the American Dietetic Association*, **68**, 143.

National dairy report: Nutrition and the elderly. *Dairy Council Digest*, **54**(4), 19.

Nutrition Canada National Survey, 1970-72. (1973). Report by Nutrition Canada to the Department of National Health and Welfare. Ottawa Information Canada.

O'Hanlon, P., & Kohrs, M.B. (1978). Dietary studies of older Americans. *The American Journal of Clinical Nutrition*, **31**, 1257.

Rae, J., & Burke, A.L. (1978). Counselling the elderly on nutrition in a community health care system. *Journal of the American Geriatric Society*, **26**(3), 130.

Read, M.H., & Graney, A.S. (1982). Food supplement usage by the elderly. *Journal of the American Dietetic Association*, **80**, 250.

Reid, D.L., & Niles, J.E. (1972). Food habits and nutritional intakes of noninstitutionalized senior citizens. *Canadian Journal of Public Health*, **68**, 154.

Weber, F., Barnard, R.J., & Roy, D. (1983). Effects of a high complex-carbohydrate, low-fat diet and daily exercise on individuals 70 years of age and older. *Journal of Gerontology*, **38**, 155.

Williamson, J., Stokoe, I.H., Gray, S., et al. (1964). The unreported needs of the elderly at home. *Lancet*, **1**, 1117.

Yearick, E.S., Wang, M.L., & Pisias, S.J. (1978). Nutritional status of the elderly: Dietary and biochemical findings. *Journal of Gerontology*, **33**, 657.

Young, C.M., & Trulson, M.F. (1960). Methodology for dietary studies in epidemiological surveys 2 strengths and weaknesses of dietary methods. *American Journal of Public Health*, **60**, 803.

PART II

Program Perspectives

9

Exercise, Sport, and Physical Activity for the Elderly: Principles and Problems of Programming

Everett L. Smith and Catherine Gilligan
UNIVERSITY OF WISCONSIN
MADISON, WISCONSIN, USA

Ancient Gerontology

Throughout recorded history, mankind has been concerned with aging. This concern focused on the causes and preventive measures for aging and continues to the present. Early views held aging to be a disease that could be prevented with special cautions. Others attributed the aging process to a decline in sexual function and devised potions and rituals to maintain sexual vigor. The concerns with the aging process may be traced back to 3000 B.C. in China, India, Egypt, and Mesopotamia. Chinese writings indicate that longevity resulted from a balance of life: That is, life harmony promotes health and longevity; aging is the result of loss of harmony with the disease of aging overcoming life. Egyptians viewed aging as a disease which could be prevented with the correct nutrients and a balanced physical and mental life. Both societies' histories report individuals living 70 to 95 years.

In the Greek period Plato wrote, "The mode of treatment by which the body and mind are to be preserved is through moderate exercises which reduces to order, according to their affinities, the particles and affections which are wandering about the body." Aristotle wrote that old age is a drying of the body and a loss of innate heat. Thus preservation of heat and moisture was necessary for vitality. In the first century A.D., Galen carried forward this Greek influence. Galen was a powerful influence in the medical world in his time and for centuries to follow. Galen used the term *gerocomy* for the medical care of the elderly (Freeman, 1979).

Modern Gerontology

The modern era of studies on aging began in 1903 when Metchnikoff at the Pasteur Institute in Paris named the biological study of sensescence *gerontology*. Six years later, Nascher of New York coined the word *geriatrics* to describe the clinical aspects of aging (Freeman, 1979). Gerontology has grown rapidly over the past 75 years, but many of the current theories of aging have historical roots. Some remnants of Aristotle's concepts are still observable in today's thoughts of aging. His concept of cooling off can be related to the decrease in metabolic rate and drying out with decrease in total body water. Even though Aristotle had no knowledge of the underlying cellular processes, his descriptions of the decrements in functional capacity were accurate.

Although only the biological facets of aging will be addressed in this text, many interactions exist between biological aging and social, psychological, and economical well-being. Many people fear aging will cause them to lose health, independence, and vigor. The goal of gerontology is to investigate methods of preserving physical and mental health and independence to the greatest extent and as late in life as possible. The role of researchers and educators is to investigate and disseminate methods to enhance life with youthfulness and well-being as long as possible through a better understanding of how an individual or population ages relative to heritage and environment.

Numerous theories try to explain the aging process on the basis of genetics or the environment and their interaction. One is that each species is genetically programmed for a specific maximum lifespan. The maximum lifespan of man has not changed much over the last 3,000 years. The average length of life, however, has increased from 35 prior to 1900, to 45 in the early 1900s, to 75 in the 1980s. This increase is due both to increased health knowledge and to the control of infectious diseases.

Understanding of the genetic controls of overall lifespan is still being sought. Research by Carrel (1912) in the early 1910s indicated that the individual cell (and thus potentially the organism) had an infinite lifespan. In the 1960s, however, Hayflick (1965) reported that the human lung fibroblast divides only a limited number of times in cell culture. After 50 (± 10) doublings, the cells cease dividing and die. His research indicated that individual organisms are programmed to die.

Two types of programmed end-points are being researched: one based on time alone and the other triggered by an external factor. An example of the first is the work of Saunders and Fallon (1967) with chick embryos. The axillary cells of the chick wing bud are programmed to die at about 4 1/2 days. It appears that within these cells there is a genetic mechanism causing self-destruction. Triggered cell death has also been demonstrated in embryological research. In the developing male embryo, Mullerian ducts are present but disintegrate with the introduction of androgen from the developing testes. If the tissue is maintained in cell culture, it will degenerate only if triggered by the presence of androgen (Donahoe et al., 1982).

Regardless of the controlling mechanisms of aging, many physiological declines with age are similar to those of disuse. Young athletes placed at extended chair rest or bedrest suffer functional decrements mirroring those of aging. At least 50% of what is commonly called aging in the population of the developed world may be attributed to disuse atrophy. If fitness were maintained across the lifespan, many of the common cardiovascular problems would be delayed and the individual would function at a much younger level than the average for his or her chronological age.

Age may be defined chronologically or physiologically. A person is often called old at the age of 65 while still having the vigor of a 45-year-old. In general, the older adult population may be separated into three groups: (a) the young old, between 55 and 75 and with a maximal capability of 5 to 7 METs; (b) the old old, 75 plus and with a maximal capability of 2 to 3 METs; and (c) the athletic old, who, regardless of their chronological age, have maintained a high degree of physical fitness and have a maximal capacity of approximately 9 to 10 METs (Morse & Smith, 1981). (A MET, or metabolic unit, is equivalent to 3.5 ml O_2/kg/min, the average oxygen consumption at chair rest.) These categories satisfy the characteristics of the general population but are not necessarily the most representative of an individual's capabilities for which physiological age is more appropriate. Physiological age is defined by one's ability to adapt to his or her environment, usually measured in terms of endurance, strength, flexibility, coordination, and work capacity. The general population peaks physiologically at about age 30 and after that sedentary persons lose functional capacity at a rate of about .75 to 1% per year. Each organ system loses capacity at a distinct rate.

In general, work capacity, cardiac output, respiratory function, muscle mass, metabolic rate, nerve conduction rate, flexibility, bone, and total body water decline while blood pressure increases with age (see Table 1). These changes are expressed by an overall loss of functional capability. Physiological aging is first observed in the decreasing ability to exercise.

Work capacity declines by 25 to 30% in the older adult and represents a decreased capability to function using large muscle grounds in sustained activity. Work capacity is comprised of many factors, including musculoskeletal, neurological, cardiovascular, and pulmonary function.

Cardiovascular

One of the major elements in work capacity is the cardiovascular system. Cardiac output declines on the average by 30% in the aging individual (between 30 and 70) as a result of changes in the characteristics of the heart and the vascular tree. The heart muscle decreases in mass and contractility. The cardiac mass is directly related to its strength, and its changes influence the duration of the systole, the volume of blood that can be expelled from the ventricles, and the pressure generated. As a result, stroke volume is decreased. In older adults, stroke volume is adequate for mild work, but maximal stroke volume is 15 to 20% lower than in the young. The decreased contractility means a decline in maximal heart rate, further decreasing maximal cardiac output.

The aging heart is thus both less efficient and weaker, limiting the amount of blood that can be delivered to sustain exertion. In addition, while the heart

Table 1. Biological functional changes between the ages of 30 and 70

Biological Function	Change
Work capacity (%)	↓25–30
Cardiac output (%)	↓30
Maximum heart rate (beats·min⁻¹)	↓24
Blood pressure (mm Hg)	
Systolic	↑10–40
Diastolic	↑ 5–10
Respiration (%)	
Vital capacity	↓40–50
Residual volume	↑30–50
Basal metabolic rate (%)	↓ 8–12
Musculature (%)	
Muscle mass	↓25–30
Hand grip strength	↓25–30
Nerve conduction velocity (%)	↓10–15
Flexibility (%)	↓20–30
Bone (%)	
Women	↓25–30
Men	↓15–20
Renal function (%)	↓30–50

Note. From "Physical Activity Prescription for the Older Adult" by E.L. Smith and C. Gilligan, 1983, from *The Physician and Sportsmedicine, 11*, pp. 91–101, Reprinted by permission.

becomes less able to move blood against resistance, there is increased resistance to blood flow. Average blood pressure increases by 10 to 40 mmHg systolic and 5 to 10 mmHg diastolic due to changes such as plaquing in the vessel walls making the walls rougher and narrower. Also, calcification of the medial layer of the arteries and arterioles limits their expansion during systole, producing higher systolic pressures and higher resistance. This is clearly observed during physical activity. These changes may precipitate conditions which limit physical activity, providing a common excuse for not exercising because it may result in injury to the older adult. Inactivity itself is dangerous to the heart; physical activity programs can be designed to prevent injury and strengthen the cardio-vascular system.

The increase in blood pressure is often called normal because it is common in our society. In many societies, and in many individuals within our society, age does not produce increases in blood pressure. Thus, changes in pressure may instead be a result of lifestyle and inactivity.

Neuromuscular

The declines in the neuromuscular system are often a limiting factor for physical activity. With age, there is wasting of muscle mass and a decline in nerve con-duction rate. These changes affect the integration of muscle action, strength, and coordination in activities of daily living or recreation. In general, both the number and size of muscle fibers decrease with age. Muscle mass declines 20 to 25% with a parallel decline in muscular strength. Burke, Tuttle, Thompson, Janney, and Lueber (1965) tested grip strength and grip strength endurance in 311 males between the ages of 12 and 79. They observed that the grip strength endurance peaked at the age of 20 to 24 and then declined at a consistent rate; grip strength also peaked in the 20 to 24 age range, but the decline was sharpened after the age of 60. Campbell, McComas, and Petito (1973) evaluated the muscular strength of the extensor digitorum brevis in 28 healthy subjects aged 60 to 69. Decreases in strength and muscle mass were observed and attributed to loss of functional motor units and a slowed muscle twitch in surviving units. While no motor unit loss was observed in the younger population (ages 3 to 58), a continual loss of functional motor units was observed in the group over 60. Whether this is unique to the specific sample or applicable to the general aging population is not clear. Moritani (1981) suggests that there may be a general anatomical change in the aging muscular system that prevents muscle hypertrophy at 60 years or older. Because of the small number of older adults he investigated, this is not conclusive, and the investigation of muscular training in older adults offers an area rich for research.

The three basic types of skeletal muscle fiber are Type I (slow twitch, high oxidative), Type IIA (fast twitch, high oxidative), and Type IIB (fast twitch, low oxidative). These change at different rates in different muscles within an individual and between individuals in the aging population. There is an overall decline in muscle diameter as a result of atrophy of all fiber types and the decreased number of Type II fibers (which are larger in diameter than Type I). An apparent preferential loss seems to be in Type IIA and IIB fibers, resulting in an increased percentage of Type I fibers. Larsson, Sjodin, and Karlsson (1978) found the ratio of Type I to Type II fibers of the quadriceps increased by 15% between the ages of 25 and 65 in men. Muscular strength loss has been significantly correlated with the loss of the Type II fibers (Larsson, Grimby, & Karlsson, 1979).

Nerve conduction velocity declines by 10 to 15% in the general population. This slowing may reflect changes at the synapse as well as in the nerve fiber itself. Changes in the neuromuscular junction of the aged include a decreased surface area because of decreased junctional folds, a wider synaptic cleft, and a decreased availability of acetylcholine packets (Smith, 1982). These changes are reflected by an increased reaction time for muscle contraction. Delayed muscle contraction may be the result of decreased nerve conduction rate, changes in the motor end plate, and/or changes in the muscle fibers. Spirduso (1980) called psychomotor speed ''a rubric describing the speed with which an individual can perform a task which involves reacting motorically to an environmental stimulus'' (p. 851). She reported that reaction time is influenced by changes in both the central and peripheral nervous systems. Spirduso (1975) reported that slower reaction times in the older adult are due more to central than peripheral nervous system changes. Birren, Carden, and Phillips (1963) compared the reaction time of pressing a key in response to a musical tone in young and old subjects. The younger adults had a time lapse of 0.18 s while the 65 + population had a .22 s delay, an increase of 22%. Increased reaction time and the decline in muscle mass often limits the older adult in activities of daily living and in a variety of recreational activities. Research has demonstrated, however, that many of these declines are due to disuse rather than aging and may be substantially reduced or prevented.

Basal Metabolism

A general decline of 8 to 12% in basal metabolic rate is observed between the ages of 30 and 70. This decline reflects changes in body composition rather than in cellular function. Tzankoff and Norris (1977) observed that while basal metabolic rate declined, its relationship to lean body mass was unchanged, showing that increased fat was responsible for the reduced total body metabolism. Thus, there is no reduction in metabolism at the individual muscle cell level.

Lung

With age, vital capacity declines 40 to 50%, and residual volume increases 30 to 50%. The lung tissue is less elastic and the thoracic cage stiffer. In conjunction with these changes, the total surface area of the lung decreases from 80 sq m to approximately 60 sq m. Declines in alveolar ventilation and blood perfusion of the lung tissue may also be observed. Close inspection of alveolar ventilation shows a reduction or cessation of capillary bloodflow to some alveoli, while in others there is a reduction in the alveolar ventilation due to the loss of tissue elasticity, thus, early closure of some alveolar sacs. Some alveoli are ventilated not at all or only during forced resistance activity or during exercise where increased pressure keeps the sac open. During rest, there is relatively little difference between young and old lung function. During exercise, however, a decreased vital capacity demands a greater breathing rate to meet the blood oxygenation demands. The greater air velocity results in greater turbulence and therefore resistance to air flow. Thus, the older adult may be limited in exercise capacity by a variety of lung function declines compromising the delivery of oxygen to body tissues.

Bone

Bone involution is pandemic in the aging population. Its manifestations are more pronounced in women than in men due to lower initial bone mass, earlier onset of loss (age 35 vs. age 50) and a higher rate of loss (1 to 2% per year vs. 0.5% per year). For a third of the female population, bone involution will lead to osteoporosis and an increased potential of fracture of the skeleton by the age of 75 (Crilly, Horsman, Marshall, & Nordin, 1978). Each year, 1.3 million fractures occur due to osteoporosis. Approximately $3 to 6 billion per year is necessary for health care related to osteoporotic fractures (National Institute of Health, 1984). The personal cost is equally high: Of these fractures, 15 to 30% are fatal, and the women who survive may be subject to chronic pain, deformity, and limited mobility and independence (Avioli, 1984). Hip fractures, vertebral crush fractures, and wrist fractures are the three most common endpoints of osteoporotic weakening.

Bone is a complex, living tissue which undergoes a continual cycle of mineral resorption and deposition. Bone remodeling is an interactive system with *osteoclasts* (bone removal) followed by *osteoblasts* (bone formation); a supply of calcium is necessary to mineralize the matrix formed. The skeleton functions both as structural support and as a mineral reservoir. Correspondingly, it is influenced by both local (mechanical) and systemic (hormonal) controls. The local factors call for bone mass to support habitual activities, while the systemic controls act to maintain serum calcium and phosphorous levels.

Systemic factors that influence bone include parathyroid hormone, vitamin D, calcitonin, estrogens and androgens, and calcium intake and absorption. The decrease in estrogen levels at menopause is particularly implicated in the development of osteoporosis: Some women have a 2.5 to 5% per year bone loss in the 4 to 5 years following menopause. Estrogen replacement therapy has been reported to almost obliterate this loss in 10-year longitudinal studies (Lindsey, Hart, Forrest, & Baird, 1980). Calcium absorption is improved by higher levels of circulating estrogen. To maintain a positive calcium balance after menopause, calcium intake must be increased approximately 500 mg/day from the 1000 mg/day premenopausal level (Heaney, Becker, & Saville 1982). The average woman, however, rarely consumes even 1000 mg/day, and there tends to be a decrease in calcium intake with aging. This results in a chronic negative calcium balance that calls for drawing calcium from the skeletal reservoir. Physical activity declines as well, and this exacerbates the imbalance between the demand for serum mineral levels and that for bone strength to support habitual activity.

Since 1892, when Wolff hypothesized that increased weightbearing produces increased bone mass, evidence has mounted that activity is vital to bone health. Bassett and Becker (1962) demonstrated that bone acts as a piezoelectric crystal, converting mechanical stress to electrical. When a load is placed on the bone, a slight deformation occurs with a resultant negative charge on the convex side and a positive charge on the concave. Calcium is deposited on the negatively charged area and resorbed from the positive.

The effects of inactivity on bone are best demonstrated in studies of weightlessness and bedrest. In short periods of time, significant amounts of bone loss can be observed in either of these conditions. Two studies found a loss rate of approximately 1% per week in the os calcis with bedrest. (Donaldson et al., 1970; Rambaut, Dietlein, Yogel, & Smith, 1972). Astronauts also experienced bone loss from this site (Mack, LaChance, Vose, & Vogt, 1967). Krolner and Toft (1983) found a corresponding decline of .9% per week in the lumbar spine of young healthy subjects placed at bedrest due to the protrusion of an intervertebral disc.

Habitual high physical activity levels are correlated with greater bone mass in athletes. Both the level of stress and the sites at which it is applied are important. Nilsson and Westlin (1971) found that weightlifters had the greatest bone mass of the athletes studied, followed by throwers, runners, soccer players, and swimmers. Dalen and Olsson (1974) found a 20% greater bone mass in the femur and humerus of cross-country runners (aged 50 to 59) than in controls of similar age, height, and weight (Dalen & Olsson, 1974). In studies of unilateral sports, greater bone mass of the dominant arm has been demonstrated in tennis players (Jones, Priest, Hayes, Tichenon, & Nagel, 1977) main active. Montoye, Smith, Fardon, and Howley (1980) found 13% more bone mass in the dominant humerus than the nondominant in 61 male tennis players at an average age of 64. In 35 male tennis players over 70, Huddleston, Rockwell, Kulund, and Harrison (1980) found an 11.4% differential. The bone mass of the nondominant arms of athletes in unilateral sports is similar to that of sedentary controls. The specificity of bone response is not confined to unilateral sports. Jacobson, Beaver, Grubb, Taft, and Talmage (1984) found that radius bone mineral content was higher in both swimmers and tennis players than in controls. Lumbar bone mineral content, however, was not enhanced in swimmers, while tennis players had 20.2% greater bone mass than controls. This shows the necessity of weightbearing activity for maintenance or hypertrophy of the spine.

The average middle-aged and older woman does not have a history of chronic physical activity. Several studies have shown, however, that intervention programs can produce higher bone mass in the formerly sedentary population as well. The radius bone mineral content of 30 elderly women (mean age 81) was monitored over a 3-year period. Twelve who participated in a 3 day per week exercise program gained 2.29% in bone mineral content, while the 18 controls lost 3.28% (Smith, Reddan, & Smith, 1981).

In a similar study of 35 to 65 year old women (mean age 51), Smith, Smith, Ensign, and Shea (1984) measured bone mineral mass of the radius, ulna, and humerus over 3 to 4 years in 200 women. The 80 control subjects and 120 exercise subjects were similar in age, height, weight, and level of fitness at the beginning of the study. The exercise program consisted of 45 min per day, 3 days per week. The control group lost 2.44% per year in left radius bone mineral. During the first year, the left radius bone mineral of the exercise group declined by 3.77%. In the following 2 years, when more emphasis was placed on upper body exercises, bone mineral content increased by 1.39% per year. After 3 years, there was a total loss of 7.2% in the control group and a 3% loss in the exercise group.

Krolner, Toft, Nielsen, and Tondevold found benefits of exercise intervention to the spine as well. They studied 31 women between the ages of 50 and 73 with a previous Colles fracture. The lumbar spine bone mineral content increased 3.5% in 8 months in 16 women who trained 1 hr per day, 2 days per week. Fifteen women who did not change their activities declined by 2.7% in lumbar spine bone mineral content.

The calcium balance reflects changes in bone mass in exercise intervention. Aloia, Cohn, Ostuni, Crane, and Ellis found a calcium balance of +42 mg/day in 9 women who began a physical activity program of 1 hr per day, 3 days per week; but the 9 control subjects lost 43 mg per day.

Evaluating Aerobic Capacity in Older Adults

Aerobic capacity is an important determinant for continuing independence in older adults. It is also a major factor in prescribing the level of intensity of exercise programs for maximum benefit. It has been shown that physical activity at a level of 40 to 70% of maximum capacity, 30 to 60 min per day, 3 to 5 days per week, is needed to increase aerobic capacity. Burning 10% of daily caloric intake in aerobic activity may be protective against cardiovascular problems. This caloric guideline can be used in determining the frequency, intensity, and duration of exercise.

The two most common instruments for evaluating aerobic work capacity are the treadmill and the bicycle ergometer. Each may be used to evaluate the maximal work capacity of a subject by progressive increments in work load. In a common treadmill protocol designed by Balke, the treadmill speed is held constant at 3 mph and the grade is raised by 2.5% every 2 minutes. This corresponds to an increase of 1 MET (3.5 ml O_2/kg/min) with each increase in grade. While this protocol can be used by some young-old subjects, it is often too rigorous for many older adults. For individuals with low-work capacity, we recommend that the speed be decreased to 2 mph and the grade increments to 2%. The increments are then about .5 METs, with a starting MET level of 2 METs (see Table 2).

The bicycle ergometer test can also be modified for older adults. The usual exercise protocol starts at 300 KGM/min (American College, 1980), but this load may exceed the maximal capacity of some older adults. A protocol modified to an initial load of about 2 METs, with increments of approximately .55 METs, is shown in Table 3.

If a treadmill or bicycle ergometer is not available, field tests of aerobic capacity are available. Our laboratory developed the chair step test for this situation (Smith & Gilligan, 1983). The subject sits in a straight-backed chair with a "step" placed in front of the chair. Each second the subject touches the front edge of the step with the arch of one foot and returns the foot to the floor, alternating right and left feet. For each step level, the test is conducted for 2 min, the subject rests, and if there are no signs of abnormality, and the heart rate is less than 75% of heart rate reserve, the level is repeated for 5 min. The subject rests between step heights and continues to the next level under the same criteria as above. The step heights are 6 in., 12 in., and 18 in. A fourth intensity level is provided with having the subject raise their arms to shoulder level simultaneously with lifting the feet to the 18 in. step. The MET levels of this test are similar to the modified Balke protocol as shown in Table 2. This protocol was designed for use as a home self-test. In the laboratory or clinic where blood pressure, ECG, and heart rate are monitored, the test can be done continuously, 2 min at each level. The test may be continued up to maximum capacity or final level in this case (Smith & Gilligan, 1984).

Several considerations are common to any exercise testing protocol. Blood pressure and ECG should be monitored. The test should be discontinued if indications of exertional intolerance (Table 4) occur. Any later prescriptions

Table 2. Comparison of 3-mph Balke Treadmill test, the Modified Balke test, and the Chair Step test

3-Mph Balke Treadmill Test*			2-Mph Modified Balke Test*			Chair Step Test†		
Grade (%)	VO_2 ($ml \cdot kg^{-1} \cdot min^{-1}$)	METs	Grade (%)	VO_2 ($ml \cdot kg^{-1} \cdot min^{-1}$)	METs	Step Ht (in.)	VO_2 ($ml \cdot kg^{-1} \cdot min^{-1}$)	METs
0.0	10.5	3.0	0.0	7.0	2.0	6	8.0	2.3
2.5	14.0	4.0	2.0	8.9	2.5	12	10.0	2.9
5.0	17.5	5.0	4.0	10.8	3.1	18	12.3	3.5
7.5	21.0	6.0	6.0	12.7	3.6	18	13.7	3.9
10.0	24.5	7.0	8.0	14.6	4.2			
			10.0	16.5	4.7			

*Energy costs calculated from formulas provided in Balke B. Ware RW: An experimental study of physical fitness of Air Force personnel. US Armed Forces Med J 10:675–688, 1959.
†Energy costs obtained from unpublished data from our laboratory tests of oxygen consumption during the chair step test.
Note. From "Physical Activity Prescription for the Older Adult" by E.L. Smith and C. Gilligan, 1983, 11, pp. 91–101. Reprinted by permission.

Table 3. Suggested bicycle ergometer protocol for older adults

Weight		Initial load[a]		Load increment[a]	
Kg	Lb	Kg/min	Watts	Kg/min	Watts
50	110	25	4.25	50	8.5
60	132	50	8.5	50	8.5
70	154	100	16.6	75	12.5
80	176	125	21	75	12.5
90	198	175	27	75	12.5
100	220	200	33.3	100	16.6

[a]Values for the met levels, based on weight and load, were determined by the formula VO_2 (1/min) = kg/min × 2 + 300 (ACSM, 1980, p. 146). The initial load is approximately 2 mets and the load increment is approximately .55 mets. Values of kg/min are rounded to the nearest 25 because of the limitations of dial settings on bicycle ergometers.

Note. From E.L. Smith, Special considerations in developing exercise programs for the older adult, In *Behavioral Health: A Handbook of Health Enhancement and Disease Prevention* (p. 535) by (Eds.) J.D. Matarazzo, N.E. Miller, S.M. Weiss, J.A. Herd, and Weiss, 1984, New York: John Wiley. Reprinted by permission.

of exercise intensity should be at a level below that of the maximum achieved on the test. The safety of the subject should be protected. For treadmill tests, it is advisable to have a low-profile treadmill with handrails. The subject should start standing on the treadmill using the handrails for support, and the speed of the treadmill should be gradually increased from 0 mph to 2 or 3 mph. A 2 to 3-min warm-up period helps the subject to get used to the treadmill before letting go of the handrails.

Subjects should be retested at intervals of 6 to 12 months. The shorter interval should be used for those who have very low capacity on the initial test. In some cases, the initial test may be terminated due to limitations other than aerobic work capacity, such as quadriceps fatigue. After some time in a physical activity program, these limitations are decreased, and moreover, aerobic work capacity is increased. The intensity of the exercise program should always be based on the subject's current fitness level.

Once the subjects fitness level is determined, the criteria of 10% of daily caloric intake and 40 to 70% intensity can be used to set the frequency, intensity, and duration of the activity program. Frequency must be at least 3 times per week in medium intensity programs to produce improvements in fitness. For older adults with low intensity, a daily or sometimes twice daily program is recommended. The intensity of a program in METs is related to its caloric cost—Excal (exercise calories) = weight (kg) × (METs-1) × 1.05 (kcals/METs/hr) per hour. Thus, to use 10% of daily calories in exercise at a particular level, duration (per day) = .1 × intake/excal. Intake per day can be estimated as weight (kg) × 1.05 (kcals/MET/hr) × 1.1 (average 24 hr MET level for older adults) × 24 (hours). Dividing 10% of this by the formula for exercise calories gives duration (hours) = 2.64/(METs-1).

Sound medical care and education and programming in physical fitness can enhance the lives of older adults. It is our responsibility to seek to understand the capabilities and needs of the older adult and to provide appropriate pro-

Table 4. Indications of exertional intolerance.

1. Signs & symptoms of Exertional Intolerance

    Dizziness or near syncope
    Angina
    Nausea
    Marked Dyspnea
    Severe claudication or other pain
    Staggering or persistent unsteadiness
    Mental Confusion
    Facial expression signifying severe distress
    Loss of sustained vigor of palpable pulse
    Cyanosis or severe pallor
    Lack of rapid erythematous return of skin color after brief firm
    compression

2. Electrocardiographic Changes

    ST-T segment horizontal or "divergent" displacement of 0.2 mV above
    or below the resting isoelectric line for at least 0.08 second duration
    after the junction ("J") point

    Ventricular Arrhythmia: Ventricular tachycardia (3 or more successive
    ectopic ventricular complexes); Continuous bigeminal or trigeminal ec-
    topic ventricular complexes; Frequent unifocal or multifocal ectopic
    ventricular complexes amounting to greater than 30% (trigeminy) of
    the total beats per minute. Due to the difficulty in differentiating bet-
    ween supraventricular and ventricular rhythms, unless well interpreted,
    supraventricular atrial complexes with aberrant ventricular conduction
    should be interpreted in the same way as extopic ventricular beats.

    Atrial-ventricular or ventricular conduction disturbances: AV Block,
    Mobitz Type I (Wenckebach); Second Degree AV Block, Mobitz Type
    II; Third Degree (complete) AV Block; Sudden Left Bundle Branch
    Block

3. *Blood Pressure Responses*

    Systolic blood pressure dropping by more than 10 mm Hg or rising
    above 250 mm Hg

    Diastolic pressure rising by more than 20 mm Hg, or above 110–120
    mm Hg

4. Malfunctioning equipment

Note. From *Guidelines for Graded Exercise Testing and Exercise Prescription* (p. 23-27) by
American College of Sports Medicine, 1980, Philadelphia: Lea & Febiger. Adapted with
permission.

grams on this basis. Currently, health care personnel are encouraging regular
exercise for older adults as a means to maintain independence and function.

Any physical activity program should have duration, frequency, and intensity chosen to maximize the physiological benefits. It should also contain
activities to stress the five major components of total fitness: endurance,
strength, flexibility, balance, and coordination. Physical activity should not
be prohibited on the basis of age. The program must, however, be designed
with the characteristics of the group in mind.

Research has demonstrated improvements in cardiovascular and muscular systems, flexibility, and bone in older adults through physical activity (American College, 1980; Shepard, 1978; Smith, 1984). The general guides to physical activity apply to both young and old, but certain modifications in programs may be necessary because of orthopedic or physiological limitations.

References

Aloia, J.F., Cohn, S.H., Ostuni, J.A., Crane, R., & Ellis, K. (1978). Prevention of involutional bone loss by exercise. *Annals of International Medicine, 80*, 356-358

American College of Sportsmedicine (1980). *Guidelines for graded exercise testing and exercise prescription* (2nd ed.). Philadelphia: Lea and Febinger.

Avioli, L.V. (1984). Calcium and osteoporosis. *Annual Review of Nutrition, 4*, 471-491.

Bassett, C.A., & Becker, R.O. (1962). Generation of electric potentials by bone in response to mechanical stress. *Science, 140*, 195-196.

Burke, W.E., Tuttle, W.W., Thompson, C.W., Janney, C.D., & Weber, R.J. (1965). The relation of grip strength and grip-strength endurance to age. *Journal of Applied Physiology, 20*, 938-947.

Campbell, M.J., McComas, A.J., & Petito, F. (1973). Physiological changes in aging muscles. *Journal of Neurology, Neurosurgery and Psychiatry, 36*, 174-182.

Carrel, A. (1912). On the permanent life of tissues outside of the organism. *Journal of Experimental Medicine, 15*, 516-528.

Crilly, R.G., Horsman, A., Marshall, D.H., & Nordin, B.E. (1978). Postmenopausal and corticosteroid-induced osteoporosis. *Frontiers of Hormonal Research, 53*, 5.

Dalen, N., & Olsson, K.E. (1974). Bone mineral content and physical activity. *Acta Orthopaedica Scandinavica, 45*, 170-174.

Donahoe, P.K., Budzik, G.P., Tralstad, R., Mudgett-Hunter, M., Fuller, A., Hutson, J.M., Ikawa, H., Hayashi, A., & MacLaughlin, D. (1982). Mullerian inhibiting substance: An update. *Recent Progress in Hormone Research, 38*, 279-330.

Donaldson, C.L., Hulley, S.B., Vogel, J.M., Hattner, R.S., Bayers, J.H., & MacMillan, D.E. (1970). Effect of prolonged bed rest on bone mineral. *Metabolism, 19*, 1071-1084.

Freeman, J.T. (1979). *Aging: The history & literature.* New York: Human Sciences Press.

Hayflick, L. (1965). The limited in vitro lifetime of human diploid cell strains. In P.L. Krohn (ed.), *Topics in the biology of aging* (pp. 83-100), New York: John Wiley.

Heaney, R.B., Recker, R.R., & Saville, P.D. (1978; 1982). menopausal changes in calcium balance performance. *Journal of Laboratory Clinical Medicine, 92*, 953-963; *Clinical Investigative Medicine, 5*, 147-155.

Huddleston, A.L., Rockwell, D., Kulund, D.N., & Harrison, B. (1980). Bone mass in lifetime tennis athletes. *Journal of the American Medical Association, 244*, 1107-1109.

Jacobson, P., Beaver, W., Grubb, S.A., Taft, T.N., & Talmage, R.V. (1984). Bone density in women: College athletes and older athletic women. *Journal of Orthopaedic Research, 2*, 328-332.

Jones, H.H., Priest, J.D., Hayes, W.C., Tichenon, C.C. & Nagel, D.A. (1977). Humeral hypertrophy in response to exercise. *Journal of Bone and Joint Surgery, 59*, 204-208.

Krolner, B., & Toft, B. (1983). Vertebral bone loss: An unheeded side effect of therapeutic bed rest. *Clinical Science, 64*, 537-540.

Krolner, B., Toft, B., Nielsen, S.P. & Tondevold, E. (1983). Physical exercise as prophylaxis against involutional vertebral bone loss: A controlled trial. *Clinical Sciences, 64*, 541–546.

Larsson, L., Grimby, G., & Karlsson, J. (1979). Muscle strength and speed of movement in relation to age and muscle morphology. *Journal of Applied Physiology: Respiratory, Environmental and Exercise Physiology, 46*, 451–456.

Larsson, L., Sjodin, B., & Karlsson, J. (1978). Histochemical and biochemical changes in human skeletal muscle with age in sedentary males, age 22–65 years. *Acta Physiologica Scandinavica, 103*, 31–39.

Lindsay, R., Hart, D.M., Forest, C., & Beird, C., (1980, November). Prevention of spinal osteoporosis in oophorectomized women. *Lancet, 29*, 1151–1153.

Mack, P.B., LaChance, P.A., Vose, G.P., & Vogt, F. (1967). Bone demineralization of foot and hand of Gemini-Titan IV, V, and VII astronauts during orbital flight. *American Journal of Roentgenology, 100*, 503–511.

Montoye, H.J., Smith, E.L., Fardon, D.F., & Howley, E.T. (1980). Bone mineral in senior tennis players. *Scandinavian Journal of Sport Science, 2*, 26–32.

Moritani, T. (1981). Training adaptations in the muscles of older men. In E.L. Smith & R.C. Serfass (Eds.), *Exercise and aging: The scientific basis* (pp. 149-166). Hillside NJ: Enslow Publishers.

Morse, C.E. & Smith, E.L. (1981). Physical activity programming for the older adult. In E.L. Smith & R.C. Serfass (Eds.), *Exercise and aging: The scientific basis* (pp. 109-120) Hillside, NJ: Enslow Publishers.

National Institutes of Health Consensus Development Conference Statement (1984). *Osteoporosis, 5*, (3).

Nilsson, B. & Westlin, N. (1971). Bone density in athletes. *Clinical Orthopaedics, 77*, 179–182.

Rambaut, P.C., Dietlein, L.F., Vogel, J.M., & Smith, M. (1972). Comparative study of two direct methods of bone mineral measurement. *Aerospace Medicine, 43*, 646–650.

Saunders, J.W., & Fallon, J.F. (1967). Cell death in morphogenesis. In *Major problems in developmental biology*. New York: Academic Press.

Shephard, R.J. (1978). *Physical activity and aging*. Chicago: Year Book.

Smith, D.O. (1982). Physiological and structural changes at the neuromuscular junction during aging. In E. Giocobini, C. Filogamo, G. Giarobini, & A. Vernadakis (Eds.), *The aging brain: Cellular and molecular mechanisms of aging in the nervous system*. New York: Raven Press.

Smith, E.L. (1984). Special considerations in developing exercise programs for the older adult. In J.D. Matarazzo, N.E. Miller, J.A. Herd, & S.M. Weiss, *Behavioral health: A handbook of health enhancement and disease prevention*. New York: John Wiley.

Smith, E.L., & Gilligan, C. (1983). Physical activity prescription for the older adult. *Physician & Sportsmedicine, 11*, 91–101.

Smith, E.L., & Gilligan, C. (1984). Physical activity for the older adult. *Family Practice Recertification, 6*(12), 89–107.

Smith, E.L., Reddan, W., & Smith, P.E. (1981). Physical activity and calcium modalities for bone mineral increase in aged women. *Medicine in Science and Sports Exercise, 13*, 60–64.

Smith, E.L., & Serfass, R.C., (Eds.) (1981). *Exercise and aging: The scientific basis*. Hillside, NJ: Enslow Publishers.

Smith, E.L., Smith, P.E., Ensign, C.J., & Shea, M.M. (1984). Bone involution decrease in exercising middle-aged women. *Calcification Tissue International, 36*, S129–S138.

Spirduso, W.W. (1975). Reaction and movement time as a function of age and physical activity level. *Journal of Gerontology, 30*, 435–440.

Spirduso, W.W. (1980). Physical fitness, aging, and psychomotor speed: A review. *Journal of Gerontology, 35,* 850–865.

Tzankoff, S.P., & Norris, A.H. (1977). Effect of muscle mass decrease on age-related BMR changes. *Journal of Applied Physiology, 43,* 1001–1006.

Watson, R.C. (1973). Bone growth and physical activity. In R.B. Mazess (Ed.), *International Conference on Bone Mineral Measurements* (DHEW Publication No. NIH 75-683). Washington, D.C.

Wolff, J. (1892). *Das Gesetz der Transformation der Knochen.* Berlin: A. Hirschwald.

10

Health and Well-Being for Older Adults Through Physical Exercises and Sport—Outline of the Giessen Model

Heinz Meusel
SPORTWISSENSCHAFTLICHES INSTITUT
KUGELBERG, GIESSEN
FEDERAL REPUBLIC OF GERMANY

Today there can hardly be any doubt that you have to lead an active life in order to maintain your physical fitness in old age (Lehr, 1974, 1978). In the field of motor performance different concepts are offered. They stress either improving flexibility (e.g., in gymnastics for senior citizens) or endurance (e.g., in sports medicine) or, in addition to these, further factors of motor mobility (Hollmann, Liesen, Rost, & Kawanats, 1978). In practice sport and exercise for the elderly mostly are a continuation of the kind of training that these people undertook as youngsters and competitors, but with reduced workloads. In most cases training programs for the elderly are confined to one sport only.

In this paper we are trying to explain why it is necessary to consider as many abilities and skills as possible when planning training programs to maintain and improve motor performance in old age (Meusel, 1982).

Physical Fitness and Personality Development

The general physical structure and condition of a person's body is designed to move. We can take this from the phylogenesis and ontogenesis of the human

Translation: StD Walter Meusel

being. The structure of our organic systems can only be fully understood if we also consider the original functions in the human species' struggle for life. Even our cerebrum has developed its present performance mainly because our motor performance has been challenged by a variety of tasks.

Before discussing the importance of physical activity and sport for the elderly, first we have to examine this specific interdependence between motor activities and personality. As a matter of fact motor activities are of the utmost importance for the development of the individual throughout his or her lifetime. The individual forms an idea of the world around him or her and a conception of society by means of psychomotor actions. A small child—as you can easily observe—"grasps" environment by "grasping" it (with his or her hands). The individual also communicates with other people and with his or her environment through motor activities (facial expressions, gestures, language). From early infancy the individual must be stimulated by diverse physical activities to develop physical and mental condition normally. Through lack of exercise and want of affection physical and mental development is restricted and delayed (deprivation syndrome caused by hospitalization).

The importance of physical activities for promoting the performance of our organic systems and for improving our general well-being can easily be substantiated. We need only observe people who have been confined to bed for several weeks. Muscles are beginning to atrophy, performance of the circulatory system is reduced, and sense of balance and other coordinative skills are impaired. We also know that many phenomena thought to be due to natural consequences of the aging process can now be traced back to conditions, some essential factors of which have been caused by lack of physical activity and exercise and not primarily by the process of growing old. If people exercise adequately, they can maintain good physical performance even after having reached old age. This has been confirmed by the performance of many old people in almost all organic systems.

In principle we can say that—with the exception of certain cases of disease or infirmity—all organic systems can be trained into old age, and their performance mainly depends on how often and how much we exercise.

Our organism is a dynamic, self-regulating system, whose functioning depends on the efficiency of numerous subsystems that depend on each other. These subsystems include: central nervous system, musculoskeletal system, cardiovascular system, autonomic nervous system, metabolism, and immune system. What matters is to influence the individual subsystems in such a way as to regain or maintain physical fitness and well-being. As everybody knows, different sport influences and develops different subsystems of our organism.

Which way of life can therefore be considered to be the most suitable for developing and maintaining all our organic systems and dispositions? It is a way of life that, based on a wide range of sport, promotes our physical fitness and keeps it on a comparatively high level. Our organism as well as its subsystems (including their psychic elements) can be trained all our lives, even in old age. Therefore, sporting activities as a means of preventing premature aging will be more effective, the more parts of our organic systems and dispositions are trained.

Such a conception of sports for the elderly must not isolate the problem of physical fitness from other problems of old age. Nor should it be confined to only improving endurance or promoting other rather limited aspects of physical fitness.

Factors of Motor Mobility

Which factors are important for physical fitness and mobility and how can they be developed through sport and exercise?

Motor mobility mainly depends on the following abilities: coordinative skills, ability of muscles to relax, joint flexibility, muscle strength, endurance, vegetative adaptability and stress tolerance, control of body weight, and resistance to infections. These factors of motor ability and physical fitness can be related to certain subsystems of our organism that serve as a physical basis (see Table 1).

Each of these subsystems can impair mobility and physical fitness considerably if it fails to work adequately. In practice, each of these factors should therefore be sufficiently considered. Good results can only be obtained by a so-called "complex" training, which consists of as many different sports and exercises as possible.

Coordinative Skills (Central Nervous System)

Coordination means the well-ordered cooperation of the central nervous system and the skeletal muscles. Coordination appears in different forms, for instance:

- in agility, as the ability to react quickly with controlled and nimble movements;
- in ability to balance, as the ability to keep some object in equilibrium or the body when standing or moving on a small area of support. Balance is a basic requirement of human posture and movement: Standing, walking, running, or climbing stairs are not possible without unimpaired balance. Protasova, Bondarevskij, and Levando (1974) examined more closely how the ability to balance develops in the course of aging. Belorusova (1965)

Table 1. Subsystems of motor mobility and their physical basis

Physical basis	Ability
Central nervous system	Coordination
Musculoskeletal system	Ability to relax the muscles Flexibility Strength
Cardiovascular and respiratory systems	Endurance
Autonomic nervous system	Stress tolerance (veg. adaptation)
Metabolism	Regulation of the body weight
Immune system	Resistance against infection

Note. From *Sport, Spiel, Gymnastik in der zweiten Lebenschälfte* by H. Meusel, (1982). Unterricht, Organisation, BAD Homburg: Limpert. Reprinted with permission.

furnished proof that the ability to balance can be trained well even in old age (see Tables 2 and 3).

These aspects of coordinative performance as well as some others are vital for the elderly. Lack of coordinative skills (e.g., inadequate agility or unsatisfactory balance) reduces a person's competence in moving, increases accident risk, adversely affects self-confidence, and confines a person's freedom of movement and living space. That is why it is most important that every fitness program contains exercises to improve agility (e.g., elements of games), static and dynamic balance, balance of objects, and the ability to determine position.

The great importance of coordinative skills in sport for the elderly becomes obvious when learning movements. A high degree of agility facilitates learning movements (e.g., acquiring new skills, learning new exercises and sports). It also enables a person to use his or her abilities economically and to relieve various organic systems. When learning new movements, an older person should first practice slowly. Working under pressure interferes with the learning process in old age. To give variety to the learning process, one should

Table 2. Static balance of 379 women between 26 and 70 years old who have participated in sport for health reasons for 1 to 5 years. Means of four exercises: standing upright with eyes open and closed, standing with head bent backwards with eyes open and closed

Age	n	Average amplitude of swayings (mm)	Amount of swayings per minute	Maximum amplitude of swayings (mm)
26-30	23	3.9	65.8	20.3
31-35	41	4.0	62.5	18.5
36-40	49	4.2	65.4	20.2
41-45	56	4.1	64.1	19.9
46-50	34	4.4	69.0	20.7
51-55	51	4.5	67.6	24.9
56-60	61	5.0	66.9	28.9
61-65	37	5.1	69.4	31.6
66-70	27	5.2	80.0	27.3

Note. From "O Vozrastnych izmenenijach ustojcivosti stojanija zenscin" by M.V. Protasova, Bondarevskij, E.Ja., and V.A. Levando, 1974, Teor. *Prakt. fiz. Kul't*, **37**, pp. 44-46. Reprinted with permission.

Table 3. Improvement of the static balance of 40 subjects, 50-73 years old, after 9 months training, evaluated by standing on a line

Age	n	Test before training average time	Test after training average time	Difference
50-59	20	11.0 s	22.6 s	+ 11.6
60-73	20	3.5 s	11.8 s	+ 7.3

Note. From Izmenenie gibkosti, Ravnovesija i bystroty dvizenji u lic srednego i pozilogo vozrasta v svjazi s zanjatijami gimnastikoj. In D.F. Cebotarev, A.V. Korobkov, and P.D. Marcuk (Eds.). Moscow: Fizkul'tura i Sport. Reprinted with permission.

make good use of the wide choice of gymnastics and rhythmic exercises with and without small apparatus, with and without a partner, and of simple forms of active games.

The Musculoskeletal System

It is a well-known fact that in the course of aging the elasticity and stability of the muscles, tendons, and ligaments deteriorate, the tonus of the muscles drops, the cross-sectional area of the muscles becomes smaller (muscular atrophy), and the mass of the muscles in proportion to body weight becomes less, thus reducing relative strength. Degenerated and damaged joints impair flexibility.

Such processes may reduce the mobility of older people considerably. Muscular atrophy increases the danger of orthopedic disabilities, and it diminishes body control. Less body control increases the risk of accident. That is why every fitness program should also contain exercises to strengthen the muscles to work against atrophy in old age. One must not begin to strengthen muscles, however, before they have thoroughly been warmed up, limbered up, and stretched sufficiently. Warm up by slowly moving large groups of muscles, not by stretching muscles as is done in many aerobic programs.

All large groups of muscles should be strengthened, those of the trunk as well as those of the extremities. Though the results of static and dynamic strength training are said to be similar, in sport for the elderly we should prefer dynamic strength training. In static strength training, holding your breath very tightly may cause considerable danger, because it is connected with great fluctuations in blood pressure. That is why in dynamic strength training, too, you should avoid working out fast against much resistance (power). That is, you should not train with a great amount of force and with sudden exertion. You should perform exercises that offer only little and later on moderate resistance. These should be repeated frequently. Push-ups and pull-ups should therefore be avoided by older people who practice only occasionally.

Flexibility denotes the range of each joint. It depends on the anatomy of the joint and how much the muscles can be stretched. Flexibility makes it easier to solve many of our everyday problems (from getting dressed to cleaning the house), and it is a most important safety factor (i.e., flexibility helps prevent accidents). To improve flexibility first warm up the muscles thoroughly and also improve their ability to relax. Older persons should be satisfied with exercises that stretch the muscles actively, that is, exercises in which the muscles are stretched by the action of their antagonists. Passive stretching exercises performed with the help of partners or weights should be avoided. Jerky and fast stretching exercises can damage muscles, tendons, ligaments, and joint capsules.

Endurance (Cardiovascular System)

The importance of endurance training as a preventive measure against diseases of the cardiovascular system is undisputed. However, what—in my opinion— has not been discussed thoroughly enough yet is the question of how to put into practice the demand that endurance training should not be neglected. A person who has exercised regularly all his or her life can still practice endurance sports even if there is a certain deterioration in the functions of the musculo-skeletal system. He or she knows by experience how much and in which way to strain. Old people, however, who have only little experience or no experience at all can—as a rule—hardly be motivated to take up long-distance running or jogging. They are not willing to bear the necessary strain. Often endurance training is made more difficult or even impossible because of overweight and orthopedic disabilities.

Many people suffering from such infirmities may still be capable of swimming. Endurance training in swimming can only be performed effectively, if special attention is paid to a proper swimming technique, which enables a person to swim smoothly and without interruption over longer distances. Endurance could best be improved by regularly alternating between different endurance sports, especially running, swimming, cycling, and long-distance skiing. The ideal endurance sport, however, is long-distance skiing, because in this sport arms and shoulders, too, are employed in an alternating rhythm when moving along. The scenic attractions of the landscape have a favorable effect on the autonomic nervous system. Even older people can still learn long-distance skiing; if they first get through an appropriate program of conditioning exercise to improve strength and coordinative skills, many are highly qualified for long-distance skiing (see table 4).

In endurance training we should definitely prefer the endurance method to the interval method. Before starting a running program, an untrained person must undertake a light program of conditioning exercise for several months to strengthen the musculoskeletal system.

Vegetative Adaptability/Stress Tolerance (Autonomic Nervous System)

In the course of aging the autonomic nervous system shows marked deterioration in its ability to adapt to changes in strain. In old age this often results in insomnia, vertigo, constipation, and other complaints. Well-balanced physical training can improve the ability of the autonomic nervous system to adapt to changing strain, thus increasing stress tolerance (i.e., a person's ability

Table 4. The average running times and best times in 1972 at Wasa-Race and at Engadine Skiing-Marathon

Age	Average running time		Best time	
	86 km	42 km	86 km	42 km
21	9:16:37	3:43:58	6:39:18	2:16:25
30	8:49:33	3:42:42	5:55:56	2:16:39
40	8:52:07	4:00:13	5:55:09	2:26:03
50	9:29:57	4:17:58	6:37:44	2:25:52
60	10:11:24	4:32:39	8:02:10	2:49:18

Note. From "Ausdauerleistung und Alter" by Ch. Schneiter, 1973, *Jugend u. Sport*, **30**, pp. 57-61. Reprinted with permission.

to withstand stress). After physical exercise the parasympathetic nervous system becomes more active than that of an untrained person. This results in a state of relaxation and well-being. That is why, besides sleep, physical exercise is helpful in accelerating recovery from stress. In this context recreative sports and remedial exercises can serve our purpose best, provided that they contain elements of play and that people enjoy them. They should also offer a great variety of activities. Such activities should not exceed moderate to average strain. Among those, there are moderate exercises from endurance sports, which have to be done for some time, as well as simple yet diversified forms of gymnastics.

Controlling Body Weight (Metabolism)

Overweight considerably reduces physical fitness and mobility. However, the influence of sporting activities on the process of controlling body weight is mostly overestimated. A high percentage of metabolism takes place in the muscles. The muscular system declines noticeably in old age, which often leads to being overweight, unless lowering caloric intake or expending calories through physical exercise. When taking physical exercise though, the consumption of energy is relatively small (see Table 5).

We can proceed on the assumption that a 60-year-old person only needs four-fifths of the food needed at the age of 20. That is why in old age a lasting reduction of weight through physical exercise can only be achieved by simultaneously lowering food intake.

Resistance to Infections (Immune System)

The influence of sport on the immune systems for older people has hardly been studied. We should like to point out, though, that outdoor sport seems to have a positive influence on reducing proneness to infection, thus helping to reduce the risk of disease. Liesen (1977) found out that the immune system of untrained persons in their 60s and 70s can be activated by endurance training.

We can conclude from this that fitness training should be performed outdoors as often as possible even in winter, provided that those taking part have previously engaged in physical activities in cold weather. The following outdoor sports can be recommended for older people: running, long-distance skiing, skiing-tours, cycling.

Speed

In this context the problem of speed will not be discussed in detail. Speed in cyclic movements (such as sprints) puts too much strain on the musculoskeletal system. The sprinter must perform anaerobic work, which cannot be recommended for older people. As far as we know, empirical studies on the aging process of the sprinting speed of older persons have only been made in the Soviet Union (see Table 6). There is, however, in such tests great risk of injuries.

Table 5. Energetic expenditure during long-distance skiing

	Speed	Power (watt/min)	Calorie consumption per min	per hour
Trained skiers	120 m/min = 7.2 km/h	100	8.0	480
	150 m/min = 9.0 km/h	125	9.5	570
	200 m/min = 12.0 km/h	175	12.5	750
Average skiers	100 m/min = 6.0 km/h	130	9.9	594
	125 m/min = 7.5 km/h	150	10.8	648

Note. From Zur Frage der körperlichen Belastbarkeit alternder und Alter Menschen, by M.J. Halhuber, 1971, *Med. d. Alternden Menschen*, 1, pp. 33-36. Reprinted with permission.

Table 6. Performance in 30-m race of 30- to 70-year-old women, depending on age and beginning of training

Age and beginning of training	n	30-m race flying M (sec)
30-39 years		
Average group performance	88	5.42
Up to 1 year	28	5.60
1-5 years	41	5.24
6-10 years	19	5.43
40-49 years (untrained 20-24 years	41	5.53)
Average group performance	111	5.52
Up to 1 year	24	6.24
1-5 years	57	5.77
11-18 years	30	5.56
50-59 years (untrained 30-34 years	52	6.24)
Average group performance	152	6.48
Up to 1 year	14	6.71
1-5 years	56	6.54
11-18 years	82	6.20
60-64 years (untrained 40-44 years	133	7.2)
Average group performance	88	6.67
1-5 years	44	6.76
11-18 years	44	6.58
65-69 years (untrained 45-49 years	67	7.2)
Average group performance	76	7.28
1-5 years	13	7.34
11-18 years	63	7.23
70 years and older		
11-18 years	45	7.93

Note. From "Vlijanie mnogoletnich zanjatij fizices koj kul'turoj na nekotorye pokazateli dvigatl'noj funkeii ljudej srednego i starsego vozrasta" by I.T. Osipov and M.V. Protasova, 1978, Teor. *Prakt. fiz. Kul't.*, **31**, pp. 45-48. The figures of the untrained are in parentheses according to Rubcov, 1974.

Speed in acyclic movements, however, is welcomed, because the ability to move fast against some resistance is a most important factor in the prevention of accidents and the exercises necessary for this purpose can easily be included in the training program.

Summary

One can only maintain and improve physical performance systematically, if training plans include as wide a range of abilities and skills and as great a variety of activities as possible. Physical training must be supplemented with further steps in health care, such as a suitable diet and limiting the so-called "risk-factors" such as smoking. The main reason why physical training should be included in geroprophylaxis is to maintain elderly people's mobility and well-being. Thus, they have a better chance of becoming independent, self-sufficient and satisfied with life.

References

Belorusova, A.V. (1965). Izmenenie gibkosti, ravnovesija i bystroty dvizenij u lic srednego i pozilogo vozrasta v svjazi s zanjatijami gimnastikoj. In D.F. Cebotarev, A.V. Korobkov, & P.D. Marcuk (Red.), *Körperkultur—Quelle der Langlebigkeit* (pp. 278-281). Moscow: Fizkul'tura i Sport.

Halhuber, M.J. (1971). Zur Frage der körperlichen Belastbarkeit alternder und alter Menschen. *mda—Medizin des alternden Menschen, 1*, 33-36.

Hollmann, W., Liesen, H., Rost, R., & Kawanats, K. (1978). Über das Leistungsverhalten und die Trainierbarkeit im Alter. *Z. Gerontol., 11*, 312-324.

Lehr, U. (1974). *Psychologie des Alterns*. Heidelberg: Quelle & Meyer.

Lehr, U. (1978). Körperliche und geistige Aktivität—eine Voraussetzung für ein erfolgreiches Altern. *Z. Gerontol., 11*, 290-299.

Liesen, H. (1977). *Metabolische Adaptationen an akute und chronische Ausdauerbelastungen (insbesondere beim älteren Menschen)*. Cologne, Germany: Deutsche Sporthochschule.

Meusel, H. (1982). *Sport, Spiel, Gymnastik in der zweiten Lebenshälfte*. Ziele, Training, Unterricht, Organisation. Bad Homburg: Limpert.

Osipov, I.T., & Protasova, M.V. (1978). Vlijanie mnogoletnich zanjatij fiziceskoj kul'turoj na nekotorye pokazateli dvigatel'noj funkcii ljudej srednego i starsego vozrasta. *Teor. Prakt. fiz. Kul't., 31*, 45-48.

Protasova, M.V., Bondarevskij, E.Ja., & Levando, V.A. (1974). O vozrastnych izmenenijach ustojcivosti stojanija zenscin 26-70 let. *Teor. Prakt. fiz. Kul't., 37*, 44-46.

Rubcov, A.T. (1974). Fiziceskaja podgotovlennost' zenscin 20-49 let, rance ne zanimavsichsja fiziceskoj kul'turoj. *Teor. Prakt. fiz. Kul't., 37*, 53-55.

Schneiter, Ch. (1973). Ausdauerleistung und Alter. *Jugend u. Sport, 30*, 57-61.

11

Exercise and the Elderly: Observations on a Functioning Program

Janice Beran
IOWA STATE UNIVERSITY
AMES, IOWA, USA

It is hard to beat the clock and the calendar. Time does take its toll. However, senior citizens in an exercise program know that exercise is as important a component of wellness as it is for those who are younger. As one of the 89-year-olds in an exercise program stated, "If you can't exercise, life just isn't worth living" (Meads, 1982). Another avid exerciser about the same age agreed that if you exercise, everything works better. These individuals and others in specially designed exercise programs for senior citizens testify to the importance of exercise in their daily lives. While the proclaimed primary benefit is physical, sociological and psychological benefits are also evident. This paper describes a long-term functioning exercise program, draws upon observed and expressed psychological and sociological benefits accrued from an exercise program, offers some suggestions regarding research, and draws conclusions regarding exercise programs for senior citizens.

Description of the Program

For the past 5-1/2 years the writer has been a volunteer exercise leader at Northcrest Retirement Community in Ames, Iowa. The thrice weekly group exercises from 8:30-9:00 a.m. in the recreation room of the retirement community. The women participants range in age from approximately 70 to 93 years.

Prior to beginning the exercise program, participants consult their physician who completes a physical assessment questionnaire, which provides information regarding history of illness, surgery, and mechanical aids.

The number in the group varies as the participants travel out of town, garden, visit friends, and participate in church and club activities. The number has been fairly consistent since its beginning in 1977, although a few have stopped because of debilitating illnesses. While there are usually 12 men among the slightly more than 100 residents, they either take their exercises in another way, do not choose to join a regular program, or are not able to exercise. Despite the enthusiastic evangelization of women exercisers, some women residents do not choose to exercise. Several do, however, participate in other forms of exercise. The exercise participants are ambulatory, although more are using canes than 6 years ago when the program began. They are a well-educated group with all having had a high school education and most having had at least some university education. They are testimony to what researchers have now demonstrated: "Certain crucial areas of human intelligence do not decline in old age among people who are generally healthy" (Goleman, 1983). They are well read, concerned about vital issues of the day, and enjoy cultural events; they do not accept the stereotype of a helpless old age. The self-fulfillment and self-worth they evidence can partially be attributed to the fact that they have sufficient resources to live comfortably, a group of retired friends to identify with, and a good attitude toward leisure and health (Atchley, 1973).

Physical Aspects

The mild low-stress exercises are done using the chair as the base. As in other exercise programs for this age group, the exercises are selected for their potential to maintain range of motion, flexibility, and strength. While some activities are designed to improve cardiovascular efficiency, this is not a primary focus. The participants in the program feel that the maintenance of flexibility is a major benefit.

The sessions typically begin with exercises for the feet and ankles and progress to other parts of the body. Attention is given to exercises designed for special problems—such as leg cramps, shoulder tenseness, loss of strength in the fingers, flabby arm muscles, protruding abdomen, and so forth. The program includes static stretching while seated as well as standing—some of it with stockings, light-weight scarves, bicycle inner tubes, bending over chairs, and stretching while seated in chairs. Exercises related to balance are also included.

Exercises designed to maintain range of motion include those for large muscles such as rowing, swimming strokes, shoulder and leg rotations, and arm pulls. Occasionally, balls are passed or bounced. Finger and toe rotations are also included. Exercises to maintain strength include squeezing tennis balls, crumpling newspapers, wall push aways, partner tugs, modified knee bends, leg lifts, and so forth. These are done to slow muscle loss most evident in the bony hands, poor posture, and general weakness of so many elderly people. Occasionally exercises for the eyes, lungs, and bladder control are included. Testimony from the participants as to the physical benefits include the following: exercise improves circulation and respiration, maintains flexibility, diminishes stress, prevents disease, delays the aging process, lessens problems of cramps—particularly in the legs—and enables participants to sleep better.

As a leader, the writer has observed that the participants have upright posture and none of the stoopedness that many elderly people evidence. Muscles have a firmness not found in all the aged. They are able to exercise more intensely, hold positions, stretch farther, and maintain continuous movement in significantly greater degrees than newcomers or casual visitors to the program even though those visitors may have been 10-20—and even 30—years younger.

While the physical benefits of exercise have been well-examined and documented, the psychological and sociological benefits are less often examined. Observation over the time span of this exercise program suggests that the latter two aspects of exercise are of vital importance, and for that reason this paper focuses principally on the psychological and sociological aspects of exercise.

Psychological Aspects

The women in the program speak of the mental lift they receive through the exercise. The music that serves as the background for exercise—be it marches, jazz, waltzes, Hawaiian, two-step, or polka—quickens the step, brings smiles, and a sense of buoyance. As an improved physical fitness heightens kinesthetic self, it also improves self-image and reduces psychologic tension (O'Keelor, 1976). An individual may arrive at the exercise session with a long face. That expression may be indicative of a physical problem such as a painful leg or an emotional problem such as a tragedy in the family or the impending death of a life-long friend. Doing exercises called chicken wings, stirring the coffee, shooting the arrow, spider doing push-ups, and so forth brings a smile and assists in putting problems into perspective. Likewise, solicitous inquiries of others in the group bring solace and support to that individual. The exercise, music, and companionship all serve to bring a new focus to life, at least temporarily if not permanently. Time and again, the writer has observed tenseness and stress in an individual that seemed to dissipate with exercise.

The leader can be sensitive to these variables. For instance, activities such as having all participants walk around the group and vigorously shake each others' hands, saying, "You look marvelous today" or "You're doing well," or joining hands, clapping hands, and giving each other hugs or even smiles can greatly reduce psychologic tension, lift spirits and heighten self-worth. Many a woman has come dragging into exercise and left almost dancing with a bounce in her step, swinging her arms, feeling she could conquer the world— or at least get through the day. While exercising can give a feeling of *joie de vivre*, if it is of appropriate intensity and duration, it can also have a tranquilizing effect. De Vries's (1972) findings that a feeling of euphoria or sense of well-being was achieved through exercise are supported by those in the exercise program.

The sessions are planned so that members have developed rapport with one another. There is a great deal of storytelling, joking about the aging process, and sharing of happenings—all of which contribute to fun and laughter. As Scher (1981) has observed, there is no magic to a program of exercise but a good workout is enjoyed, and it provides a feeling of freedom and of being in control.

To senior citizens the capacity to go places and do things without being dependent upon others provides a strong psychological lift conducive to good mental health. Exercise is viewed by the women in the program as an aid to maintaining independence, a quality most prized in later years. The women in the group feel that through exercise they have some control over the aging process. Regular participation in the exercise program also serves to reduce boredom and monotony. Exercises provide a change of pace. A regular time to exercise with others gives structure to the day. It brings variety and a degree of stimulation. It promotes camaraderie that can serve to refocus attention on things beyond one's own immediate life. As one member said, "If I don't go to exercise, I don't know what's going on" (Schneider, 1984).

Another member of the group, when asked the reason for exercise, noted that if she exercises with others, she compares her abilities with others' and sets goals for herself. Among the exercisers there is a spirit of gentle competition wherein the women are self-motivated to try to extend themselves a bit (i.e., to reach as high as they were able to the previous year, to maintain a held position longer than their neighbor, or to do as many bicycle circles as the entire group). While aware they should proceed at an individual pace, the still evident desire to compete or excel is present and desirable. It encourages people to keep on trying. For example, the group does cycling or leg extensions in the seated position. As leader I do enough repetitions until I'm tired. Most of them pluckily try to keep up even though they are 25-40 years my senior. I'll comment, "that makes my legs tired" or "that pulls." They will agree but will not give up.

Additional observations are that the participants, regardless of age, are still very concerned about personal appearance and physical attractiveness. A protruding abdomen, flabby applause (upper arm) muscles, and saggy skin are some of the concerns. There are frequent questions to the leader regarding specific exercises for such problems. A second observation is that seniors, at least in this group, are uninhibited. They are not embarrassed to prance like a drum majorette leading a band, swivel their hips to "clean the barrel," or try a dance step like the Charleston or Huki-Lau. This invites frivolity and enhances conviviality. Likewise, they are not hesitant to question the value of a particular exercise or speak their minds regarding some of the TV exercise gurus. From time to time university students have assisted in the program. They welcome contact with young people and are very kind to give interviews to students doing special projects. They smugly note that at times they have been more flexible than football players or have a greater range of motion than some of the young people.

Sociological Benefits

As one of the participants noted, "It's more fun to exercise with others, it's hard to do it alone, perhaps I'm lazy . . ." (Wright, 1982). The touching, smiling, and laughing are part of the sociability aspect of exercising. A person who lives alone is given a boost by vigorously pumping hands with someone while mutually wishing each other a good day. Even laughing together heartily is companionable and at the same time good for the lungs and terrific for the mental well-being.

Researchers have found that activities that are primarily social and/or physical in nature have the most positive effect upon life satisfaction (Peppers, 1976; McAvoy, 1977; Neugarten, Havighurst, & Tobin, 1961). The optimal arrangement is to combine the two. The music for exercise is purposefully background music so that conversation can take place. (Some of the group are hard of hearing and want to hear what is being said.) At one point a person who had lost her sight participated so descriptive, precise instructions were used. A vigorously paced exercise is followed by a slower one so that the exercise doesn't always preclude conversation. We enjoy each other. One witty member enjoys puns. Another often brings a joke to share. Others share incidents relative to their aging that enables the whole group to laugh at itself. While some have relatives in town, others do not, so we do things to promote a feeling of caring. We do a fair amount of touching; we give each other big smiles, terrible frowns, and pretend punches. Members are generally solicitous of one another but are not inclined to dwell on their physical aches and pains because everyone has those. The experience of group exercise helps to improve attitudes, behavior, and interpersonal relations of older persons as much as it does for younger people.

We sometimes eat together. Whenever a student associate assists as a practicum experience, the exercise group hosts a very nice dinner in our honor at the termination of the practicum. This contact between students and the senior exercisers is prized because it serves to break down what Rosabel Koos (1982) has noted as the "polarization of the generations." It enables the seniors to have a firsthand experience with someone they might not otherwise encounter—it serves to keep them engaged with university and community life. They enjoy going out—potlucks at the leader's house and participation in exercise workshops. They also have given demonstrations at conventions and have hosted an out-of-state exercise group. These activities have served to bring satisfaction and a sense of being able to contribute something worthwhile. As this group experiences a constant series of substitutions and exchanges, they value being of service to others. Many in the group have, and some still do, participate in voluntary community and church service activities. Exercising enables them to continue in that in a limited way, both in proclaiming the value of exercise to nonexercisers and also in formally participating in presentations.

Research and the Elderly

It has been observed that getting access for field research with the elderly is difficult (Sinnott, Harris, Block, Collesano, & Jackson, 1983). An exercise group over the long term provides a fountain of information on the physical changes that are part of the aging process. It also, of course, furnishes insight into the lives and actions of this population. The Northcrest group has participated in research. Most of them did it willingly, even though it meant going to an arranged location several times for evaluation. They are most likely to participate in research as subjects if the particular researcher involves them in developing the questions. They insist that the research be practical, applicable, and have potential for solving problems relative to aging. They have little patience with esoteric academic projects, even though many of them have been in the education profession. They are vitally interested in the findings of the research project and want it presented to them in an understandable language.

While some enjoy attention and welcome being research subjects, others strongly resent researchers assuming they have nothing else to do and can participate as research subjects at any time and on short notice. Such procedures, in their opinion, imply that senior citizens have nothing important to do with their time. To people for whom work, and other worthwhile endeavors, has had a central place all their lives, it is belittling to be considered always available and having nothing to do.

Conclusions

Participation as a leader in a thrice weekly long-term exercise program at a retirement community has shown that the success of a program is as dependent upon the psychosociological setting as upon the type and duration of the exercises. The physical aspect of our being is so affected and related to the other dimensions of life that all aspects need to be considered in planning and implementing an exercise program. Knowledge of exercise physiology is important but of equal importance is knowledge of the psychosociological realities of aging. Researchers and exercise leaders who are aware of all of these dimensions are most effectively able to work together to enable the aged in our society to add years to their lives and, perhaps even more importantly, add life to those years.

References

Atchley, R. (1973). Retirement and leisure participation: Continuity or crises. *Gerontologist,* **11**(1), 13-17.

de Vries, N.A., & Adams, G. (1972). Electromyographic comparison of single doses of exercise and meprobomate as to effects on muscular relaxation. *American Journal of Physical Medicine,* **51**(3), 43-46.

Coleman, D. (1984, March 18). Old age. *Des Moines Register.*

Koss, R.S. (1982). *Aging and health changing life styles.* Houston, TX: American Alliance for Health, Physical Education, Recreation and Dance.

McAvoy, L.H. (1977, March). Needs of the elderly: An overview of the research. *Parks and Recreation,* **90**(3), 31-34, 55.

Meads, G. (1982). [Interview]. Videotape, Iowa State University Extension Service, Ames, IA.

Neugarten, B., Havighurst, R., & Tobin, S.S. (1961). The measure of life satisfaction. *Journal of Gerontology*, 16.

O'Keelor, R. (1976). The rule of physical fitness in reducing health and long term care of the elderly. Federal, State and Community Relations. Testimony to the Select Committee on Aging. Washington, DC.

Peppers, L.G. (1976). Patterns of leisure and adjustment to retirement. *Leisure,* **16**(5), 441-446.

Scher, C. (1981). Calisthenics for seniors, synopsis of the national conference on fitness and aging. Washington, DC, 36.

Schneider, U. (1982). [Interview]. Videotape. Iowa State University Extension, Ames, IA.

Sinnott, J.D., Harris, C.S., Block, M.R., Collesano, S., & Jackson, S.G. (1983). *Applied research in aging, a guide to methods and resources.* Boston: Little, Brown and Company.

Wright, M. (1982). [Interview]. Videotape, Iowa State University Extension, Ames, IA.

12

Diagnosis and Optimization of Selected Components of Physical Fitness in Elderly Sport Participants

Stephan Starischka
UNIVERSITÄT DORTMUND
DORTMUND, FEDERAL REPUBLIC OF GERMANY

Dieter Böhmer
UNIVERSITÄT FRANKFURT
FRANKFURT, FEDERAL REPUBLIC OF GERMANY

Fitness training has been recommended for adults for many years for preventive reasons. It provides alternatives for leisure time, and it can be used to compensate for job stress. For more than 10 years the German Sports Federation (DSB), an association with more than 18 million members, has tried to encourage nonsporting adults to take part in leisure fitness sports. Campaigns named "trim yourself by sports, "jogging without breathing heavily," "join in the game and get to know your neighbor," and "sport and health" are examples.

When analyzing these programs it can be shown that adults between 20 and 30 years of age are especially addressed. However, the latest trials are given to encourage older adults to leisure fitness sports. These efforts can be illustrated by the "Trimming-130" campaign of the DSB (Palm, 1982; 1983) aimed at attracting adults between the ages of 35 and 60. The slogan "Trimming-130" is an invitation to participate in leisure sports in an easygoing way (i.e., a pulse rate of 130 minutes should be maintained for 10 minutes or more). The exercises should involve as many muscles and joints as possible and should consist of at least two sessions a week so that a total time of at least 60 minutes

This study was supported by a grant from the German Sports Federation (DSB).

a week is achieved (Starischka, 1982:4). These leisure-sport activities should be conducted according to the ideas of the DSB in their 58,091 sport clubs (DSB, 1984) and should be initiated and organized by DSB honorary training supervisors. An analysis of the instruction courses for honorary training supervisors (DSB, 1978) revealed a lack of knowledge in the aspects of fitness diagnosis (resp. performance, resp. motor ability diagnosis). This deficit complicates the task of planning and guiding an effective fitness training program. Knowledge within the field of fitness diagnosis is however desired by those honorary teachers whose duty it is to transfer the Trimming-130 idea to the honorary training supervisors of the sport clubs. Interviews with 45 honorary teachers (multipliers) of German elite sport associations revealed a desire to increase their knowledge within the field of fitness diagnosis:

1. To assess the fitness level more precisely,
2. To simplify the grouping of fitness training teams,
3. To make clear the effectiveness of fitness programs, and
4. To motivate the leisure sports participants to a continuous Trimming-130.

To assist the honorary teachers of the DSB in their efforts in fitness training, a team of scientists (sport medicine and training theory) from the universities of Dortmund and Frankfurt investigated several simple fitness tests when preparing the Trimming-130 campaign.

Pilot Study 1

Pilot study 1 was conducted to examine selected variables of the fitness level of elderly endurance athletes.

The aim was to diagnose selected sportmotoric variables of the physical fitness level of endurance athletes (joggers) between the ages of 30 and 59.

The subjects were 42 participants of 1983 senior jogging meeting in Bad Soden. For detailed characteristics of the subjects see Table 1.

The test procedures for the sportmotoric tests carried out are reported in Table 2.

Table 1. Subjects from Bad Soden 1983

Age (Years)	Sex (Male, Female)	Age of Training (M, Years)	Jogging (M, Hours Per Week for 6 Months)
30–39	5	4.1	2.1
	1	8.2	2.3
40–49	8	5.4	2.3
	11	2.3	2.1
50–59	10	6.8	1.9
	7	4.0	2.4

Table 2. Test Procedures, Bad Soden

Number	Name	Purpose	Procedure*	Scoring
1	Darting	Eye-hand-coordi-nation	10 throws 230 cm distance	Score (max. 40 points)
2	Stick catching	Motor ability to react Speed of movement	Catching of a falling stick	Distance (cm)
3	One leg standing	Equilibrium (static)	One leg stand on board edge (2 cm)	Time (1/10 sec)
4	Agility (Slalom) run	Agility	Run between 10 sticks, 20 m	Time (1/10 sec)
5	Stick removing	Flexibility (shoulders)	Remove stick over head	Grip width—shoulder width (cm)
6	Trunk bend forward	Flexibility	Reach forward along a measuring scale (knee extended)	Distance (cm)
7	Bend-twist-touch	Flexibility (dynamic) Speed of movement	Touch floor and wall	Number in 20 sec.
8	Motor connection	Ability to transfer impulse (trunk-upper extremities)	Long distance throw (soccer ball, standing) Long distance throw (medicine ball, 1500 gr) a) standing b) kneeling c) sitting	Distance (m)
9	Standing long jump	Power (leg muscles)	Jump horizontally	Distance (cm)
10	Abalakow-Test	Power (leg muscles)	Jump vertically	Distance (cm)
11	Sit-ups	Strength endurance (trunk muscles)	Curl to the sitting position (elbow-knee) a) without load b) with load of 2.5 kg	Time (1/10 sec)
12	Push-ups	Strength endurance (upper extremities)	Flex and extend arms, trunk, and legs stretched	Number in 30 sec.
13	Leg-lifts	Strength endurance (trunk muscles)	On back, lift legs into vertical position	Number in 20 sec

*For detailed instructions see Beuker (1976) and Grosser and Starischka (1981).

Test process

After individual warming-up of 3 to 5 minutes, the subjects completed the 13 sportmotoric tests (1 trial). Each test station was controlled by two physical education (PE) students trained to administer the entire test battery. Afterward the subjects were tested by sportsmedicine specialists (i.e., ergometry, skinfold measurement). About 45 minutes later the subjects completed the test battery a second time during which the controlling PE students were replaced by others. Each trial ran about 25 to 30 minutes. Before leaving the gym the subjects were asked for their opinions of the test items (i.e., authenticity, difficulty, character of demand, transfer to the training process). Finally, the senior athletes participated in an endurance run (12-minute run, respectively, 3.0 to 8.5 km, depending on age). The sportmotoric tests were filmed (Super-8) and offered to a rating team.

Results

Table 3 includes the levels of sportmotoric test performances with reference to age and sex.

There is no comparative discussion of results for methodological reasons (i.e., problem of norms, extent of sampling) (Letzelter & Letzelter, 1983; Neumaier, 1983). Correlation coefficients of objectivity-reliability (see Letzelter & Letzelter, 1979) could be calculated. They differed from "acceptable" (Rho = 0.83. Item motor connection) to "excellent" (Rho = 0.97. Item trunk bend) (Barrow & McGee, 1979:38). The films were rated by a team of four sport scientists (theory of training, sport medicine). Criteria of judgment were: comparison of movement, completion of task by elderly subjects, risk of injuries, and degree of organization.

On the basis of conclusions drawn from the rating process and the analysis of the interviews, and taking into account the fitness model of the Trimming-130 campaign, the test battery was reduced from 13 to 9 items, for Pilot Study 2.

Pilot Study 2

Pilot study 2 examined selected variables of the fitness level of elderly gymnasts.

The aim was to diagnose selected sportmotoric variables of the physical fitness level of gymnasts between the ages of 30 and 65.

The subjects were 185 participants of the 1983 German Gymnastic Festival held in Frankfurt/Main. For detailed characteristics of the subjects see Table 4:

On the average (1982) the subjects practice 2½ to 3 hours a week: gymnastics and tumbling, 70%; track and field events and ball games, 18%; jogging, swimming, and cycling, 12%.

Test Procedures

The procedures for the sportmotoric tests are compiled in Table 5:

The subjects completed the 9 sportmotoric tests in 3 mornings. Test stations were controlled by 10 trained PE students. Item Number 8 ("horizontal

Table 3. Sportmotoric test results from Bad Soden 1983

Age (years)	Number(N) M=Male F=Female	Darting (Score)	Stick catching (cm)	One leg standing (sec)	Agility run (sec)	Stick removing (cm)	Trunk bend (cm)
30-39	M 5	25.5 ± 6.2	19.6 ± 4.6	23.0 ± 22.2	6.6 ± 0.4	63.2 ± 12.2	6.8 ± 5.0
	F 1	14	16	60.0	6.6	44.0	20.0
40-49	M 8	24.9 ± 6.2	21.8 ± 6.0	16.5 ± 17.9	6.5 ± 0.7	71.6 ± 9.7	1.3 ± 5.3
	F 11	21.8 ± 4.1	22.5 ± 4.6	16.8 ± 18.2	8.0 ± 0.9	54.6 ± 9.5	7.3 ± 6.2
50-59	M 10	24.9 ± 4.4	21.8 ± 7.2	8.5 ± 5.9	7.2 ± 0.5	70.9 ± 14.5	4.0 ± 6.9
	F 7	20.9 ± 6.9	22.1 ± 5.6	9.0 ± 8.5	7.4 ± 0.5	58.9 ± 7.6	5.6 ± 4.4

Age (years)	(Number)	Bend-twist-touch (number)	Soccerball (standing)	Motor connection (m) (standing)	Medicine ball (kneeling)	(sitting)	
30-39	M 5	14.4 ± 3.5	13.80 ± 1.40	9.40 ± 2.10	8.20 ± 2.80	5.30 ± 0.50	
	F 1	15	12.70	7.90	6.90	4.80	
40-49	M 8	12.0 ± 2.1	13.80 ± 1.60	9.30 ± 1.10	7.80 ± 1.10	5.20 ± 0.80	
	F 11	12.6 ± 3.5	7.50 ± 1.00	5.20 ± 0.70	4.10 ± 0.50	3.40 ± 0.40	
50-59	M 10	12.0 ± 2.9	11.90 ± 2.60	8.50 ± 1.10	6.60 ± 1.10	4.70 ± 0.50	
	F 7	10.5 ± 2.3	8.40 ± 1.20	5.90 ± 0.80	4.70 ± 1.10	3.50 ± 0.50	

Age (years)	Number	Standing long jump (cm)	Abalakow test (cm)	Sit-ups (sec) without load	Sit-ups (sec) + 2.5 kg load	Push-ups (number)	Leg-lifts (number)
30-39	M 5	193.8 ± 18.2	43.0 ± 8.8	17.7 ± 6.9	20.8 ± 8.1	19.7 ± 11.2	12.8 ± 2.0
	F 1	200.0 ±	41	14.5	16.3	24	15
40-49	M 8	181.9 ± 40.4	44.6 ± 9.4	17.6 ± 5.0	17.4 ± 3.5	17.8 ± 6.7	14.0 ± 1.3
	F 11	138.6 ± 23.6	30.3 ± 6.0	17.6 ± 5.4	17.2 ± 2.4	15.7 ± 2.6	12.4 ± 1.4
50-59	M 10	169.0 ± 32.0	40.3 ± 8.3	17.0 ± 4.4	20.0 ± 7.8	16.7 ± 4.5	13.8 ± 3.0
	F 7	130.1 ± 20.5	27.3 ± 7.0	24.9 ± 7.6	—	14.5 ± 2.4	11.7 ± 2.7

Mean ± SD data

Table 4. Subjects by sex and age group, German Gymnastic Festival

Age	30–34	35–39	40–44	45–49	50–54	55–59	60–64	>65
Male	9	9	22	14	10	5	5	8
Female	12	19	26	18	10	8	6	4

Table 5. Test procedures, German Gymnastic Festival

Name	Purpose	Procedure*	Scoring
1 One leg standing	Equilibrium (static)	One leg stand on board edge (2 cm)	Time (1/10 sec)
2 Stick moving	Flexibility, (shoulder)	Move stick over head	Grip width— shoulder width (cm)
3 Trunk bend forward	Flexibility, stretching ability	Reaching forward along a measuring scale (knees extended)	Distance (cm)
4 Standing long jump	Power (leg muscles)	Jumping horizontally	Distance (cm)
5 Differentiation jump	Motor ability to differentiate	Jumping horizontally 2/3 of maximum standing long jump performance	Distance 5 trials (cm)
6 Sit-ups	Strength endurance (trunk muscles)	Curling to the sitting position (elbow-knee)	Time (sec) a) for 10 b) for 20 sit-ups
7 Leg-lifts	Strength endurance (trunk muscles)	On back, lift legs into vertical position	Time (sec) a) for 10 b) for 20 leg-lifts
8 "Horizontal skipping"	Strength endurance (upper extremities)	Skipping horizontally with hands in push-up position	Time (sec) a) for 10 b) for 20 skippings
9 Step-test	Short-time endurance	Stepping on a box (40 cm) 90 times within 180 sec	Pulse rate (min) a) initial pulse b) load pulse c) recovery pulse (+1 min)

*For detailed instructions see Beuker (1976) and Grosser and Starischka (1981).

skipping") was videorecorded. There was no second test trial due to organization.

Results

Table 6 includes the levels of sportmotoric test performances with reference to age and sex.

A detailed discussion of the results is in preparation (Starischka, in press; see also Beuker, 1976; Jokl, 1954; Meusel, 1980.)

Attention is drawn to the high degree of motor learning ability of elderly athletes within the field of coordination abilities (see Table 6, characteristic motor ability to differentiate during standing long-jump trials (item 5). Difference from the set point, comparison of first and fifth attempt. See also Blume, 1981; Baltes & Willis, 1981.

Analysis of the test items (rating) and calculations of correlation coefficients (Ewerle, 1984; see Table 7), led to an additional reduction of the test battery. Item 8 ("horizontal skipping") proved to be less standardized, Item 7 (leg-lifts) was withdrawn due to economical reasons (see also Table 7, intercorrelations).

Conclusions

From the results and the recommendations of an additional rating (four sport scientists, four skilled honorary teachers of sport clubs, elite associations) two test batteries were offered for the diagnosis of selected variables to obtain the fitness level of those elderly subjects who express the desire to participate in the Trimming-130 leisure fitness sport campaign (see Figure 1).

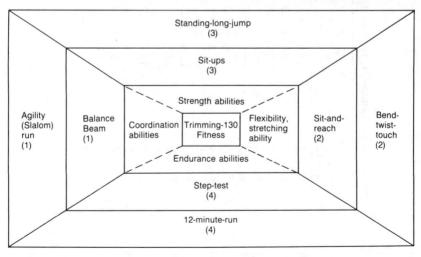

Figure 1. Fitness-tests of the Trimming 130 campaign

Table 6. Sportmotoric test performances, German Gymnastic Festival

Age (years)	Number (N) M = Male F = Female		One leg Standing (sec)	Stick removing (cm)	Trunk bend (cm)	Standing long jump (cm)
30–34	M	9	24.6 ± 6.0	62.2 ± 6.0	6.1 ± 2.5	219.1 ± 13.7
	F	12	19.3 ± 3.9	43.1 ± 6.4	10.3 ± 1.8	173.6 ± 3.9
35–39	M	9	31.0 ± 7.5	49.7 ± 3.1	5.1 ± 1.5	218.6 ± 4.2
	F	19	25.2 ± 3.9	50.5 ± 4.1	8.4 ± 1.6	172.3 ± 5.4
40–44	M	22	29.5 ± 3.7	62.1 ± 2.9	6.4 ± 1.9	218.0 ± 3.2
	F	26	21.4 ± 3.3	51.8 ± 2.7	7.0 ± 1.8	167.8 ± 3.2
45–49	M	14	26.4 ± 4.6	64.3 ± 3.3	4.5 ± 1.4	208.5 ± 4.2
	F	18	22.3 ± 3.8	48.9 ± 4.2	13.7 ± 1.4	165.7 ± 5.4
50–54	M	10	22.9 ± 3.5	73.1 ± 2.9	5.3 ± 1.9	201.8 ± 5.6
	F	10	7.9 ± 1.1	70.4 ± 4.3	8.5 ± 2.1	148.6 ± 4.8
55–59	M	5	15.1 ± 2.6	87.8 ± 2.9	7.2 ± 2.0	197.2 ± 8.6
	F	8	12.8 ± 2.7	55.5 ± 6.7	9.5 ± 2.3	147.0 ± 6.9
60–64	M	5	8.4 ± 1.9	80.0 ± 13.3	−1.6 ± 2.0	170.2 ± 10.5
	F	6	6.3 ± 0.9	59.2 ± 7.6	4.7 ± 4.0	132.2 ± 11.8
>65	M	8	7.0 ± 1.2	83.0 ± 5.0	1.4 ± 2.9	161.1 ± 6.9
	F	4	4.0 ± 0.5	69.5 ± 9.6	10.3 ± 0.7	107.2 ± 9.3

Mean ± SD data

Table 6. Sportmotoric test performances, German Gymnastic Festival (cont.)

Age (years)	Number (N)		Differentiation Jump (cm)		Sit-ups (sec)		Leg-lifts (sec)	
			1st trial	5th trial	10	20	10	20
30–34	M	9	4.1	1.1	11.6 ± 1.6	27.8 ± 2.8	11.5 ± 0.7	23.2 ± 1.3
	F	12	3.7	0.1	14.8 ± 0.8	30.3 ± 2.1	12.7 ± 1.1	24.7 ± 1.2
35–39	M	9	4.4	1.0	12.3 ± 0.7	25.4 ± 1.1	11.4 ± 0.3	22.1 ± 0.9
	F	19	3.3	0.7	16.0 ± 1.1	31.8 ± 1.2	13.3 ± 0.7	26.0 ± 1.2
40–44	M	22	2.9	0.3	15.2 ± 1.0	31.8 ± 3.0	12.6 ± 0.6	24.8 ± 1.2
	F	26	1.5	0.2	16.6 ± 0.8	38.7 ± 3.2	12.8 ± 0.5	26.4 ± 1.3
45–49	M	14	2.9	2.1	14.5 ± 0.7	30.6 ± 1.4	13.1 ± 0.9	24.0 ± 0.9
	F	18	4.7	2.4	17.3 ± 1.1	31.1 ± 2.1	13.7 ± 0.7	26.4 ± 1.5
50–54	M	10	0.8	0.3	14.3 ± 0.7	31.0 ± 1.0	13.1 ± 0.8	24.5 ± 1.0
	F	10	4.9	2.7	18.8 ± 1.3	41.0 ± 2.8	13.5 ± 0.5	26.7 ± 0.8
55–59	M	5	10.6	0.4	15.1 ± 2.1	36.4 ± 3.7	13.8 ± 0.6	28.2 ± 0.6
	F	8	3.0	1.0	22.7 ± 2.2	38.9 ± 4.7	13.1 ± 0.7	25.9 ± 1.7
60–64	M	5	13.4	3.2	18.3 ± 1.8	32.2 ± 4.8	14.8 ± 1.5	26.7 ± 1.5
	F	6	5.8	4.5	—	—	15.6 ± 1.3	29.7 ± 1.5
>65	M	8	3.6	3.1	21.9 ± 2.6	36.1 ± 5.5	16.6 ± 1.1	29.8 ± 5.2
	F	4	11.5	6.7	—	—	—	—

Table 6. Sportmotoric test performances, German Gymnastic Festival (cont.)

Age (years)	Number (N)		Push-ups (sec) 10	Push-ups (sec) 20	(Pulse rate/min) initial pulse	Step-test load pulse	Recovery pulse
30–34	M	9	8.9 ± 0.7	17.1 ± 1.0	76.8 ± 5.5	136.3 ± 4.8	103.3 ± 4.6
	F	12	10.0 ± 0.5	19.4 ± 1.1	76.9 ± 3.6	123.4 ± 4.8	87.1 ± 6.2
35–39	M	9	8.6 ± 0.5	16.4 ± 0.5	75.1 ± 3.4	121.8 ± 4.9	94.1 ± 5.3
	F	19	9.9 ± 0.5	19.3 ± 1.1	75.9 ± 3.2	126.1 ± 3.4	93.9 ± 4.2
40–44	M	22	9.2 ± 0.4	17.0 ± 0.5	75.9 ± 2.6	124.4 ± 3.2	90.5 ± 3.4
	F	26	10.4 ± 0.4	19.9 ± 0.7	79.4 ± 2.5	130.3 ± 3.2	95.1 ± 2.9
45–49	M	14	9.3 ± 0.4	17.5 ± 0.5	78.1 ± 3.9	124.4 ± 4.1	92.1 ± 5.9
	F	18	10.4 ± 0.6	20.0 ± 0.9	76.3 ± 2.6	126.7 ± 3.7	93.7 ± 3.9
50–54	M	10	11.0 ± 0.7	20.0 ± 0.9	76.9 ± 2.7	122.4 ± 5.5	93.9 ± 5.0
	F	10	11.9 ± 0.5	22.3 ± 1.3	76.6 ± 3.2	124.4 ± 5.4	93.4 ± 5.7
55–59	M	5	11.4 ± 0.8	22.5 ± 1.1	76.4 ± 7.6	124.8 ± 9.7	95.2 ± 12.3
	F	8	11.0 ± 0.8	21.1 ± 1.6	87.1 ± 6.9	146.9 ± 6.3	108.0 ± 6.7
60–64	M	5	11.3 ± 0.6	23.2 ± 2.8	77.0 ± 8.8	117.0 ± 7.5	95.2 ± 10.0
	F	6	11.8 ± 1.1	21.8 ± 1.5	78.7 ± 4.8	125.8 ± 4.3	97.0 ± 5.1
>65	M	8	12.1 ± 0.6	24.5 ± 1.4	80.9 ± 3.8	131.0 ± 6.8	109.4 ± 6.8
	F	4	14.5 ± 0.8	—	76.0 ± 4.7	118.0 ± 6.0	97.2 ± 4.5

Table 7. Intercorrelation coefficients (Rho) of selected sportmotoric tests

Age	Sex/Number M = Male F = Female		Stick moving/ truck bend	Sit-ups (10)/ leg lifts (10)	Sit-ups(20)/ leg lifts (20)
40–44	M	22	− 0.468	0.403	0.804**
45–49	M	15	− 0.345	0.622**	0.359
40-44	F	24	0.686**	0.622**	0.286
45–49	F	17	0.108	0.423	0.593*

*$p<0.001$ **$p<0.001$

Trimming Test 1 includes the items, walking forward on the balance beam, sit-and-reach, sit-ups, and step-test. The balance beam was given preference to item 1, leg-stand, because of the latest results on the structure of coordination abilities (see Bös & Mechling, 1983; Roth, 1982).

Trimming Test 2 includes the items, agility (slalom) run, bend-twist-touch, standing long jump, and 12-minute-run. Trimming Test 2 can supplement or be continued from trimming Test 1 after a 3-month Trimming-130 training program (see Starischka, 1982 for minimum Trimming-130 programs).

The initial results of ongoing research with untrained adults (40- to 48-year-old workers in steel factories) point to the utility and acceptance of the two trimming-tests offered (see Reekers & Schmidt, 1985).

References

Baltes, P.B., & Willis, S.L. (1982). Plasticity and enhancement of intellectual functioning in old age. Penn State's Adult Development and Enrichment Project. In F.J.M. Craik & Trehúb (Eds.), Aging and cognitive processes. New York: Pleniùm Press.

Barrow, H.M., & Mc Gee, R. (1979). *A practical approach to measurement in physical education*. Philadelphia: Lea & Febinger.

Beuker, F. (1976). *Leistungsprüfungen im Freizeit-und Erholùngssport*. Leipzig: J.A. Barth.

Blume, D.D. (1981). Kennzeichnung koordinativer Fähigkeiten und Möglichkeiten ihrer Herausbildung im Trainingsprozeß, Wiss. *Zeitschrift Deutsche Hochschule Körperkultur Leipzig,* **22**, 3, 17–41.

Bös, K., & Mechling, H. (1983). *Dimensionen Sportmotorischer Leistungen*. Schorndorf: Hofmann.

DSB, Hrsg. (1978). *Rahmen-Richtlinien für die ausbildung im bereich des deutschen sportbundes*. Frankfurt: Haßmüller.

DSB, Hrsg. (1984). *Jahrbuch des Sports*. Niedernhausen: Schors.

Ewerle, A. (1984). *Zur Diagnostik ausgewählter Variablen des körperlich-sportlichen Fitness-Zustandes älterer Menschen*. Dortmund: Staatsarbeit.

Grosser, M., & Starischka, S. (1981). *Konditionstests*. München: BLV.

Jokl, E. (1954). *Alter und Leistung*. Berlin: Springer.

Letzelter, H., & Letzelter, M. (1979), Zur Aussagekraft von Konditionstesten: "Der allgemeine Konditionstest von Nordrhein-Westfalen." *Sportunterricht,* **28**, 13–21.

Letzelter, H., & Letzelter, M. (1983). *Leistungsdiagnostik. Beispiel Eisschnellauf.* Niedernhausen: Schors.

Meusel, H. u.a. (1980). *Dokumentationsstudie: Sport im Alter.* Schorndorf: Hofmann.

Neumaier, A. (1983). Sportmotorische Tests in Unterricht und Training. Schorndorf: Hofmann.

Palm, J. (1982). Die Formel zur Prävention, die jeder versteht: Trimming 130. *Moderne medizin,* **10**, 1040–1045.

Palm, J. (1983). Was ist Trimming 130? In H. Pieper (Ed.), *Triming 130: Die neue Richtgeschwindigkeit für Ihre Gesundheit.* Frankfurt: Búsche.

Roth, K. (1982). Strukturanalyse koordinativer Fähigkeiten. Bad Homburg: Limpert.

Starischka, S. (1982). Gesundheit durch Trimming 130. Giessen: Werbedrúck.

Starischka, S. in press (1984). *Fitness-tests zur Begleitung der Trimming 130-Aktion.* Dortmund: Forschungsbericht DSB.

Reekers, H., & Schmidt, R. (1985). *Fitness-Taining-Trimming 130 am Arbeits-platz. Erste Erfahrúngen únd Verschläge.* In S. Starisschka, B., Gschwender, & W. Hellwing (Eds.). Dortmùnder: Schiften Sport 1. Aspekte von Lehre ùnd Forschùng. Erlensee: S-F-T Verlag.

13

Research for Independent Living Among the Elderly

Marlene J. Adrian
UNIVERSITY OF ILLINOIS AT URBANA-CHAMPAIGN
URBANA, ILLINOIS, USA

The search for the fountain of youth is the goal of many dreamers and many romanticists, but the goal for scientists might well be the research for independent living among the elderly.

One perspective of this research, biomechanical analysis of activities of daily living (ADL), is probably one of the most important determinants of improved quality of life for the elderly because independent living means independence in ADL, or survival in the basics of life. The fringe benefits or luxuries of life, such as sport, are dependent upon achievement of ADL. Independence and, therefore, improvement of the quality of life may be discussed with respect to three categories: locomotion, manipulation, and combination of manipulation and locomotion. Walking is the most widely recognized locomotion pattern. As other locomotor patterns, it is influenced by financial constraints, environmenal factors, such as the weather, and many physiological, and sociological factors. Other patterns include ascending and descending stairs and entering vehicles.

Manipulative skills include such patterns as eating skills, writing, macrame, crocheting, hoeing, and playing the piano. Many older persons use these skills to eliminate pain and problems with stiffness accompanying arthritis.

Thus, manipulative skills are an excellent means of extending activities of daily life into home recreational pursuits. In addition, these skills provide an avenue for work. Many persons continue to work through the ages of 70, 75, 80, 85 years, and older and use writing, typing, and other manipulative skills in their jobs.

The third category, the combination of locomotion and manipulative skills, includes such activities as walking while using an edger or other garden tools and walking while manipulating a tennis racquet.

The basic research in these categories is to assess the fundamental ADL patterns, determine causes of dysfunction, improve the patterns, and suggest alternate forms of performance. Patterns may be compared with those of younger persons, longitudinal assessments may be conducted, and assessment of patterns with constraints placed upon them can aid in the identification of causes of dysfunction.

Walking

The first topic to review is walking because it is the fundamental pattern to expand one's life space. Murray, Kory, and Sepic (1970) have conducted extensive studies of the kinematics of walking by adults in the United States. The walking patterns of older persons show only minor differences from those of younger persons. However, these data are not from longitudinal studies. Generally, researchers have compared the patterns of different age groups, that is, cross-sectional data and not the same persons across ages (Nelson, 1981). Older persons show greater magnitudes in their vertical pathways and slightly more toeing-out of the feet than do younger populations. However, these results are not consistent with respect to all studies, or all older individuals.

Using a countrywide cross-sectional individualized sample of 2,500 noninstitutionalized persons greater than 65 years of age, Azar and Lawton (1964) interviewed and observed pedestrian patterns. Only 12% were noted to have abnormal gaits. These abnormalities were characterized as follows:

- Bow-leggedness in approximately one third of this group
  marked—(3.5%)
  moderate—(12%)
  slight—(15.5%)
- Increasing bow-leggedness with age
- Narrow walking and standing bases
- Waddling gait, with moderate or marked bow-leggedness.

Walking ability and speed were studied by Aniansson (1980) using several hundred 70-year-old men and women. Independent walking was achieved by 90% of the men and 93% of the women. Walking aids, including wheelchairs, were required by 12% of the men and 7% of the women. Aniansson (1980) suggested a criterion measure for success in walking across an urban intersection. The criterion is a walking speed of 1.4 m/sec and was used to assess skill in walking by her population. This criterion speed of 1.4 m/sec was not achieved by the population. The average speed of walking for the men was 1.3 m/sec when asked to walk at their normal speed. Approximately 24% of the men walked at 1.4 m/sec or faster. The average speed of walking for the women was 1.1 m/sec. Less than 15% achieved the criterion value. With respect to the male population the slowest walkers were also the least physically active. One might hypothesize reasons for these slow speeds, but Dahlstedt (1978) has given us a clue when he reported older people's perceptions of speed.

A speed of 0.9 m/sec was identified as a comfortable walking speed. A 1.1 m/sec was a hurried type of walk and 1.3 m/sec was the speed at which people would catch a bus. Thus, 1.4 m/sec speed to cross a traffic intersection may not be associated with the speed which an older population might do naturally or is capable of performing.

Research by Murray et al. (1970) and Nelson (1981) included data as a result of asking subjects, not only to walk at their normal comfortable pace, but to walk as fast as they could safely walk. In the latter condition these persons walked 1.6 and 1.8 m/sec, respectively. It is evident that depending upon what research design is used, what questions are posed, and what goals are set, the researchers could state misleading conclusions. For example, one might conclude the walking pattern is deficient or excellent. I believe that most healthy individuals can walk fast enough to meet the speed criterion suggested by Aniansson if they are asked to do so.

Ascending and Descending Patterns

Because falls rank first among accidental deaths of the elderly, and constitute 67% of deaths of persons over 75 years of age, the investigation of locomotor patterns involving ascents and descents is important. Not only is balance important, but also muscular leg strength and range of motion (flexibility). Very little quantitative research has been conducted with respect to stair ascents and descents of the elderly. Azar and Lawton (1964) state that women over 75 years of age are apt to step down from curbs in a falling fashion with less control than normal. Aniansson (1980) assessed the difficulty of stepping up and down from elevations of 40, 30, 20, and 10 cm heights among her previously described population. None of the population had difficulty with the 10, 20, or 30 cm heights. Table 1 depicts the success and difficulty of the step tests. In general, these healthy 70-year-olds experienced little difficulty if a handrail could be used.

Women had greater difficulty than men. However, these women showed more failures in ascending than descending. This might be related to leg length/leg strength/body weight interactions.

Single correlational techniques were used to investigate possible causes of failure/success. Significant r's were found between healthy women, maximum height of success and dynamic quadriceps strength (.59) and isometric quadriceps strength (.59). No other correlations were above .41. Although step heights in Sweden are not standardized, most of these men and women would be successful in ADL. For example, the maximum bus step is 35 cm, train step is 37.5 cm, and railway step is 30 cm.

Investigation of the ability of the elderly to negotiate bus entry steps in Leylend, England was conducted with 208 subjects with an average age of 69 years. Eighty percent were greater than 60 years old (Brooks, 1979). Although approximately 50% of the population suffered from osteoarthritis, other orthopedic disabilities, and neurological difficulties, more than 85% of the population stated that they had problems with the height of bus entry steps.

Table 1. Ability of healthy 70 year-old men and women to negotiate steps of various heights

Step height condition	Success (up and down)	
	Men (n = 90)	Women (n = 110)
10–30 cm	All	All
40 cm	UP — all with handrail / all but 4 without	UP — all but 1 with handrail / all but 23 without
	DOWN — all with handrail / all but 5 without	DOWN — all but 1 with handrail / all but 10 without
50 cm	UP — all with handrail / all but 10 without	UP — all but 9 with handrail / all but 71 without
	DOWN — all but 2 with handrail / all but 9 without	DOWN — all but 6 with handrail / all but 34 without

Note. Adapted from "Evaluation of functional capacity in activities of daily living in 70-year-old men and women," by A. Aniansson, A. Rundgren, and L. Sperling, 1980. *Scandinavia Journal Rehabilitative Medicine*, **12**, 145-154.

A mock-up bus entry was used to test the subjects on ease of negotiating different heights of an entry step. Results are depicted in Table 2.

The lower the step, the greater the percent of success. Contrary to the Aniannson data a step of 43 cm was easily negotiated by less than 10% of this population.

Thus, it is evident that age is not a valid basis for predicting success in negotiating stairs or steps. Disease and other factors influence abilities in this activity. Researchers must be cautioned to avoid stereotyping the ADL capabilities of the elderly as a group.

Research now being conducted in the Biomechanics Research Laboratory at the University of Illinois, Urbana-Champaign, goes beyond the kinematics of walking and stepping patterns. Force platforms have been embedded in a staircase to obtain ground reaction forces during descent of stairs. Differences have been noted in magnitudes of these forces between persons carrying excess weight and no excess weight. Greater vertical forces occur with the former. This research is continuing in an effort to gain information concerning trauma-producing movements and architectural design of housing.

Fundamental Patterns

Another approach to movement analysis is to investigate the fundamental patterns: running, jumping, and throwing. Motor development specialists have done so with children, why not with the elderly? Nelson (1981) determined the kinematic changes occurring with changes in speed and gait pattern of women aged 58 years and older. The women engaged in swimming, but not running or jogging. Step length and frequency increased from a slow walk to a fast walk; and between a slow run and a fast run. These results were expected because young populations perform in this manner. However, when comparing the older women's patterns with those of younger women there was much longer support time, less flexion at the knee during the swing through of leg, and a lower arc of swing of the foot during the "run as fast as you safely can" condition. The older women's fast run resembled the younger

Table 2. Ability of older persons (men = 69 years) to negotiate steps of various heights

| Height of Step (cm) | % Success | | | |
	With ease without handrails	Just possible without handrails	With ease without handrails	Just possible without handrails
9	83	99	99	100
18	61	77	92	100
27	36	56	73	94
36	18	29	42	71
43	9	18	22	44

Note. Adapted from "An investigation into aspects of bus design and passenger requirements," by B.M. Brooks, 1979. *Ergonomics*, **22**, 175-188. Reprinted with permission.

women's slow run. Because the speed of the older women's run was equivalent to that of the younger women's slow run this would be expected. Both lack of speed in moving body segments and an uwillingness to shift the line of gravity forward of the base of support may be contributors to the older women's performances. Most of the women, however, had coordinated patterns.

Similar results were found with my unpublished research into the jumping patterns of women age 58 years and older. Each subject was videotaped while performing 3 trials of vertical jumps for maximal height while standing on a force platform. An electrogoniometer was attached to the knee to record angular displacements at the knee. The performances were videotaped and assessed qualitatively. Although the patterns were coordinated, the speed of leg extension was too low to cause the subject to jump more than a few inches. Either the fast twitch fibers were lacking or the strength/body weight ratio was too small. The use of the force platforms thus appears to be a viable approach to determining quantitative data with respect to gross movement patterns involving impacting forces with the feet.

Throwing patterns of a group of elderly men and women were studied by Reifsteck (1982). In general, the men threw overhand better than did the women, but all were able to perform the proper coordinated movements with the lower extremities. The one common deficiency was lack of full trunk rotation about the vertical axis. This factor needs further investigation if we are to provide guidelines for sports participation in which trunk rotation is necessary. Activities of daily living often utilize such trunk movements as well.

The last category in which research has been conducted is in the area of manipulative skills. Although much of the research has been basic research into reaction time (Spirduso, 1975; Mowatt, Evans & Adrian, 1984), some specific ADL manipulative tasks have been studied. For example, Aniansson, Rundgren, and Sperling (1980) reported that less than 13% of their population of 70-year-old men and women had difficulty in performing one or more of the upper extremity functional tests. The tests consisted of grasping the ear lobe with the hand anteriorly and posteriorly, fitting the hand between buttock and seat of chair while sitting, touching the finger tips to opposite big toe, pouring water from a jug to a glass and back, reaching for a 1 kg packet on shelves of varying heights, pulling out and inserting a key in lock, unscrewing and screwing an electric light bulb, inserting a coin into a slot, and dialing telephone numbers. Approximately 17% of the women had difficulty or could not perform the reaching tasks involving a shelf 180 cm high. The authors suggested that the short stature of the women may have been a dominant factor in the performance.

Those women who handled the key and light bulb tasks with difficulty were found to be significantly weaker in strength than healthy women studied by Sperling (1980). The light bulb test was performed more slowly by the women than the men. Healthy subjects performed faster than others, but they performed more slowly than a reference group of 20–30 year olds (Sperling, 1980).

The research pertaining to movement patterns of elderly persons can be summarized as follows:

1. Healthy elderly persons perform differently than less healthy older persons.

2. There is as much variance in performance within an elderly population as within a young population.
3. Research to improve performance in ADL may be an avenue to improvement in the quality of life for the elderly person.
4. Interrelationships of range of motion, level of strength, disease, speed of muscular contraction, and other factors with performance abilities need to be investigated.

References

Aniansson, A., Rundgren, A., & Sperling, L. (1980). Evaluation of functional capacity in activities of daily living in 70-year-old men and women. *Scandinavia Journal Rehabilitative Medicine,* **12**, 145-154.

Aniansson, A. (1980). Muscle function in old age with special reference to muscle morphology, effect of training and capacity in activities of daily living. *Department of Rehabilitation Medicine and Geriatric and Long-Term Care Medicine,* University of Goteburg, Goteburg, Sweden.

Azar, G.J. & Lawton, A.H. (1964). Gait and stepping as factors in the frequent falls of elderly women. *Gerontologist,* **4**, 83.

Brooks, B.M. (1979). An investigation into aspects of bus design and passenger requirements. *Ergonomics,* **22**(22), 175-188.

Dahlstedt, S. (1978). *Slow pedestrians—walking speeds and walking habits of old-age People (Report R2).* Stockholm: The Swedish Council for Building Research.

Mowatt, M., Evans, g., & Adrian, M. (October, 1984). Assessment of perceptual-motor abilities of healthy rural elderly men and women. *Physical Educator,* **41**(3).

Muray, M.P., Kory, R.C., & Sepic, S.B. (1970). Walking patterns of normal women. *Archives of Physical Medicine,* **51**, 639-654.

Nelson, C.J. (1981). Locomotor patterns of women over 57. Unpublished master's thesis, Washington State University.

Reifsteck, J. (1982). *Cinematographical analysis of overarm throwing patterns of elderly men and women.* Unpublished thesis, Washington State University.

Sperling, L. (1980). Evaluation of upper extremity function in old age. *Scandinavian Journal Rehabilitative Medicine,* **12**, 39.

Spirduso, W. (1975). Reaction and movement time as a function of age and physical activity level. *Journal of Gerontology,* **30**, 435-440.

14

Exercise: An Effective Strategy to Activate Seniors

David R. Stirling, Guy Miller, Phillip Barker,
Gail Rowden, and Stephen Meehan
SIMON FRASER UNIVERSITY
BURNABY, BRITISH COLUMBIA, CANADA

Melvin Ralston
WHITE ROCK BAPTIST CHURCH
WHITE ROCK, BRITISH COLUMBIA, CANADA

One characteristic in our modern urban society that has increased is the number of people living in core areas of our cities in condominiums and apartment housing complexes. Along with this increase in the number of apartment dwellers is the proportion of those persons who are handicapped and/or elderly. Of concern to many health care and social work agencies is contact with these persons within their apartment complexes in a meaningful way, while still maintaining the necessary level of security and privacy.

A number of communities in North America, like the community of White Rock used in the study, experience persons relocating into their communities for retirement. This results in a large number of senior citizens relative to the rest of the population. For example, in White Rock, a retirement center in Western Canada, over 50% of the community are retired. With relocation, seniors can experience varying degrees of social and emotional stress (Blenker,

This study was supported by grant funds from Employment and Immigration Canada. The authors would like to acknowledge the assistance of Mr. and Mrs. A. Graham, Mrs. J. Poelvoorde, Mr. and Mrs. D. Sherwin, Mr. and Mrs. F. Griggs, and Mrs. R. Ralston in completing this project.

1967). In the period of adjustment, if social contacts are not made, they can become isolated unto themselves. This can mean an increase of inactivity in an already sedentary lifestyle.

Changes in lifestyle are not easy to initiate, particularly when there is no urgent health care need present (Brunner, 1969). The need to maintain some level of activity for health and personal well-being has long been recognized (Shephard, 1978). The techniques that successfully activate seniors living in apartments, however, are not as well recognized.

Purpose

The purpose of this study was to develop a number of different Active Health programs that could be used to activate seniors living in various apartment complexes in White Rock, British Columbia, and to identify which program or programs would be most effective.

Method

One hundred and twenty-eight seniors from six apartment blocks were activated by the programs of "Active Health for Seniors," a community service project sponsored by the White Rock Baptist Church and the Department of Kinesiology of Simon Fraser University. Other programs established by this project included: visitation; audiotape distribution; literature and library resource distribution; transportation service; telephone contact; special interest courses; and exercise programs.

In order to initiate any aspects of the Active health programs, initial contact into the specific apartment complex had to take place. Figure 1 illustrates the process that was used during this study.

Selection of the apartments for study was completed using two criteria: The apartment must primarily be occupied by seniors, and the apartment should have an activity room or similar space where either activity or exercise classes could be held. Apartments with large numbers of young and middle-aged adults present a management problem for the fitness leader. Programs for younger adults emphasize more cardiovascular conditioning, whereas the program developed here for seniors focused on stretching and flexibility. Finally, without an activity space there would be no place to hold the activity or exercise class. With these two criteria being met, the apartment manager was then contacted and a meeting was arranged that included the manager and a committee of residents to explain the purposes of the program. Appropriate advertisements were placed throughout the building for the first organizational class. Mutually convenient times were arranged for the subsequent exercise classes. For the first four weeks, classes were held once a week and then expanded to twice

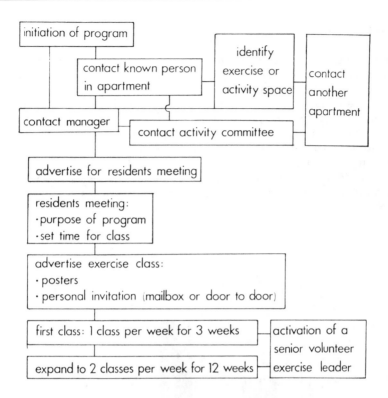

Figure 1. Strategies for implementing active health programs into apartment complexes

a week for the remaining time period. Once the program had begun in a particular apartment block, advertisements for each type of program were placed in the apartments, with compliance and retainment data collected. The effectiveness of each of the programs was established using the following formulas:

Program Compliance

$$\frac{\text{number-registered}}{\substack{\text{number contacted by} \\ \text{specific program}}} \times 100 = \substack{\text{compliance effectiveness} \\ \text{(CE)}}$$

Program Retention

$$\frac{\text{number-retained-in-programs}}{\text{total number initially recruited}} \times 100 = \substack{\text{retention} \\ \text{effectiveness} \\ \text{(RE)}}$$

Results

In the six apartment blocks selected for study, 582 persons living in the 479 units were contacted, and 128 persons were recruited, this resulted in an effectiveness rating of 20.3 ± 8.2%.

Of five Active Health programs, the biweekly exercise program attracted the largest number of people and had the largest retention rating. These data are shown in Figure 2. The retention ratings of the programs ranged from 3% for the telephone to 91% for the exercise program. Of the 128 who initially registered for the exercise program, 116 attended all of the classes or missed only one. At the end of the exercise program, the participants were asked which features of the program they liked the most and what factors influenced their remaining in the program (refer to Table 1).

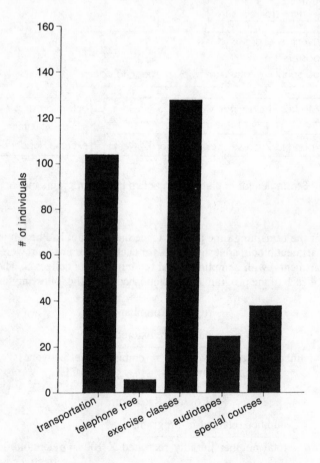

Figure 2. Activity strategies used in six-apartment complexes.

Table 1. Results of the questionnaire administered to the seniors participating in the biweekly exercise program

Program feature	Percent of participants
Enjoyment of class	36
Regularity of exercise class	32
Enjoy scialization	22
Feels good	20
Instructor	18
Instructive	5
Qualities of Instructor	
Good personality	36
Clear instructions	22
Easy to follow	14
Interest in group	12
Knowledge of fitness	12
Conscientious	2

Discussion

From a recent review of the literature no reports have been published concerning the compliance and adherence of seniors to an exercise program. Data from this study have several implications for the approach, organization, and management of such programs.

Seniors have a wide range of abilities and interests. In order to attract these people a wide range of activity choices are necessary. With this in mind, the programs that were developed attempted to foster and encourage physical, social, emotional, and spiritual health and well-being.

The fact that the biweekly exercise program was the most effective strategy to activate the seniors was an unexpected finding. The adherence rate observed during our exercise program was high compared to other reports found in the literature. Adherence ratings reviewed ranged from 222 to 35.6% (Faulkner & Stewart, 1977; Gettman, Pollock, & Ward, 1983). The reasons for the striking differences observed in this study are not entirely clear yet may, in fact, be due to several factors.

The exercise classes were convenient with respect to time and location. Each class was run within the particular apartment complex at the most convenient time for residents. Transportation to an outside location was eliminated. Time was taken to contact each potential participant, and to outline carefully the objectives of the program. The exercise classes were individually prescriptive, emphasizing stretching, flexibility, and strength exercises, with a de-emphasis on cardiovascular exercises. All classes began at a low level of intensity with gradual increases where appropriate.

The personalities of the three instructors were rated highly on the questionnaire administered following the progam (refer to Table 1). The rapport that was established with each participant appears to be a significant factor in retaining seniors in the program. Results reported in Table 1 show sincere interest in the group of individuals was considered as important as background knowledge of fitness and fitness concepts.

Following each class, time was taken to talk to each participant to assess the appropriateness of each class, to offer individual counseling relating to health and fitness concerns, and to identify any physical discomforts as a result of the exercise stress. This time at the end of each class provided an opportunity for the instructors to express their interests in each person, as well as an opportunity to obtain essential information as to their state of wellness. This aspect of follow-up can, however, become time-consuming and can require anywhere from 15 to 45 minutes in addition to regular class time. For seniors registered in this program it was time well spent.

Summary

A biweekly exercise program was the most effective program run by a seniors' activation project (Active Health for Seniors). In this broad spectrum activity program, a biweekly exercise program was 91% effective in activating and retaining older adults. Several elements stressed during this program have led to these results and may have implications for the organization and management of other apartment or condominium exercise programs for seniors. The elements emphasized in this program are as follows:

1. Exercise classes are run in the particular apartment complex.
2. Emphasis is placed on stretching and strength exercises.
3. Initial intensity levels are minimal and increases are gradual.
4. The program includes activities that address and encourage social and emotional interaction between the participants and the fitness leader.
5. Follow-up after each exercise class is emphasized.
6. The personalities of the instructors are an important factor.
7. Interest in individual seniors is expressed throughout the program.

References

Belkner, M. (1967). Environmental change in the aging individual. *Gerontologist,* **7,** 101.

Brunner, B.C. (1969). Personality and motivating factors influencing adult participation in vigorous physical acivity. *Research Quarterly,* **40,** 467.

Faulkner, R., & Stewart, G. (1977). Exercise management: Recruitment and retention. Employee Fitness Program Occupational Health Service, B.C. Ministry of Health, Victoria, B.C.

Gettman, L.R., Pollock, M.L., & Ward A. (1983). Adherence to unsupervised exercise. *The Physician and Sports Medicine,* **11,** 57.

Heinzelmann, F., & Bagley, R.W. (1970). Response to physical activity programs and their effects on health behavior. *Public Health Reports,* **85**, 905.

Roth, W.T. (1974). Some motivational aspects of exercise. *Journal of Sports Medicine and Physical Fitness,* **14**.

Shepard, R.J., (1978). *Physical activity and aging.* Wanzel, B., & Danielson, R., (1977). Improve adherence to your Fitness programs, Part III., *Recreation Management.*

15

Health Education and Physical Fitness for Older Adults

Exercise and fitness are attracting the interest of many older adults in the United States today. However, according to the 1983 Statistical Abstract of the United States, only 42.3% of people over 65 exercise regularly. Franks, Lee, and Fullarton (1983) point out that exercise plays an important role in the prevention and treatment of many health problems common to older adults, such as coronary heart disease, hypertension, obesity, diabetus mellitus, anxiety/depression, arthritis, and osteoporosis. Smith and Gilligan (1983) estimate that as much as one-half of physical and mental decline, heretofore associated with aging, is due to muscular disuse.

Price and Luther (1980) report additional benefits in the psychosocial realm from exercise. They include greater ability to cope with stress, overall improved mood, reduced levels of anxiety, improved body image, better perceived health, and increased self-sufficiency. Exercise can build up an individual's working capacity, endurance, and stamina necessary for independent living (Franks, 1983).

Knowing that a large number of positive benefits can be received from regular exercise by older adults, the Center for Health Promotion at George Mason

University developed the Health Education and Physical Fitness Project for Older Adults (HEP) to increase the number of older adults in the community who exercise on a regular basis. The 3-year project is funded by the Virginia State Health Department, Division of Health Education and Information as part of the Prevention Block Grant. The project also investigated factors affecting compliance with exercise behavior in the older adult age group.

Methods

Three program strategies were developed (Center for Health Promotion, 1983)

1. to inform older adults in the community about the benefits of exercise;
2. to develop a model exercise program for older adults; and
3. to educate recreation specialists, health care professionals, and others about the need for fitness activities for older adults.

The remainder of this paper addresses the second strategy.

A pilot exercise program was conducted over a 10-week period in the winter of 1983. One hundred and five men and women volunteered to participate in the 10-week program. Ninety-two participants answered both the pretest and the posttest questionnaires; they form the study population. Thirty-one percent of the study population were men and 69% were women. All were white. They ranged in age from 55 to over 80 (mean age was 63). Mean annual income was $27,000. Seventy-two percent were college educated.

Most participants (92%) indicated that they were in good to excellent health (Center for Health Promotion). Based on self-report, 44% had arthritis, bursitis, or rheumatism, 23% had hypertension, and 64% considered themselves to be overweight. Only 5% of exercise program participants noted that regular exercise had been recommended to them by a physician.

Physical assessments were taken at the beginning and end of the 10-week study. Assessments included measures of grip strength, flexibility, weight, resting heart rate, blood pressure, and aerobic capacity as measured by distance walked in 12 minutes.

Based on a review of the literature and a survey of older adults in the community, the following strategies were incorporated into the model program:

• Education about the reasons for following a regular program of physical activity because this motivates them to continue.
• Education about safe and effective techniques for exercising.
• Instruction in monitoring pulse rates during exercise.

HEP participants spent 2 hours twice a week at the university in activities such as walking, racquet sports, dance, aerobic exercise to music, calisthenics, weight lifting, and health education seminars. Blood pressure screening was conducted at the beginning of each session for persons with borderline or high blood pressure and for others who desired it.

Results

Variables Related to Program Attendance

Participants were classified according to their attendance in the program. "High attenders" participated in 15 or more of 20 2-hour sessions. High attenders were more likely to be male and younger than those who were "low attenders." High attenders were more likely to rate their health status as excellent. They had more favorable expectations of the benefits of exercise, perceived fewer barriers to future exercising, and were more likely to state that they intended to be exercising 1 month and 3 months after the initial program. Low attenders were less confident of their physical abilities and more worried about injuring themselves.

Physical and Emotional Changes in HEP Exercise Participants

Ninety-two percent of participants in the study said after 10 weeks that they felt better in general and more physically fit. Fifty-seven percent reported sleeping better and 61% said they felt less stress. The high attendance group

- showed a drop in systolic blood pressure (76% of women, 68% of men);
- showed a decrease in diastolic blood pressure (33% of women, 53% of men);
- showed increases in flexibility (68% of women, 71% of men);
- lost weight (45% of men and women); and
- increased aerobic endurance (40% of women, 67% of men).

Discussion

Exercise programs planned for older adults should include interventions (Center for Health Promotion, 1983) that

- educate participants about benefits to be achieved through exercise and about what is a realistic time frame in which to achieve those benefits;
- build self-confidence through a progressive program of exercises which promotes success at every stage;
- demonstrate correct exercise techniques and exercise information in order to reduce injury and fear of injury; and
- address related concerns of the elderly such as weight control, chronic disease management, hypertension control, and the need for opportunities to socialize.

References

Center for Health Promotion. (September 1983). *Health education and physical fitness project for older adults (HEP): Final report.*

Franklin, B.A. (June 1978). Motivating and educating adults to exercise. *Journal of Physical Education and Recreation, 49*, 13-17.

Franks, P., Lee, P.R., & Fullarton, J.E. (April 1983). *Lifetime fitness and exercise for older people*. San Francisco: Aging Health Policy Center, University of California.

Price, J.H., & Luther, S.L. (September 1980). Physical fitness: Its role in health for the elderly. *Journal of Gerontological Nursing, 6*, 517-521.

Smith, E.L., & Gilligan, C. (August 1983). Physical activity prescription for the older adult. *The Physician and Sports Medicine, 11*, 91-101.

Statistical Abstract of the United States. (1982-1983). Washington, D.C.: U.S. Department of Commerce, Bureau of the Census.

16

Diagnostic and Therapeutic Aspects of Physical Exercise and Sport in Clinical Health Care of the Aging

Raymond Harris
ST. PETER'S HOSPITAL
ALBANY, NEW YORK, USA

Physicians, physical educators, and other allied professionals concerned with the elderly have accepted as normal the reduced physical capacities of inactive, sedentary aging people limited by poor physical condition and/or subclinical or clinical disease. They have overlooked the therapeutic and preventive potential of physical exercise and sport, which when properly prescribed, enable the well and the sick aged to function at a higher optimal level. The modalities also provide a cost-effective therapy to maintain better physical fitness, prevent illness, and reduce health costs.

However, appropriate physical training and sport regimens for the elderly must be adapted to their particular needs. This paper discusses some of these modifications and the value of clinical exercise stress testing to measure physiologic cardiovascular fitness, to pinpoint the presence of cardiovascular disease, and to detect occult cardiac arrhythmias.

The Physical Potential of the Aging Person

Performances in the Boston marathon, American Senior Olympics, and similar world-wide sport competitions testify to the physical potential of aging people. They reveal physical capacities in geriatric superstars that most physicians and others concerned with the sick and infirm aged have generally overlooked. They demonstrate that in the absence of disease and illness, physically conditioned, trained older men and women are as fit or even more fit than untrained younger individuals (Harris, 1981).

Consider, for example, John E. Kelley of East Dennis, Massachusetts, who ran the 26-mile, 385-yard Boston course for the 50th time in 1981. This 73-year-old veteran runner, who for physical reasons dropped out of his first race in 1928 at the age of 20, finished the 1981 marathon in 4:01:25 and said, "It was the easiest race in years!" At 77, he finished the 1985 Boston marathon in 4:31 and said, "I ran it because it was the 50th anniversary of my first Marathon victory, but I had to walk over the hills."

Or, the 75-year-old weight lifter in the American Senior Olympics who lifted 790 pounds—3 times his own body weight. His ability to perform this feat is due to the physiologic fact that although agility and flexibility are lost at an earlier age, strength and power are usually the last to be lost with age and weight lifting can increase physical fitness, stamina, and strength.

Cardiac disease need not be a barrier to better fitness. Seventy-one-year-old Jim Thomas completed 26 miles in the American Senior Olympics. At age 64 he developed severe angina due to triple coronary artery disease. Seriously handicapped, he started walking the best he could. After a few years of persistent walking, he was finally able to walk 4 miles in 1 hour. He then tried jogging for 15 steps before he had to stop because of angina. Then he was able to jog a full 5 miles without walking and gradually conditioned himself to complete 26 miles without adverse cardiovascular effects despite his coronary heart disease.

Too many of us who work with the elderly have set our sights too low. We have accepted inactive, sedentary older people who are incapacitated by subclinical or occult disease as normal. Even an outstanding researcher like Dr. Nathan Shock fell into this error in his classic work showing the decline of cardiac output with age. More recent similar studies at the same institution, the Baltimore Gerontological Research Center, show the decline in cardiac output is absent in physically fit older people without occult coronary artery disease. This study employed noninvasive studies with radioactive thallium, nuclear and echocardiographic studies unavailable at the time of the earlier study (Rodeheffer, Gerstenblith, Becker, Fleg, Weisfeldt, & Lakatta, 1984).

In practice we tend to overlook the great therapeutic potential of physical exercise. As Professor Ernst Jokl (1981) has noted:

> The theoretical basis for understanding the unimpaired adaptability to exercise with aging was provided more than 100 years ago by the great pathologist, Julius Cohnheim. He pointed out that irrespective of age, physiological challenges of all kinds are reliable in that they invariable result in an enhanced functional status. Training for strength increases strength; training for endurance increases endurance; training for skill increases skill.

Physical exercise and nutrition provide a solid foundation for a sound and healthy old age and can delay the inevitable deterioration due to the aging process. However, the body's adaptability to exercise is admittedly less reliable when pathologic processes are present.

Diagnostic Uses of Physical Activity

Physical activity is an important diagnostic noninvasive tool in the clinical evaluation of elderly people. This can be performed in the gymnasium, office, hospital, or nursing home. The Kraus-Weber muscular fitness tests are invaluable to appraise the minimum muscular fitness of older people to determine which muscles are weak and why some people find it difficult to get out of a chair, walk up stairs, or even do ordinary walking. Although originally developed to detect muscular weakness in young people, the same diagnostic criteria apply to young and old people (Kraus, 1977b). Once the weak muscles responsible for the defect have been identified, proper muscle strengthening exercises can be prescribed.

The treadmill and bicycle exercise stress tests have become important to determine the physiologic, muscular, and cardiovascular fitness of people, and as a guide for exercise prescription. The treadmill exercise test is also useful to analyze the patient's ability to walk or to run at different rates of speed and to detect gait and movement disturbances that may not show up when people walk slowly. Before vigorous exercise is permitted, people over the age of 40 should have a treadmill or other exercise tolerance test to determine their physical and cardiovascular fitness and to make sure exercise causes no dangerous electrocardiographic changes or serious disturbances of their heart rhythms. The results of these tests can be used to prescribe a safe effective amount of aerobic exercise at a rate that promotes cardiovascular fitness (Shepard, 1981; Morse & Smith, 1981; Davison, 1977).

The exercise stress test is also valuable to detect occult cardia arrhythmias, which may be absent on the routine resting electrocardiogram. Ambulatory Holter monitoring in which a patient wears a small recording electrocardiogram unit for 24 hours or longer is a useful technique to detect arrhythmias during exercise and daily activity to see if exercise and activity produce heart irregularities.

Therapeutic Prescription of Physical Activity and Exercise

Animal and human studies show that exercise and training can improve cardiovascular function and fitness (Harris, 1977, 1981). For example, aging in rats decreases the concentration of capillaries of the old rat heart, which chronic exercise can improve (Tomanek, 1974). Swimming training prevents the myosin isoenzyme redistribution found with age in spontaneously hypertensive rats (Rupp & Jacob, 1982) and actually makes the heart biochemically younger.

Although aging reduces the working capacity, the maximum $\dot{V}O_2$, endurance, power, strength, agility, flexibility (Adrian, 1981), and coordination, physical exercise, and training can counterbalance these age-related changes in work capacity and physical performance. They can also improve the fitness and physical capacity of older people and promote a healthier old age (deVries

1977; Harris, 1977), mainly because the body's adaptability to exercise remains unimpaired by aging (Jokl, 1981).

Physical training programs can reduce the damage and disability from cardiovascular, musculoskeletal, and other impaired organ systems of aging people and benefit people with coronary artery disease, diabetes mellitus, hypertension, pulmonary disorders, and other illnesses by reducing overweight, high blood sugar, blood fat, high blood pressure, and improving circulation (Shepard, 1978). Exercise also compensates for some genetically programmed trends that adversely affect the body's responses to stress and disease (Harris, 1981).

Exercise has been particularly useful in patients with coronary artery disease. Exercise and training enhance oxidation capacity in trained muscles and increase the arteriovenous oxygen differences rather than producing changes in pump function and perfusion. Training for cardiovascular fitness neither alters collateral circulation of the heart, scintigraphic findings, or left ventricular function at rest, nor affects coronary sinus blood flow or left ventricular oxygen consumption during exercise (Iskandrian, Hakki, DePace, Manno, & Segal, 1983).

Exercise training programs for the aged have practical importance although the physiologic gains they produce are relatively smaller than in younger people. Regular physical training and exercise promote endurance, improve cardiovascular and muscular fitness, eliminate fatigue, stimulate metabolism, and enhance specific neuromuscular coordination and skills in people up to the age of 65 and even in some older people (Harris, 1977; deVries, 1977; Kraus, 1977a; Jokl, 1981; Shepard, 1978; 1981; Adrian, 1981; Moritani, 1981). Exercise programs for the aged enable both the ambulatory well and ambulatory or institutionalized sick to function at more optimal levels and provide a cost-effective therapeutic modality that prevents illness and improves medical care (Rodstein, 1977).

Physical activity has not proven to extend the life span in human subjects. However, proper physical exercise improves the physical capacity and abilities of many normal healthy older people, enriches their quality of life, and increases the duration and happiness of their good years so they can enjoy active retirement.

A good medical examination should be performed to assess medical limitations, exercise tolerance, and activity potential before vigorous exercise is prescribed. People over the age of 40 should have a treadmill or another type of exercise tolerance test to evaluate their physical and cardiovascular fitness. Such a test might have prevented the recent death of James Fixx who didn't practice what he preached. His autopsy showed two of his coronary arteries were blocked, and he suffered from silent heart disease. It was reported that Mr. Fixx avoided doctors and check-ups, possibly because he feared doctors would discover heart disease.

The results can be used to prescribe a safe but effective amount and rate of aerobic exercise that promotes cardiovascular fitness. Asymptomatic elderly patients with ischemic heart disease manifested only by minor electrocardiographic abnormalities and no angina should be reassured concerning their prognosis, should be cautioned aganst overeating, and should be advised to

keep physically fit by walking, dancing, bowling, swimming, yoga, and golf-
ing, if a good medical examination and exercise treadmill stress tests disclose
no significant cardiovascular contraindications against exercise.

Symptomatic patients with coronary artery disease require the use of medications and properly prescribed exercise in carefully supervised cardiac rehabilia-
tion programs. Some may benefit from coronary artery bypass operations
followed by more active, supervised exercise (Harris, 1981).

The Exercise Prescription

Exercise programs for normal older people should begin at a low level of activity and be raised by gradually increasing the number of repetitions, distance,
and rate of exercise. Heart rate response to exercise and the absence of significant symptoms and signs should be used as reasonably good indicators for
the overall reaction to exercise.

The exercise program should include an initial warm-up period of 10–15
minutes during which stretching, light calisthenics, and leisure walking are
performed to loosen muscles and joints, to slowly accelerate the heart rate,
and to improve circulation.

Gentle stretching exercises promote flexibility, neuromuscular coordination,
balance, and relaxation. Yoga, under the supervision of a qualified instructor
with experience in exercise for the elderly, is safe to promote muscle tone
and prevent musculoskeletal injuries.

Aquatic exercises performed in water at a comfortable temperature of 75
to 80°F enable many stiff, arthritic, or otherwise handicapped older in-
vidividuals to become more agile, flexible, and relaxed. Physical therapy exercises prescribed by a physiatrist or a qualified physical therapist are especially
useful for individuals with serious disability. Range-of-motion stretching
movements and other exercises to build up muscle power help the bedfast patient
progress from bed to chair.

Calisthenics and light weight training can improve muscular strength and
lean muscle mass of many older persons. Weight-bearing exercises against
the force of gravity can prevent or reduce osteomalacia and osteoporosis. When
hypertension or other medical problems are present, it is best to check first
with the patient's physician for permission before starting these programs. One
can begin by lifting a 1-2 pound weight and then gradually increasing it up
to 15-20 pounds as strength and endurance improve. When a weight can be
lifted 12 times without difficulty, the weight can be increased to an amount
that can be comfortably lifted 8 times without straining. The interval between
each weight lift should be long enough to avoid substantial rise of blood pressure
and to permit the oxidation of metabolites that accumulate in the body during
exercise. Older people should not lift heavier weights unless they are in good
physical shape and have done it most of their lives.

Walking is the best and safest all-around warm-up exercise for people 60
years of age and over. Elderly people can begin by walking their usual distance
at a rate they can comfortably perform without becoming overly tired or

distressed. Then, over a period of several weeks to several months, the distance can be gradually increased to 1 or more miles daily and the rate of walking accelerated to 3 or 4 miles per hour, if possible (Wear, 1977).

A vigorous exercise period of 20 minutes or more to condition the heart, lungs, and blood vessels, to induce relaxation, and to reduce weight is desirable for many well elderly.

For good cardiovascular fitness, a person must exercise vigorously and aerobically for at least 20 to 30 minutes 3 or more times weekly at his or her age-related target training heart rate (Brunner, 1977; Wear, 1977). This rate can be calculated by first subtracting the individual's age from 220 to get the age-adjusted maximum heart rate and then multiplying the result by 60-70% to obtain his or her optimal target training heart rate. Exercise that keeps the heart rate at this level for 20 to 30 minutes improves cardiovascular fitness. For safety, this rate should not be exceeded during exercise. It is important to check the heart rate during exercise to make sure that it is not higher and that no heart irregularities occur during exercise.

A carefully planned regimen of walking, walking-jogging, swimming, bicycling, or a combination may also be prescribed, according to the physical and orthopedic fitness and personal desires of the individual (Wear, 1977). People with orthopedic or other barriers to walking or running will benefit from bicycling, swimming, and water sports that involve major groups of muscles. Many elderly persons find hydroslimnastics (exercise in water) and swimming an ideal conditioning program (Harris, 1977). Outdoor exercise is another enjoyable source of exercise. A cool-down period of 5 to 10 minutes during which light exercise is performed and the body returns gradually to its normal resting state should follow the vigorous exercise period.

Summary

Proper physical exercise and activity programs can counterbalance the age-related decrease in work capacity and physical performance; develop, maintain, and improve range of motion, muscle strength, flexibility, balance, and endurance; and reduce the damage and disability of associated cardiovascular, musculoskeletal, and other organ systems in aging people. It also improves the independence, quality and enjoyment of life (Shepard, 1978; deVries, 1977). Exercise programs to develop lifetime fitness and performance skills are best begun early in life, but at no age are they contraindicated (Kraus, 1977a). Physical activity not only enhances physical capacity but also maintains and improves wellness, lifestyle, and health at all ages.

References

Adrian, M.J. (1981). Flexibility in the aging adult. In E.L. Smith & R.C. Serfass (Eds.), *Exercise and aging: The scientific basis*. Hillside,NJ: Enslow.

Brunner, D. (1977). Physical exercise and cardiovascular fitness. In R. Harris & L.J. Frankel (Eds.), *Guide to fitness after 50* (pp. 143–150). New York: Plenum.

Davison, E.T. (1977). Multi-stage cardiovascular testing. In R. Harris & L.J. Frankel (Eds.), *Guide to fitness after 50* (pp. 151–161). New York: Plenum.

deVries, H.A. (1977). Physiology of physical conditioning for the elderly. In R. Harris & L.J. Frankel (Eds.), *Guide to fitness after 50* (pp. 47–52). New York: Plenum.

Harris, R. (1977). Fitness and the aging process. In R. Harris & L.J. Frankel (Eds), *Guide to fitness after 50* (pp. 3–11). New York: Plenum.

Harris, R. (1981). *Therapeutic and diagnostic aspects of physical exercise in geriatric care. Implications for "the rectangular society."* XII International Congress of Gerontology, Hamburg, Germany.

Iskandrian, A.S., Hakki, A.H., DePace, N.L., Manno, B., & Segal, B.L. (1983). Evaluation of the left ventricular function by radionuclide angiography during exercise in normal subjects and in patients with chrnoic coronary heart disease. *Journal of American College of Cardiology, 1,* 1518.

Jokl, E. (1981). Abstract. XII International Congress of Gerontology, Hamburg, Germany.

Kraus, H. (1977a). Preservation of physical fitness. In R. Harris & L.J. Frankel (Eds.). *Guide to fitness after 50* (pp. 35–38). New York: Plenum.

Kraus, H. (1977b). Principles of exercise for musculoskeletal reconditioning and fitness. In R. Harris & L.J. Frankel (Eds.), *Guide to fitness after 50* (pp. 247-251). New York: Plenum.

Moritani, T. (1981). Training adaptations in the muscles of older men. In E.L. Smith & R.C. Serfass (Eds.), *Exercise and aging: The scientific basis.* Hillside, NJ: Enslow.

Morse, C.E., & Smith, E.L. (1981). Physical activity programming for the aged. In E.L. Smith & R.C. Serfass (Eds.), *Exercise and aging: The scientific basis.* Hillside, NJ: Enslow.

Rodstein, M. (1977). Changing the habits and thought patterns of the aged to promote better health through activity programs in institutions. In R. Harris & L.J. Frankel (Eds.), *Guide to fitness after 50* (pp. 215–220). New York: Plenum.

Rodeheffer, R.J., Gerstenblith, G., Becker, L.C., Fleg, J.L., Weisfeldt, M.L., & Lakatta, E.G. (1984). Exercise cardiac output is maintained with advancing age in healthy human subjects: Cardiac dilatation and increased stroke volume compensate for a diminished heart rate. *Circulation, 69,* 203-213.

Rupp, H., & Jacob, R. (1982). Response of blood pressure and cardiac myosin polymorphism to swimming training in the spontaneously hypertensive rat. *Canadian Journal of Physiology and Pharmacology, 60,* 1098.

Shepard, R.J. (1978). *Physical activity and aging.* Chicago: A Croom Heim Book. Distributed by Year Book Medical Publishers.

Shepard, R.J. (1981). Cardiovascular limitations in the aged. In E.L. Smith, & R.C. Serfass (Eds.), *Exercise and aging: The scientific basis.* Hillside, NJ: Enslow.

Tomanek, R.J. (1974). In *Structure and chemistry of the aging heart* (pp. 172–186). New York: MSS Information Corp.

Wear, R.E. (1977). Conditioning exercise programs for normal older persons. In R. Harris & L.J. Frankel (Eds.), *Guide to fitness after 50* (pp. 253–270). New York: Plenum.

PART III

Psychological Perspectives

17

Athletes and Nonathletes in the Middle Years of Life

William P. Morgan
UNIVERSITY OF WISCONSIN–MADISON
MADISON, WISCONSIN, USA

There has been a continuing debate concerning the influence of athletics on longevity. More recently, there has been a focus on physical activity per se and its ability to prevent disease, as well as to assist in rehabilitation once illness occurs. The first investigations (J. Morgan, 1893; Meylan, 1904; Hill, 1927; Cooper, O'Sullivan, & Hughes, 1937; Hartley & Llewellyn, 1939) suggested that adult males who had participated in sports such as rowing, cricket, and skiing while in college were observed to live longer than control groups comprised of insured men or the general population. Research by Dublin (1932), Rook (1954), Montoye, Van Huss, Olson, Pierson, and Hudec (1967), Polednak and Damon (1970), and Olson, Montoye, Sprague, Stephens, and Van Huss (1978), who compared former college athletes with nonathletes, failed to support the view that participation in college athletics enhances life expectancy. A group comprised of college graduates would, of course, seem to be the most appropriate control in such studies. While the number of years lived (quantity of life) may not correlate with athleticism, it is quite possible that the *quality* of years lived may be influenced by physical activity patterns. In view of the reported association between physical activity on the one hand, and reduced anxiety, depression, suicide, and heart disease on the other, it seems reasonable to hypothesize that *quality of life* (Flanagan, 1978) would be higher in aging individuals who remain physically active. However, it must be acknowledged that the underlying factors responsible for adoption of, and adherence to, a physically active lifestyle are not well understood. There is

The preparation of this paper was supported in part by NIH Grant Number HL-25786 from the National Heart, Lung and Blood Institute.

conflicting evidence, for example, regarding the question of whether former athletes and nonathletes resemble or differ in their exercise patterns during later life. At any rate, the issue of "life quality" has only begun to be addressed during recent years. Investigators have historically focused on the "quantity," not the "quality," of years lived.

One possible explanation for the failure to observe a protective influence of athletics is that investigators have not traditionally viewed athletes and nonathletes in a multidimensional context. It has been assumed that individuals can be classified into one of the two groups, and all other variables remain fairly static. Such an assumption, however, is rather difficult to accept. First of all, the research of Paffenbarger, Wing, and Hyde (1978) suggests that physical activity per se, not athleticism, decreases the risk of heart attack. These investigators evaluated the self-reported energy expenditure of 16,936 Harvard alumni, aged 35–74 years, and compared exercise behavior with risk of heart attack. There were 572 heart attacks in this sample, and risk was found to be opposed by physical activity patterns. A physical activity index below 2,000 Kcal per week placed subjects at a 64% higher risk than classmates who had higher indices. Also, former varsity athletes only had a lower heart attack risk if they maintained a high level of physical activity after graduation. Paffenbarger et al. (1978) concluded that:

> The persistent corroborations encountered in these data strongly support a protective role for vigorous exercise in the reduction of heart attack risk. Alumni who had not been especially athletic as students, but rated high physical activity starting at middle age, were at lower risk of heart attack than former athletes whose later exercise level was in the low index category. (p. 173)

These findings are particularly significant in light of the earlier report by Montoye et al. (1957) that former college athletes were significantly more active than nonathletes following graduation, and this difference persisted up to 45 years of age. Self-reported activity patterns were identical for the two groups in the 45–49 age span, but the nonathletes became significantly more active from the fifth decade on. Montoye et al. (1957) cautioned, however, that "...it may be that differences in judgments regarding the intensity of activity... are responsible for the results" (p. 81).

It appears obvious that comparisons of former athletes and nonathletes must take various factors into consideration. It is clear at both a theoretical and empirical level, for example, that postgraduate activity level must be taken into account.

Acceptable scientific proof of the hypothesized relationship between physical activity and longevity, and especially the efficacy of physical activity in preventing coronary disease and death, may not be available for many years. It is also imperative that basic information be generated relative to the role of physical activity and sport in the development and maintenance of mental health, as well as physical health, because quality of life would intuitively be influenced in part by various affective states. Available literature concerning the role of sport and physical activity in the development and maintenance of mental health will, therefore, be examined in the following sections.

Psychological Impact of Sports

Most of the research involving the psychological impact of involvement in athletics has been of a cross-sectional nature, and this research has been reviewed by Morgan (1977b, 1981, 1982, 1984). Athletes and nonathletes have consistently been found to differ, and these differences have emerged regardless of the age group investigated or the psychological model(s) employed. A fundamental question raised by such research relates to the issue of whether or not the observed differences reflect an effect due to involvement in sport. A great deal of longitudinal research has not been conducted on this topic, but the existing evidence does not support a causal explanation. This is an important issue because personality structure has been proposed as one of the factors that may influence the onset of coronary heart disease (Morgan, 1979b); that is, the reported personality differences between athletes and nonathletes could influence health status and quality of life independently of exercise patterns.

Several studies carried out at the U.S. Military Academy bear directly on this topic. In the first study, Werner (1960) administered the 16 Personality Factor Inventory (16 PF) to entering cadets at West Point, and it was found that former high school athletes differed from nonathletes on 8 of the 16 factors at the time of admission. This observation is in agreement with the majority of the cross-sectional research described in the preceding paragraph. In a subsequent study, Werner and Gottheil (1966) administered the 16 PF to 340 entering freshmen who had participated in high school athletics. They differed significantly from the nonathletes on 7 of the 16 factors, including Factors A and H, which are thought to be governed largely by heredity. These students were also tested at the time of graduation and found to differ even though the former nonathletes had now participated in 4 years of required athletics at the U.S. Military Academy.

It might be argued that sport actually was responsible for the differences between athletes and nonathletes in the West Point studies, but the effects were realized in high school prior to admission at the Academy. This argument is indirectly challenged by the work of Schendel (1970) who administered the California Psychological Inventory (CPI) to 50 male athletes and 41 male nonathletes in grade 9 and again in grade 12. The cross-sectional phase of this study revealed that the athletes and nonathletes differed on 9 of the 18 CPI scales from the outset. A comparison of the two groups 3 years following the initial testing indicated they differed on 4 of the 18 CPI scales at the later date. The athletes, however, remained rather stable across time, whereas the nonathletes tended to change appreciably.

A similar study has been reported by Lukehart and Morgan (1969) who evaluated 12-year-old boys prior to their involvement in organized sport. The Junior Eysenck Personality Inventory was administered to the boys at the beginning of the seventh grade. Approximately one-half of the boys subsequently elected to participate in competitive football on an interscholastic basis, while the remainder elected not to become so involved. There were no opportunities for other forms of age group athletics in the rural setting where these boys lived; and, therefore, it was not possible for the nonathletes to become involved in organized athletics outside the school setting. Those boys who elected to join the team were significantly more extroverted than those who did not, and this difference existed from the outset. These young football players did not experience a change in extroversion following this initial season of competitive athletics, and the nonathletes did not change either. In other words, psychological differences existed from the outset, and this observation supports the view that individuals with particular psychological characteristics gravitate toward sports.

Research involving still younger boys supports the above view. Seymour (1956), for example, conducted a study of 10- to 12-year-old boys prior to and following a season of Little League baseball. These boys were compared to boys who did not take part in the activity, and it was found that:

> The boys who took part in Little League had somewhat more desirable traits before the baseball season than nonparticipants and they retained these traits during and after participation. More important for our consideration here, little changes in personality traits and social acceptance were noted in each group. (p. 97)

There is also limited cross-cultural support for the findings reviewed in this section. Yanada and Hirata (1970), for example, administered the Tokyo Personality Inventory (TPI) to students who participated in sport clubs at the University of Tokyo. Those who dropped out of their sport clubs were found to be significantly more neurotic, depressive, and manic from the outset than those who continued.

It should also be noted that athletes in sports such as distance running, wrestling, and rowing who continue to participate beyond college are consistently found to differ from the general population (Morgan & Pollock, 1977). The differences, however, are primarily noted for psychological states rather than enduring personality traits. These athletes have been found to score significantly lower on affective measures such as tension, depression, fatigue, and confusion and higher on psychic vigor. This stereotyped pattern has been dubbed the "iceberg" profile, and all the differences favor the athlete samples from the standpoint of positive mental health. The Profile of Mood State (POMS) has been used to measure mood in this research (McNair, Lorr, & Droppleman, 1971).

The available research, both longitudinal and cross-sectional, suggests that athletes and nonathletes differ significantly on selected psychological states and traits, and these differences have consistently been observed to favor athletes in terms of positive mental health (W.P. Morgan, 1980). Furthermore, these differences appear to exist from the outset rather than being changed by involvement in sport. It is also known that numerous physiological differences exist between athletes and nonathletes from the outset as well. Maximal aerobic power, for example, a crucial prerequisite for success in many sports, has been reported to be about 86% generic (Klissouras, 1970). Other largely hereditary variables such as height, somatotype, and muscle fiber type are all recognized determinants of success in certain sports. These observations pose methodological problems that must be considered by investigators concerned with the psychologic impact of sport in health maintenance and disease prevention.

Indirect evidence supporting the view that college athletes possess a more favorable mental health profile comes from the work of Carmen, Zerman, and Blaine (1968) and Pierce (1969) who have reported that athletes use college psychiatric services less than nonathletes do. These investigators have proposed, however, that one possible explanation for lower usage of the psychiatric service by athletes stem from the abundant source of informal counseling opportunities available to them. An athlete with minor problems, for example, might seek assistance from the coach, team physician, trainer, or teammates, and only resort to the psychiatric service when these outlets have been exhausted. On the other hand, Paffenbarger & Asnes (1966) reported that significantly fewer ($p<.01$) former athletes at Harvard committed suicide than did nonathletes. Ten percent of the controls and 4% of the former athletes were suicides. This led Paffenbarger & Asnes (1966) to propose that participation in college athletics may have an influence on emotional stability. These same investigators have reported that the incidence of self-reported anxiety and depression was significantly higher ($p<.01$) in University of Pennsylvania's male students who later became suicides (30%) in contrast to randomly selected controls (10%).

While 16% of the subsequent suicides, in comparison with 11% of the controls, reported that they were not in good health at the time of college casetaking, they did not differ in the number of clinical visits and hospitalizations during college. Nor did the two groups differ in their usage of the guidance or psychiatric services at Harvard. In other words, college students who subsequently became suicides reported more health problems and anxiety-depression than controls, but they did not seek or receive more or less assistance at the health, psychological, or psychiatric services (Paffenbarger & Asnes, 1966). These observations seem to challenge the view advanced by Carmen et al. (1968).

It has also been emphasized by Carmen et al. (1968), however, that athletes who require therapy are consistently found to have *less* favorable prognoses. One possible explanation for this finding is that athletes only turn to the psychiatric service for help when their problems become quite severe. Another consideration is Pierce's (1969) proposal that athletes are simply less verbal and typically have a difficult time "playing the role of patient" while undergoing therapy. These general observations have also been supported by Little (1969). Most of the athletes studied by Little were hospitalized for psychiatric treatment in connection with some form of threat to physical self. This research also suggests that athletes possess better mental health than nonathletes, but the prognosis for athletes is much less favorable when therapy is required.

The position assumed by Little (1969, 1979) has profound implications with respect to psychological comparisons of athletes and nonathletes, and this would be particularly the case in prospective studies. While athletes are consistently observed to possess better psychological adjustment scores than nonathletes, it appears that athletes are susceptible to neurotic illness following physical injury. In other words, the "fitness fanatic" seems to experience a deprivation crisis when injured and unable to continue regular exercise. This phenomenon has been described as "negative addiction" in runners. At any rate, the psychological advantage enjoyed by young athletes may only persist in older age where continued exercise is possible. This possibility would best be evaluated in a prospective study involving athletes and nonathletes who were tested psychologically in the early years and then reexamined in the middle and later years. Three exploratory studies involving a comparison of athletes and nonathletes will be reviewed next.

Exploratory Study I

Most of the epidemiological research involving comparisons of athletes and nonathletes has been restricted to college graduates, and comparisons are usually not carried out on the subjects after 30 years of age or older. In the first exploratory study to be discussed, former high school athletes ($n=83$) and nonathletes ($n=70$) were compared at 24 and 25 years of age, respectively (Morgan, Vogel, & Patton, 1975). The groups were formed on the basis of the number of varsity letters earned in high school. The mean number of letters earned by the athlete group was 3.34, and none of the subjects classified as nonathletes reported the earning of a varsity letter while in high school. A summary of the questionnaire data appears in Table 1.

Attitude toward physical activity and estimation of physical ability were assessed with the Physical Estimation and Attraction Scale (PEAS) developed by Sonstroem (1974) and modified by Morgan et al. (1975) for use with adults. Frequency and duration of exercise were measured with forced choice items, and exercise intensity was assessed with Borg's perceived exertion scale (Borg, 1973). Former athletes possessed a significantly higher score on both attitude toward physical activity and estimation of physical ability. It is of interest, however, that various emotional states such as anxiety and depression were not associated with self-reports of exercise behavior. This finding held for frequency, duration, and intensity of exercise. In other words, the former athletes possessed more favorable attitudes (affect) toward physical activity, but their actual exercise behavior did not differ from that of the nonathletes. It is not uncommon in such research to observe a discrepancy between the effective and behavioral components of attitude. While the validity of self-report data is often questioned, Breslow (1972) has pointed out that, "...it appears possi-

Table 1. Attitude toward physical activity, estimation of physical ability, and exercise behavior in former high school athletes ($n = 83$) and nonathletes (n = 70)

Variable	Athletes		Nonathletes		
	M	SD	M	SD	p
Age	25.12	5.43	26.04	5.51	NS
Physical Activity Attitude	35.68	8.73	27.75	10.71	<.001
Estimation of Physical Ability	21.98	7.02	17.12	6.78	<.001
Exercise (days/weeks)	3.41	2.36	3.39	2.36	NS
Exercise (minutes/days)	27.97	21.27	24.71	18.86	NS
Exercise (intensity)	10.07	5.73	9.38	5.76	NS

ble to measure health status through questions that only individuals can answer about themselves." (p. 347)

The physiological data collected in this study are presented in Table 2, and these data can be used as an indirect validity check for the self-reports of exercise behavior. In other words, because the exercise behavior of the two groups did not differ, it would be predicted that body weight, percent body fat, and maximal aerobic power would not differ either. The former athletes were found to have an aerobic power of 48.1 ml/kg•min that was identical to that of the former nonathletes, and this observation can be interpreted to mean that the two groups probably did not differ in their actual levels of physical activity. This finding is also in agreement with the percent body fat of 18.5 and 18.0 for the former athletes and nonathletes, respectively. The similarity of body composition, aerobic power, and self-reports of exercise behavior suggests that these former high school athletes and nonathletes were quite similar on these variables when measured at 25 years of age. Extensive literature demonstrating that athletes in training differ from nonathletes exists (Åstrand & Rodahl, 1977).

It is important to recognize that not only did former athletes possess a higher score on attitude toward physical activity, but they also estimated their physical ability to be superior ($p<.001$) to that of other men their age. It is conceivable that former athletes, when asked to rate their physical abilities, base their judgments on perception of self at an earlier point in time; that is, their reference points may not involve the here and now. Therefore, the validity of certain self-report data remains open to question. It should be noted, however, that subjects with high conformity or lie scores, as measured by the Eysenck Personality Inventory (Eysenck & Eysenck, 1962), were not included in these analyses. Therefore, response distortion should not have been a significant problem.

From the standpoint of mental health, previous investigations of junior high school, high school, and college athletes have all revealed psychological differences favoring the athletes. In the present study, a series of psychological inventories was also administered to the samples of former high school athletes and nonathletes. It will be recalled that the mean age of the two groups was

Table 2. Body composition and aerobic power of former high school athletes ($n = 83$) and nonathletes ($n = 70$)

Variable	Athletes M	Athletes SD	Nonathletes M	Nonathletes SD	p
Age	25.12	5.43	26.04	5.51	NS
Height (cm)	176.12	6.96	174.61	6.18	NS
Weight (kg)	76.51	12.69	73.08	11.81	NS
Body Fat (%)	18.48	5.92	18.02	5.44	NS
$\dot{V}O_2$max (1/min)	3.62	0.45	3.47	0.44	NS
$\dot{V}O_2$max (ml/kg•min)	48.08	6.88	48.08	6.57	NS

24 and 25 years, respectively, and therefore, they averaged about 6–7 years beyond graduation at the time of testing. The State-Trait Anxiety Inventory (Spielberger, Gorsuch, & Lushene, 1970) was employed to assess state and trait anxiety; the Profile of Mood States (McNair, Lorr, & Droppleman, 1971) yielded scores on tension, depression, anger, vigor, fatigue, and confusion; extroversion, neuroticism, and conformity were assessed with the Eysenck Personality Inventory (Eysenck & Eysenck, 1962); and field dependence was measured with the Embedded Figures Test (Scheier & Cattell, 1958). The results of this comparison are presented in Table 3.

The two groups were found to be remarkably similar on all the psychological variables. A stepwise discriminant function analysis (BMDO7M) was carried out on these data, and it was found that the best predictor of group affiliation was vigor. The athletes scored higher, but not significantly so, on this psychological mood state. It will be recalled that these same athletes scored significantly higher ($p < .001$) than did the nonathletes in their estimations of physical ability. A second stepwise discriminant function analysis was carried out, and it included estimation of physical ability and attitude toward physical activity as measured by the PEAS (Sonstroem, 1974), as well as the psychometric variables summarized in Table 4. The best predictors of group affiliation were found to be estimation of physical ability (PEAS), attitude toward physical activity (PEAS), and vigor (POMS). Estimation of physical ability accounted for most of the variance followed by attitude toward physical activity and vigor. It is rather intriguing that these former athletes possessed exercise attitudes and estimations of physical ability and psychological vigor which were not congruent with their actual physical abilities and exercise patterns. Evidence shows that estimation of physical ability, as measured by the PEAS (Sonstroem, 1974), is significantly correlated with various measures of self-esteem (Sonstroem, 1984). However, with the exception of the PEAS variables, this pilot study suggests that any differences, psychological or physiological, that may have existed between these former high school athletes and nonathletes were not present 6–7 years following graduation. This, of

Table 3. Psychological states and traits of former high school athletes ($n = 83$) and nonathletes ($n = 70$)

Variable	Athletes M	SD	Nonathletes M	SD	p
State Anxiety	39.41	10.99	40.53	10.71	NS
Trait Anxiety	39.00	9.98	39.01	8.73	NS
Tension	8.25	6.15	9.07	6.73	NS
Depression	10.60	10.68	10.63	11.37	NS
Anger	8.58	8.90	8.07	8.32	NS
Vigor	17.27	6.82	14.91	7.05	NS
Fatigue	4.79	5.20	6.40	6.70	NS
Confusion	5.65	4.91	5.94	5.04	NS
Extroversion	12.40	3.10	12.34	3.23	NS
Neuroticism	9.44	5.14	8.49	5.01	NS
Conformity	3.64	1.87	3.60	1.78	NS
Field Dependence	16.96	7.53	16.76	7.23	NS

course, should not be viewed as being at odds with earlier investigations involving samples of college athletes and nonathletes.

Summary

The results of this exploratory research (Morgan, et al., 1975) suggest that these former high school athletes and nonathletes had adopted similar exercise patterns by 25 years of age. This similarity in patterns was found to be consistent for frequency, duration, and intensity of exercise. Furthermore, the self-reported exercise patterns of the two groups were indirectly validated by means of body composition and maximal treadmill testing (Patton, Morgan & Vogel, 1977), and the two groups were found to be remarkably similar on measures of body composition and maximal aerobic power. It was also observed, however, that former athletes possessed a higher score on a measure of attitude toward physical activity than did the former nonathletes, and the athletes also rated themselves higher on estimation of physical ability (i.e., self-esteem).

Individuals who estimate their physical ability to be greater than it actually is, might be more likely to overexert themselves and experience a higher incidence of illness as a consequence. These former athletes appear to base their subjective judgments of physical ability on an earlier reference point. While the former athletes and nonathletes can both be viewed as nonathletes by the middle of the third decade of life, it appears that the former athletes still regard themselves as athletes. Investigations dealing with the health of former athletes and nonathletes must obviously consider factors other than athleticism during the early years (Paffenbarger et al., 1978).

Exploratory Study II

A second exploratory investigation, which is still underway, has involved a comparison of athletes and nonathletes at the university level. Details describing this pilot work appear in Morgan & Johnson (1977, 1978) and Johnson & Morgan (1981), and the major findings from this pilot work will be examined in the present section.

The Minnesota Multiphasic Personality Inventory (MMPI) was routinely administered to each entering class at the University of Wisconsin–Madison for a number of years. These data have been preserved in the University Counseling Service so that research studies might be conducted with the profiles. The MMPI profiles of all male athletes who earned numerals in a freshman sport during the period 1960–1965 were included as subjects. This resulted in a sam-

Table 4. Overall design of the study and summary of samples

MMPI and Athletic Evaluation	Follow-up Study	Athletes n	Nonathletes n
1960	1980	54	62
1961	1981	50	47
1962	1982	56	44

ple of 865 athletes. Invalid profiles were eliminated according to the criteria established by Dahlstrom, Welch, & Dahlstrom (1972–1975) and Pearson & Swenson (1967). The result was rejection of 22 profiles, and therefore, 85% (n=735) of the original group of 865 were included in the study. Ninety-five percent of all incoming students completed the MMPI during the period from 1960 to 1965. A random sample of 100 male nonathletes was selected from each of the five classes (n=500). A student was not included in the comparison sample if he had earned a freshman numeral in 1 of the 14 intercollegiate sports, or if his profile was found to be invalid according to the criteria referred to above.

A series of multivariate and univariate analyses of variance were performed. Comparisons of

1. athletes and nonathletes,
2. athletes in the 12 sport groups,
3. team athletes versus individual sport athletes, and
4. successful versus unsuccessful athletes were made (Johnson & W.P. Morgan, 1981).

However, the present discussion will be limited to a summary of the comparison between athletes and nonathletes.

The mean MMPI profiles for the athletes and nonathletes were found to differ significantly as measured by the Wilk's Lambda test ($F=2.80$, $p<.0004$). The nonathletes were found to score significantly higher than athletes on unusual feelings or behavior (F scale, cultural-aesthetic interests (Mf scale), social introversion (Si scale), and depression (D scale). The actual mean differences were quite small, and none of the differences exceeded one-quarter of a standard deviation unit. This, of course, raises the question of statistical versus practical or clinical significance. However, despite small mean differences, the MMPI scales proved to be effective in differentiating between athletes and nonathletes with extreme scores.

A T-score equal to 70 or greater is regarded as the upper limit in the normal range. Statistical analysis revealed that nonathletes scored above the T-score of 70 on the Mf and Si scales 2 to 3 times as often as athletes. In other words, the nonathletes possessed more cultural-aesthetic interests, and they were characterized by a higher frequency of social introversion. These findings indicate that the psychological characteristics of athletes were significantly different from those of nonathletes at the time of their entrance to the University of Wisconsin–Madison. The extent to which these initial differences persist across time and the influence of psychological adjustment and athleticism on health status and quality of life have been examined 20 years later in these same subjects. This pilot work will be examined in the next section (Morgan, Montoye, & Brown, 1983).

Exploratory Study III

Overview

The primary objectives of this longitudinal investigation were to compare former college athletes and nonathletes with special reference to perceived quality of life, current exercise patterns, and physical and mental health, and to determine the ability of personality measures obtained in the early years to predict health status, health behaviors, and quality of life in the middle years. The Minnesota Multiphasic Personality Inventory (MMPI) was completed by approximately 95% of all entering students at the University of Wisconsin–Madison during the years 1960–1964, and the results have been preserved by the University of Wisconsin Counseling Service for research purposes. The present study dealt with the entering classes of 1960, 1961, and 1962, and it was limited to those alumni who

1. completed the MMPI during the first week of school as freshmen,
2. subsequently graduated from the University of Wisconsin–Madison,
3. were locatable 20 years later in 1980, 1981, and 1982, and
4. signed informed consent statements indicating a willingness to take part in the study.

Procedure

Questionnaires were sent to all former athletes, as well as random samples of nonathletes from each entering class. All participants in the study met each of the criteria for inclusion cited above, and a summary of the overall design appears in Table 4. It was possible to locate current addresses for 56% of the potential participants. Approximately 88% of these individuals volunteered to be in the study, and they completed the questionnaires described in the next section. The remaining 12% either declined to volunteer, or they elected to not return the questionnaires. The questionnaire packet consisted of the following 5 parts:

1. *Personal Data Questionnaire (PDQ).* The PDQ was designed to measure factors such as age, estimated height and weight, present occupation, marital status, sleep patterns, alcohol and tobacco usage, use of prescription medication, and frequency and nature of hospitalizations over the past 20 years. The rationale for measuring these variables was that each one is directly or indirectly associated with health status and quality of life.
2. *Needs Questionnaire.* This questionnaire was adapted from the research of Flanagan (1978) and was designed to measure the variable known as "quality of life." Related research has focused almost entirely on the issues of disease and length of life, but more and more health professionals are coming to realize that the "quality" of years lived is equally, if not more, important.
3. *Physical Activity Questionnaire (PAQ).* The PAQ was developed with an aim toward quantifying exercise patterns. There is evidence that regular exercise of a vigorous nature has both mental and physical benefits.
4. *Profile of Mood State (POMS).* The POMS yields measures of tension, depression, anger, vigor, fatigue, and confusion, as well as a global measure of mood based upon a combination of these six states. This scale provided a measure of current mood.
5. *Minnesota Multiphasic Personality Inventory (MMPI).* All participants in the present research had completed the MMPI 20 years earlier during orientation week at the University of Wisconsin–Madison. This information was employed in evaluating the extent to which pesonality structure in the early years (e.g., 18 years was effective in predicting mood state and quality of life in the middle years (e.g., 38 years).

Results

A series of statistical analyses was carried out in this study, but the present discussion will be limited to the results of the stepwise discriminant function analyses. This analysis permits evaluation of the extent to which a given set of variables are effective in classifying individuals into recognized criterion groups (e.g., athletes and nonathletes). The overall results are presented in Tables 5 and 6.

The accuracy of classifying former athletes and nonathletes on the basis of currently available data ranged from 67% to 78%, and the average accuracy across the three samples was 72%. This suggests the possibility that athleticism in the early years may influence behavior in the middle years. Another possibility is that such differences always existed, and involvement in sport is not a mediating variable. Partial support for this alternative view is that body size was significantly different in the athletes and nonathletes at follow-up, as well as 20 years earlier as determined by self-report recall. Also, while the former athletes tended to be comparable to the former nonathletes in their exercise patterns, they judged themselves to be superior in physical ability. The two groups did not differ in

1. health status,
2. health behavior (e.g., exercise, smoking, alcohol, and drug habits),
3. quality of life, or
4. job status.

This suggests that former athletes and nonathletes are more alike than unalike in the middle years. For this reason, it was decided that a comparison of currently active and sedentary alumni, irrespective of earlier athletic histories, would be appropriate. This analysis revealed that active individuals possessed more desirable mood scores than did the sedentary subjects, but the two groups did not differ on health status or quality of life. Since health status was inferred on the basis of prescription medication and hospitalization records, this finding should be viewed as tentative until testing under controlled, laboratory conditions is carried out. It was possible, however, to accurately classify 87% of the active and sedentary alumni, and the predictions for the three years ranged from 86% to 91%. This finding suggests that activity patterns during the middle years are more important than athletic patterns in the early years.

Table 5. Use of current biological and behavioral characteristics in discriminating between groups differing in athletic patterns at 18 years of age and exercise patterns at 38 years of age

| Comparison Groups | Cases correctly classified in follow-up studies | | | |
	1960–80	1961–81	1962–82	Mean
Former Athletic Patterns (Athlete vs. nonathlete)	78%	67%	72%	72%
Current Exercise Patterns (Active vs. sedentary)	88%	86%	91%	87%

Another important consideration in this study was the question of whether or not personality structure in the early years could be effective in predicting mood state, quality of life, and exercise patterns in the middle years. A series of stepwise discriminant function analyses was carried out in order to answer this question, and the results are presented in Table 6. It was found that MMPI data collected at 18 years of age was effective in predicting mood states at 38 years of age. The classification accuracy averaged 76%, and predictions ranged from 69% to 85%. Quality of life (high vs. low) was predicted with 73% accuracy, and the predictions ranged from 68% to 79%. This can be interpreted to mean that the extent to which perceived needs are being met at 38 years of age is associated with personality structure at 18 years of age. The accuracy of these predictions ranged from 75% to 83%, and the average accuracy was 78% across the three years. Since the MMPI is regarded as being made up largely of psychological traits that are thought to be stable across time, this finding implies that the decision to be active or inactive in the middle years is associated with personality structure in the early years.

Discussion and Conclusions

The following conclusions are presented on the basis of findings from the initial 20-year longitudinal study carried out in 1980 and the replications performed in 1981 and 1982:

1. Significant differences exist between former athletes and nonathletes when evaluated in the middle years (Mean=38 years), but the observed differences tend to be of the type one would predict to exist during the early years as well. Former athletes, for example, are heavier, taller, and judge themselves to be more physically fit in comparison with individuals who did not participate in organized sports while attending the University of Wisconsin–Madison. It is of considerable interest, however, that former athletes tend to be no more active in the middle years than are former nonathletes. There is also a consistent trend for former athletes and nonathletes to be similar on measures of health status, quality of life, mood state, job status, tobacco usage, and alcohol consumption. There was a trend for former athletes to rate themselves as feeling more refreshed in the morn-

Table 6. Use of MMPI data collected in the early years to predict quality of life (perceived needs), mood state, and exercise patterns in the middle years

| Comparison Groups | Cases correctly classified in follow-up studies | | | |
	1960–80	1961–81	1962–82	Mean
Mood States (POMS) (Normal vs. elevated)	75%	85%	69%	76%
Quality of Life (Needs) (High vs. low)	71%	79%	68%	73%
Exercise Patterns (Active vs. sedentary)	75%	77%	83%	78%

ing or sleeping longer than did former nonathletes, and this needs to be explored since sleep patterns are known to be associated with health status in later years. With the exception of these differences, which probably existed in the early years at mean age 18, *it is concluded that the former athletes and nonathletes in this investigation were more alike than unlike in the middle years at mean age 38.*

2. Personality structure, as measured by the Minnesota Multiphasic Personality Inventory (MMPI) during the early years (Mean=18 years), was found to be correlated with mood state, quality of life, and exercise patterns in the middle years (Mean=38 years). It was possible to classify individuals differing in mood state, life quality, and exercise patterns with 76%, 73%, and 78% accuracy. *It is concluded that personality structure in the early years is associated with mood state and quality of life, as well as the decision to be physically active or sedentary in the middle years.*

3. It was found that individuals differing in physical activity patterns in the middle years differed on a number of variables judged to be of importance. The first study carried out in 1980 revealed that active individuals scored higher than did sedentary individuals on a measure of perceived physical ability, and this finding was replicated in the 1981 and 1982 replications. As a matter of fact, this was the first variable to enter the stepwise discriminant functions in all three studies, and this variable is usually regarded as a measure of self-esteem. Active and sedentary groups were also found to differ on sleep patterns, mood state, job status (Duncan index), quality of life (needs), and weight gain over the previous 20 years. The active individuals were characterized by preferred scores on each of these variables. *It was concluded that many of the biological and behavioral measures thought to be influenced in the middle years by personality structure in the early years are subject to modification through physically active life styles.*

Physical Activity Research

The preceding discussion has focused on the interaction of sport and psychological health. The value of nonathletic, physical activity in disease prevention and health maintenance, however, may possess far greater potential. It is important to understand the role of athleticism in this process, however, because it is quite probable that involvement in *sport* during the first 2 to 3 decades of life influences later involvement in *physical activity*, at least to some degree. The importance of studying the interaction of early athletic patterns with exercise behavior during the aging process is reinforced by the reports of Montoye et al. (1957), Morgan et al. (1983), and Paffenbarger et al. (1978).

Two contemporary health problems, anxiety and depression, appear to respond quite well to programs of vigorous physical activity. It has been reported that 10 million Americans suffer from anxiety neurosis at the present and that as many as 30% of all patients seen by general practitioners are anxiety neurotics. It also has been estimated that between 30 to 70% of all patients examined by general practitioners and internists are suffering from conditions that have their origins in unrelieved stress. Vigorous physical activity of an acute nature has been observed to consistently result in a decrease in tension or state anxiety (Morgan, 1979a) and this decrease in anxiety is comparable to that observed for other therapies such as pharmacologic therapy (deVries & Adams, 1972), systematic desensitization (Driscoll, 1976), and noncultic meditation (Bahrke & Morgan, 1978).

There is also strong evidence to support the view that vigorous physical activity of a chronic nature is capable of reducing depression in moderately depressed individuals (Morgan, Roberts, Band, & Feinerman, 1970). Furthermore, it has been reported that physical working capacity, as measured on a bicycle ergometer test, is implicated in the pathogenesis of depression (Morgan, 1969). In this latter investigation, depressed psychiatric patients were observed to posses significantly lower levels of physical working capacity than nondepressed patients on the same psychiatric service. This finding is consistent with the observation that level of physical fitness at the time of admission to a psychiatric facility is negatively correlated with length of hospitalization (Morgan, 1970). This research has been largely of a correlational nature, and it has not addressed the more fundamental issue of causality. However, the recent research of Greist, Klein, Eischens, Faris, Gurman, and Morgan (1979) makes a strong case for the potential role of running therapy in the treatment of patients with minor depressions. Indeed, this study revealed that exercise was equal to time-limited psychotherapy in its ability to reduce depression. Furthermore, a 12-month follow-up revealed that members of the running group were still free of depression, whereas the time-unlimited psychotherapy group had experienced a far more uneven recovery period. Recent reviews by Folkins and Sime (1981) and Morgan (1981, 1983) present summaries of the extant literature involving the psychological benefits of physical activity. These reviews demonstrate that individuals who exercise regularly are *characterized* by more desirable mental health profiles than nonexercisers, but there is essentially no evidence that exercise *causes* such differences.

Summary

The present review indicates that athletes have consistently been observed to possess more desirable psychological profiles than their nonathletic classmates. This particular finding has been reported by various investigators who have often relied on different psychological models, and have included diverse samples ranging from Little League athletes (10- to 12-year olds) to elite or world-class performers. A reasonable conclusion seems to be that individuals with certain personality characteristics gravitate toward sport, rather than involvement in sport modifying personality. There is substantial cross-sectional data to support such a conclusion, and the limited longitudinal research is in agreement with this view.

The debate as to whether or not athletes live longer than nonathletes continues, but the existing evidence suggests that involvement in athletics, at the college level, does not enhance longevity. There is evidence, however, that former high school athletes and nonathletes have adopted similar exercise patterns by 25 years of age, and there is some evidence that former college athletes may become less active than individuals who were nonathletes in college as the two groups become older. Former athletes, however, seem to evaluate their physical ability as being superior to that of former nonathletes even though the two groups have been found to possess comparable exercise habits and levels of physical fitness by age 25. Most of the longitudinal studies conducted to date on the issue of involvement in athletics and psychological change have been limited to periods of 1 to 4 years. These studies have shown that athletes possess more desirable psychological profiles from the outset, and very little change has been noted across time.

Evidence suggests that college athletes who do not continue to be physically active following graduation are just as likely to develop heart disease as former nonathletes are. As a matter of fact, former nonathletes who become active following graduation from college have been reported to have less likelihood of developing heart disease than former athletes who adopt sedentary lifestyles. While it is hazardous to generalize to the psychological domain from such evidence, it would seem reasonable to propose that groups of former athletes and nonathletes who possess comparable exercise patterns would not differ in their psychological structrures. This is precisely what was found in the first pilot study described in this review. Some evidence also suggests that former athletes who are no longer able to be physically active are more likely to develop psychological problems than are sedentary former nonathletes.

Recent research has demonstrated that vigorous physical activity is comparable to pharmacologic therapy, systematic desensitization, and mediation in its ability to reduce anxiety. Also, aerobic exercise of a chronic nature has been found to be effective in the treatment of minor depression, and physical exercise of this type is associated with an increase in self-esteem. These changes covary with alterations in body composition, physical work capacity, and effort sense. All these changes theoretically enhance quality of life. While regular exercise may not alter longevity, evidence suggests that quality of years lived can be enhanced through the adoption of a physically active lifestyle. It is not clear, however, why some individuals elect to be active and others choose a sedentary life style.

In view of the psychological and physiological correlates of physical activity and the potential role of exercise in the prevention of disease and maintenance of health, it is important that basic information becomes available on the nature of athleticism and exercise adherence in the aging and aged. While there appears to be widespread agreement within the exercise sciences that regular physical activity increases the *quality* of years lived (Milvy, 1977), there is an absence of objective evidence in support of this view. Also, it is not clear why some individuals prefer sedentary to active lifestyles, why some individuals elect to become physically active, and why some individuals adhere to vigorous exercise programs once they are adopted whereas others discontinue. Also, most of the research involving adherence to physical activity has been of relatively short duration (seldom for longer than a year), retrospective in nature, seriously limited by attenuation due to volunteerism effects, and typically physiological in nature with little or no attention paid to psychological variables. A need exists for

1. a prospective study lasting for 20-years or more,
2. an investigation not limited from the outset to a group of volunteers who may bias the initial sample,
3. a study focusing on the psychological characteristics of those individuals who adopt active versus sedentary lifestyles, and
4. research directed toward an understanding of the role played by athleticism in early life on exercise involvement in later life.

An investigation of this type is currently underway, and it was summarized earlier (Morgan, et a., 1983).

The interaction of various antecedent and consequent variables should be examined in future research involving physical activity and aging. It is unlikely that continued utilization of cross-sectional research designs will advance our knowledge in this area of inquiry, and it is imperative that longitudinal designs be employed in the study of exercise, personality, and the aging process.

References

Åstrand, P.O., & Rodahl, K. (1977). *Textbook of work physiology* (2nd ed.), New York: McGraw Hill.

Bahrke, M.S., & Morgan, W.P. (1978). Anxiety reduction following exercise and meditation. *Cognitive therapy and research, 2,* 322-333.

Borg, G.A.V. (1973). Perceived exertion: A note on "history" and methods. *Medicine and Science in Sports, 5,* 90-93.

Breslow, L. (1972). A quantitative approach to the World Health Organization definition of health: Physical, mental and social well-being. *International Journal of Epidemiology, 1,* 347-355.

Carmen, L.R., Zerman, J.l., & Blaine, G.B., Jr. (1968). Use of the Harvard psychiatric service by athletes and nonathletes. *Mental Hygiene, 52,* 134-137.

Cooper, E.L., O'Sullivan, J., & Hughes, E. (1937). Athletics and the heart: An electrocardiographic and radiological study of the response of healthy and diseased heart to exercise. *Medical Journal of Australia, 1,* 569-579.

Dahlstrom, W.G., Welsh, G.W., & Dahlstrom, L.E. (1972-1975). *An MMPI handbook* (2 vols.). Minneapolis: University of Minneapolis Press.

deVries, H.A., & Adams, G.M. (1972). Electromyographic comparison of single doses of exercise and meprobamate as to effect on muscular relaxation. *American Journal of Physical Medicine, 51,* 130-141.

Driscoll, R. (1976). Anxiety reduction using physical exertion and positive images. *Psychological Record, 26,* 87-94.

Dublin, L.I. (1928). Longevity of college athletes. *Harper's Magazine, 157,* 229-238.

Eysenck, H.J., & Eysenck, S.B.G. (1962). *Manual for the Eysenck Personality Inventory.* San Diego, CA: Educational & Industrial Testing Service.

Flanagan, J.C. (1978). A research approach to improving our qauality of life. *American Psychologist, 33,* 138-147.

Folkins, C.H. & Sime, W.E. (1981). Physical fitness training and mental health. *American Psychologist, 36,* 373-389.

Greist, J.H., Klein, M.H., Eischens, R.R., Faris, J., Gurman, A.S., & Morgan, W.P. (1979). Running as treatment for depression. *Comprehensive Psychiatry*, **13**, 238-297.

Hartley, P.H.S., & Llewellyn, G.F. (1939). Longevity of oarsmen: Study of those who rowed in Oxford and Cambridge boat races from 1829-1928. *British Medical Journal*, **1**, 657-662.

Hill, A.B., (1927). Cricket and its relation to the duration of life. *Lancet*, **2**, 949-950.

Johnson, R.W., & Morgan, W.P. (1981). Personality characteristics of college athletes in different sports. *Scandianvian Journal of Sports Science*, **3**, 41-49.

Klissouras, V. (1970). Heretability of adaptive variation. *Journal of Applied Physiology*, **29**, 358-367.

Little, J.C. (1969). The athlete's neurosis—A deprivation crisis. *Acta Psychiatricia Scandinavica*, **45**, 187-197.

Little, J.C. (1979). Neurotic illness in fitness fanatics. *Psychiatric Annals*, **9**, 49-56.

Lukehart, R.E., & Morgan, W.P. (1969). Effect of a season of interscholastic football on the personality of junior high school males. In F.Z. Cumbee (Ed.), *Abstracts of Research*, Washington, D.C.; American Association for Health, Physical Education, and Recreation.

McNair, D.M., Lorr, M., & Droppleman, L.F. (1971). *Profile of Mood States Manual*. San Diego, CA: Educational & Industrial Testing Service.

Meylan, G.L. (1904). Harvard University oarsmen. *Harvard Graduate Magazine*, **12**, 363-376.

Milvy, P. (Ed.). (1977). *The Marathon: Physiological, Medical, Epidemiological and Psychological Studies*. (Vol. 301). New york: New york Academy of Sciences.

Montoye, H.J., Van Huss, W.D., Olson, H.W., Pierson, W.R., & Hudec, A.J. (1957). *The Longevity and Morbidity of College Athletes*. Indianapolis:: Phi Epsilon Kappa Fraternity.

Morgan, J. (1893). *University Oars*. London: MacMillan.

Morgan, W.P. (1969). A pilot investigation of physical working capacity in depressed and nondepressed psychiatric males. *Research Quarterly*, **40**, 859-861.

Morgan, W.P. (1970). Physical fitness correlates of psychiatric hospitalization. In G.S. Kenyon (Ed.), *Contemporary Psychology of Sport*.

Morgan, W.P. (1977a). Anxiety reduction following acute physical activity. *Psychiatric Annals*, **9**, 36-45.

Morgan, W.P. (1977b). Psychological consequences of vigorous physical activity and sport. In M.G. Scott (Ed.), *Academy Papers*. Iowa City: American Academy of Physical Education.

Morgan, W.P. (1979a). Negative addiction in runners. *Physician and Sportsmedicine*, **7**, 57-70.

Morgan, W.P. (1979b). Psychological aspects of heart disease. In M.L. Pollock (Ed.), *Symposium on Heart Disease and Rehabilitation: State of the Art*. New York: Macmillan.

Morgan, W.P. (1980). The trait psychology controversy. *Research Quarterly for Exercise and Sport*, **51**, 50-76.

Morgan. W.P. (1981). Psychological benefits of physical activity. In F.J. Nagle & H.J. Montoye (Eds.), *Exercise, Health and Disease*. Springfield, IL: Charles C. Thomas.

Morgan, W.P. (1982). Psychological effects of exercise. *Behavioral Medicine Update*, **4**, 25-30.

Morgan, W.P. (1984). Physical activity and mental health. In H.M. Eckert & H.J. Montoye (Eds.), *Exercise and health*. Champaign, IL: Human Kinetics.

Morgan, W.P., Montoye, H.J., & Brown, D.R. (1983, August). *Quality of life and health status of aging athletes and nonathletes: A twenty-year longitudinal study*. Paper presented at the annual convention of the American Psychological Association, Anaheim, CA.

Morgan, W.P., Vogel., J.A. & Patton, J.F. (1975). *Psychological aspects of physical activity.* Unpublished Annual Report, U.S. Army Research Institute of Environmental Medicine, Natick, MA.

Morgan, W.P. & Johnson, R.W. (1977). Psychological characterization of the elite wrestler: A mental health model. *Medicine and Science in Sports,* **9**, 55–56.

Morgan, W.P., & Johnson, R.W. (1978). Personality characteristics of successful and unsuccessful oarsmen. *International Journal of Sport Psychology,* **9**, 119–133.

Morgan, W.P., & Pollock, M.L. (1977). Psychologic characterization of the elite distance runner. In P. Milvy (Ed.), *Annals of New York Academy of Science.* New York: New York Academy of Science.

Morgan, W.P., & Pollock, M.L. (1978). Physical activity and cardiovascular health: Psychological aspects. In F. Landry & Wordan (Eds.), *Physical Activity and Human Well-Being,* (pp. 163–181). Miami, Fl: Symposia Specialists.

Morgan, W.P., Roberts, J.A., Brand, F.R., & Feinerman, A.D. (1970). Psychological effects of chronic physical activity. *Medicine and Science in Sports,* **2**, 213-217.

Olson, H.W., Montoye, H.J., Sprague, H., Stephens, K., & Van Huss, W.D. (1978), The longevity and morbidity of college athletes. *Physician and Sportsmedicine,* **6**, 62–65.

Paffenbarger, R.S., Jr., & Asnes, D.P. (1966). Chronic disease in former college students: III. Precursors of suicide in early and middle life. *American Journal of Public Health,* **56**, 1026–1036.

Paffenbarger, R.S., Jr., Wing, A.L., & Hyde, R.T. (1978). Physical activity as an index of heart attack risk in college alumni. *American Journal of Epidemiology,* **108**, 161–175.

Patton, J.F., Morgan, W.P., & Vogel, J.A. (1977). Perceived exertion of absolute work during a military physical training program. *European Journal of Applied Physiology,* **36** 107-114.

Pearson, J.S., & Swenson, W.M. (1967). *A user's guide to the Mayo Clinic Automated MMPI Program.* New York: Psychological Corporation.

Pierce, R.A. (1969). Athletes in psychotherapy: How many, how come? *Journal of American College Health Association,* **17**, 244–249.

Polednak, A.P., & Damon, A. (1970). College athletics, longevity and cause of death. *Human Biology,* **42**, 28–46.

Rook, A. (1954). An investigation into the longevity of Cambridge sportsmen. *British Medical Journal,* **1**, 773–777.

Scheier, I.H., & Cattell, R.B. (1958). *Embedded Figures Test.* Champaign, IL: Institute for Personality and Ability Testing.

Schendel, J.S. (1970). The psychological characteristics of high school athletes and nonparticipants in athletics: A three year longitudinal study. In G.S. Kenyon (Ed.), *Contemporary Psychology of Sport.* Chicago, IL:

Seymour, E.W. (1956). Comparative study of certain behavior characteristics of participant and nonparticipant boys in Little League baseball. *Research Quarterly,* **27**, 338-346.

Sonstroem, R.J. (1974). Attitude testing examining certain psychological correlates of physical activity. *Research Quarterly,* **45**, 93–103.

Sonstroem, R.J. Exercise and self-esteem (1984). In R.L. Terjung (Ed.), *Exercise and sport sciences reviews* (Vol. 12). Lexington, MA: Collamore Press.

Spielberger, C.D., Gorsuch, R.L., & Lushene, R.E. (1970). *The State-Trait Anxiety Inventory Manual.* Palo Alto, CA: Consulting Psychologists Press.

Werner, A.C. (1960). Physical education and the development of leadership characteristics of cadets at the United States Military Academy. Unpublished doctoral dissertation, Springfield College.

Werner, A.C. & Gottheil, E. (1966). Personality development and participation in college athletics. *Research Quarterly,* **37**, 126–131.

Yanada, H., & Hirata, H. (1970). Personality traits of students who dropped out of their athletic clubs. *Proceedings of the College of Physical Education*, University of Tokyo.

18

The (In)Stability of Attitudes Toward Physical Activity During Childhood and Adolescence

Robert W. Schutz
UNIVERSITY OF BRITISH COLUMBIA
VANCOUVER, BRITISH COLUMBIA, CANADA

Frank L. Smoll
UNIVERSITY OF WASHINGTON
SEATTLE, WASHINGTON, USA

The construction of Kenyon's (1968b, 1968c) inventory to assess attitudes toward physical activity (ATPA) is regarded as a major advance in the area of sport psychology (Martens, 1975). The inventory is based on a conceptual model characterizing physical activity as a multidimensional phenomenon (Kenyon, 1968a). Since its introduction in the literature, Kenyon's inventory has been used with adults and high school students in innumerable studies concerning the status and change of ATPA. Recognizing the salience of middle childhood in the formation of basic attitudes (Ausubel & Sullivan, 1970; Medinnus & Johnson, 1976), Simon and Smoll (1974) developed a children's version of Kenyon's (1968b) semantic differential instrument for use with elementary school students. The equivalence of these two inventories was confirmed by Schutz and Smoll (1977). The availability of an instrument for assessing children's ATPA subsequently stimulated a moderate amount of attitude research with this age group (e.g., Carre, Mosher, & Schutz, 1980; Eastgate, 1975; Meyers, Pendergast, & DeBacy, 1978).

Appreciation is extended to Julie Zylstra for assistance in data collection and to the students of King's Senior High School, Seattle, Washington, for their cooperation throughout the study.

With respect to formulations of the attitude concept, the notion of an *enduring* behavioral disposition is a common element in the multitude of definitions available (e.g., Kenyon, 1968b; Krech, Crutchfield, & Bellachey, 1962; Leventhal, 1974; Rokeach, 1968). Consequently, ATPA is assumed to be a relatively stable attribute. Interest in the nature and characteristics of ATPA prompted us to test this assumption for children's physical activity attitudes (Smoll & Schutz, 1980). Analysis of multiple longitudinal data indicated stability of *group* attitude scores across Grades 4 to 6. However, between grades correlation analyses and factor analyses revealed a lack of stability of ATPA within *individuals* over time. In light of the absence of stable grade-to-grade attitude relationships, it is not surprising that earlier research (Smoll, Schutz, & Keeney, 1976) failed to detect a consistent across grades pattern in the relationship between children's ATPA and their involvement in physical activities.

The findings of these two studies gave rise to two conclusions; namely, physical activity attitudes are not stable for young children, and attitude-behavior (i.e., involvement) relationships are moderate (at best) with this age group. Furthermore, we have shown that, for a sample of young athletes, responses to the ATPA inventory are not related to the sport and/or activities that they perceive as being most representative of specific subdomains but rather are differentiated on the basis of sport involvement (Schutz, Smoll, & Wood, 1981a). These heuristic results gave rise to a number of speculative hypotheses:

1. The lack of consistency in ATPA over time is a developmental phenomenon, and one can expect such attitudes to stabilize with age, *ceteris paribus*.
2. The instability in ATPA is a function of changes in the nature and the degree of involvement in physical activity.
3. The absence of strong attitude-behavior relationships can be attributed to instability in ATPA and/or involvement in physical activity.

The present study was undertaken to examine these hypotheses (but does not purport to provide a direct test). This entailed a longitudinal analysis of physical activity attitudes and involvement of high school students, with a comparative interpretation of these findings to those of the earlier studies.

Method

Subjects

Data were obtained for two groups of students attending a private high school in Seattle, Washington (hereafter referred to as Classes A and B for convenience). Class A consisted of 37 males and 38 females who were in Grade 10 when the study was initiated. Attrition due to change in residence during the first or second year of the study resulted in 61 subjects (33 males, 28 females) with complete data. Of the 77 students in Class B, 71 (28 males, 43 females) participated over the 2-year course of the study. Thus 87% of combined Classes A and B comprised the final sample of 132 subjects.

For Class A, means and standard deviations of chronological age for the males and females at Grade 10 were 198.1 (±3.8) and 196.8 (±4.6) months, respectively. Those for the males and females of Class B were 198.4 ($\pm$3.7) and 195.5 ($\pm$4.2), respectively. Both classes participated in the same physical education programs taught by the same instructor. Written informed consent was obtained from the students and their parents for participation in the study.

Measures of Physical Activity Attitudes and Involvement

ATPA Inventory

Through a series of studies, Simon and Smoll's (1974) inventory was restructured, resulting in a revised instrument, which is both shorter and psychometrically superior to the original (Schutz, et al., 1981b). The ATPA inventory provides a measure of attitudinal dispositions toward seven physical activity subdomains. More specifically, the inventory assesses the perceived instrumental value held for physical activity as a social experience (i.e., for social growth and social continuation), as health and fitness, as a pursuit of vertigo, as an aesthetic experience, as catharsis, and as an ascetic experience. Attitudes for each dimension are quantified through use of a 5-point semantic differential scale for each of five bipolar adjectives *(good-bad, of no use-useful, not pleasant-pleasant, nice-awful, happy-sad)*. For scoring purposes, "5" is always associated with the positive adjective and "1" with the negative adjective of the word pairs. The scores are added to yield a total score out of 25 for all subdomains except Health and Fitness. This subdomain is scored as Health and Fitness: Value (with a maximum score of 10, based on the word pairs *good-bad* and *of no use-useful*), and as Health and Fitness: Enjoyment (with a maximum score of 15, based on the remaining three word pairs). For intersubdomain comparisons, these two Health and Fitness components are rescaled to a value out of 25 by multiplying the scores by 2.5 and 1.67.

Physical Activity Questionnaire

A questionnaire was devised to assess the degree of primary involvement or actual participation in various forms of physical activity. For each of the physical activity subdomains, the students indicated the frequency (number of days per month) in which they were involved in activities that to them reflected the dimensions in question. For example, the following item was responded to for the subdomain Aesthetic:

> Think of examples of physical activities which have beautiful and graceful movements. How many days per month do you take part in physical activities *as the beauty in human movement*, when they are in season?

Procedures

The ATPA inventory and physical activity questionnaire were administered during half-hour classroom sessions following standard procedures (Schutz, Smoll, Carre, & Mosher, in press). The data collection was conducted by the same person during the months of October and April, while the students were attending Grades 10 and 11. Thus, over a 2-year period of time, four repeated measurements were made at 6-month intervals, hereafter referred to as Terms 10a, 10b, 11a, and 11b, respectively.

The two groups of students (Classes A and B) were assumed to be equivalent in all demographic and situational characteristics and thus could be collapsed for the purpose of analysis. This assumption was statistically tested by a Class (2) by Sex (2) by Term (4) MANOVA on the ATPA measures. Because the main purpose of this study was to examine ATPA stability over time, the class by term interactions were the effects of primary interest with respect to the validity of collapsing over classes. The results showed a nonsignificant class by sex by term interaction ($p = .21$) but a significant class by term effect ($p = .024$). Further analyses on the significant interaction revealed no significant class by term effects within Grade 10 ($p = .17$) nor within Grade 11 ($p = .24$). The significant class by term interaction resulted from a difference between the classes in the nature and magnitude of change in ATPA scores from Term 10b to Term 11a. Two subdomains were responsible for this effect—Health and Fitness: Value ($p = .014$) and Aesthetic ($p = .02$). For both variables, attitudes for Class A declined slightly (approximately 1 unit) from Term 10b to 11a, whereas for Class B the mean values increased (approximately 0.5 units) over this time period. In light of the nonsignificant class by sex and term effect, the nonsignificant class by term effects within Grades 10 and 11, and the fact that only 2 of the 8 ATPA variables distinguished between Classes A and B for Terms 10b to 11a, it was concluded that the two classes represented a common population. Thus, data for Classes A and B were combined for all subsequent analyses involving change over time.

The internal consistency and validity of the ATPA inventory are well established (Schutz et al., in press; Schutz, Smoll, & Wood, 1981b). However, reliability analyses were performed on this data set to examine any possible changes in internal consistencies over the measurement sessions. Alpha coefficients were uniformly high (.85–.95) for both males and females and remained stable over the four terms. Because reliability information was not available for the involvement questionnaire and test-retest ATPA reliabilities were not available for this age group, a reliability study was conducted. Another Grade 10 sample of 32 males and 30 females completed the attitude and involvement inventories on a test-retest basis with a 2-week interval. ATPA scores yielded test-retest coefficients of .47 to .96, with median values of .57 and .79 for males and females, respectively. Test-retest reliabilities for the involvement data ranged from .38 to .91, with medians of .62 (males) and .72 (females). These reliabilities, although not as high as one would like, fall within the range acceptable in most sociophysical research.

Results and Discussion

The Stability of ATPA

ATPA subdomain means are presented in Table 1. Standard deviations for seven of the subdomains exhibited stability over the four terms, with all values in the 3.0 to 4.0 range (the Aesthetic subdomain being somewhat higher, with standard deviations ranging from 4.0 to 6.0). The standard deviations for Health and Fitness: Value, however, were low and showed an almost linear increase over the four terms (approximately 1.5 in 10a to 3.3 in 11b). This interesting

Table 1. ATPA subdomain means at each term separately by sex

	Term			
Subdomain	10a	10b	11a	11b
Males (n = 61)				
Social growth	20.7	20.8	21.2	21.5
Social continuation	21.9	21.4	21.4	20.9
Health & fitness: Value	24.2	23.5	23.4	23.3
Health & fitness: Enjoyment	18.8	18.6	18.5	17.9
Vertigo	21.0	20.7	20.6	20.1
Aesthetic	17.1	15.6	16.7	16.9
Catharsis	21.4	21.3	21.1	20.1
Ascetic	14.9	15.8	16.3	16.2
Females (n = 71)				
Social growth	22.0	22.4	21.8	22.2
Social continuation	23.2	23.1	22.3	22.5
Health & fitness: Value	24.5	24.5	24.1	24.0
Health & fitness: Enjoyment	20.5	20.1	19.7	19.5
Vertigo	18.4	18.7	17.9	18.0
Aesthetic	20.1	21.3	20.5	20.6
Catharsis	21.0	21.5	20.9	21.2
Ascetic	16.2	17.5	16.4	16.9

effect, peculiar to the Health and Fitness: Value subdomain, is important for interpretation of subsequent analyses.

A Sex (2) by Term (4) MANOVA was performed on the 8 ATPA scores to test for group stability of attitudes over the 2-year period. Neither the Term ($p = .10$) nor the Sex by Term effect ($p = .58$) was significant, indicating that, averaged over subjects, the mean attitudinal values were stable across the testing period. These findings of *group* stability are in agreement with the results found with younger children (Smoll & Schutz, 1980).

The canonical correlation analyses provided evidence suggesting that *individual* as well as group stability was characteristic of the present sample. In other words, not only were group means for ATPA consistent over time, but individuals demonstrated relative stability within their age groups over each of the three consecutive 6-month intervals. Table 2 is representative of these analyses, giving specific statistics for males on relationships between ATPA at Terms 10a and 10b. Canonical analysis for this data set yielded four significant canonical relationships, which accounted for 31.9% shared variance (total redundancy) between attitudes at Term 10a and at Term 10b. Each pair of canonical variates represents a pattern of stability specific to one or more attitudinal subdomains. Canonical variate #2 is the most unique, showing a relatively strong relationship in Social Continuation between Terms 10a and 10b. Canonical variates #3 and #4 are each comprised of two subdomains; variate #3 showing attitude consistency in Vertigo and Catharsis, and variate #4 reflecting the stability of the Health and Fitness: Enjoyment and Aesthetic

Table 2. Canonical correlation analyses: Loadings and correlations for males, terms 10a-10b

| | Canonical Variate | | | | | | | |
| | #1 | | #2 | | #3 | | #4 | |
Subdomain	10a	10b	10a	10b	10a	10b	10a	10b
Social growth	.46	.73						
Social continuation			.62	.67				
Health & fitness: Value								
Health & fitness: Enjoyment	.71	.65					.56	.57
Vertigo					.75	.64		
Aesthetic	.45	.52			.53	.72		
Catharsis	.49	.62			.45	.47		
Ascetic	.75	.57						
R^c		.83		.73		.61		.56
p		<.001		<.001		.004		.043
Redundancy		16.3%		6.2%		5.7%		3.7%

Note. Only loadings ≥.45 are presented.

subdomains. The strongest variate pair (#1) is representative of a more general relationship, being composed of five subdomains. However, the strength of the relationship is due to each of the five subdomains showing consistency within themselves over the two terms. Seven of the eight subdomains contributed to at least one of the significant canonical relationships, Health and Fitness: Value being the only one that did not emerge as a stable attribute. The virtual absence of any interindividual variability in the subdomain severely restricted the possibility of detecting any significant term-to-term relationships here. Canonical analyses on the other two pairings for the males (Terms 10a–10b, 11a–11b) and all three pairings for the females resulted in a comparable pattern of results. That is, each analysis yielded 4–6 significant canonical correlations, with one canonical variate pair representing a somewhat general relationship and the remaining pairs being subdomain specific.

The results indicated that ATPA is relatively stable for subjects at the particular age/developmental level in question. This might be contrasted with the greater degree of interindividual variability reported for children of elementary school age (Smoll & Schutz, 1980). In our initial longitudinal investigation conducted with students in Grades 4 through 6, one or more significant canonical correlations emerged for each grade pair, but their magnitude was considerably lower (R_C's ≅ .65). More importantly, with the younger children, there was no consistency in the structure of the relationships. More precisely, there was an absence of a pattern of any type insofar as any specific subdomain contributing to the relationship. The present data set, contrariwise, yielded coefficients in the first canonical variate that were associated with exactly the same subdomain as those generated in the second canonical variate.

That is, the relationship is due to stability within each of the specific subdomains.

A comparison of redundancy statistics is additionally illuminating. The total redundancy associated with each canonical analysis provided a single quantitative measure, which indicated the degree of stability for that particular subject group (males, females) and time period (adjacent terms) (see Table 3). These values, ranging from 27.6% to 43.8%, are considerably higher than those obtained for younger children. Specifically, redundancies for the canonical variate of adjacent pairings of the earlier longitudinal study (Grades 4-5 and 5-6) were 11% and 26% for males, and 17% and 16% for females. The ascending pattern for the total redundancy statistics indicated that ATPA stability was more pronounced in Grade 11 than in Grade 10. Thus, the higher canonical correlations, the presence of subdomain specific relationships, and the greater redundancies associated with the data of the present study all support the conclusion that ATPA is a more stable attribute in Grades 10 and 11 than in Grades 4, 5, and 6.

In the Smoll and Schutz (1980) study with elementary school children, a factor analysis (data collapsed over sex) revealed that the relationship among ATPA scores over time was grade-dependent rather than subdomain-dependent. Three of the five factors were composed of all subdomain scores for a specific grade, and only two factors represented the repeated measures of specific subdomains (Aesthetic, Vertigo) over time. These findings supported the conclusion regarding lack of intraindividual stability of ATPA across grades. The present data set was subjected to a similar analysis (principal component analysis with varimax rotation). Because the factor patterns were alike for the males and females, the data were collapsed over sex, yielding the factor solution presented in Table 4.

The factor analysis produced eight factors and accounted for 68.8% of the total variance. Five of these factors were clearly subdomain specific with all

Table 3. Summary of canonical correlation analyses: Redundancies, number, and range of significant coefficients

Data set	Canonical analysis pairing		
	10a and 10b	10b and 11a	11a and 11b
Males			
Total redundancy[a]	31.9%	36.9%	43.8%
No. of sig. R_c's ($p<.05$)	4	5	6
Range of sig. R_c's	.56 - .83	.61 - .82	.41 - .87
Females			
Total redundancy	27.6%	30.7%	41.3%
No. of sig. R_c's ($p<.05$)	4	4	5
Range of sig. R_c's	.50 - .80	.62 - .78	.55 - .82

[a]The redundancy index presented is the percent variance of ATPA scores in one term (e.g., 10b) extracted by the canonical variates in the preceeding term (e.g., 10a). The reciprocal redundancies (e.g., 10a variance accounted for by 10b R_c variate) were almost identical and are not presented.

Table 4. Factor analysis of ATPA: Males and females, terms 10a to 11b

Subdomain	Term	Factor 1	2	3	4	5	6	7	8
Aesthetic	10a	.65							
	10b	.77							
	11a	.73							
	11b	.77							
Social continuation	10a		.65						
	10b		.78						
	11a		.86						
	11b		.52						
Health & fitness: Enjoyment	10a			.69					
	10b			.67					
	11a			.81					
	11b			.69					
Vertigo	10a				.79				
	10b				.81				
	11a				.83				
	11b				.74				
Catharsis	10a							.82	
	10b							.79	
	11a							.75	
	11b							.50	
Ascetic	10a						.58		
	10b						.79		
	11a								
	11b						.58		
Health & fitness: Value	10a								.62
	10b						.58		
	11a					.59			
	11b					.80			
Social Growth	10a								
	10b						.51		
	11a								
	11b					.53			
Percentage of variance[a]		10.4%	10.3%	9.3%	9.2%	8.7%	8.6%	7.7%	4.6%

Note. Only loadings > ± .50 are presented.
[a]This value represents the percentage of total variance among the attitudinal subdomains accounted for by the factor.

four term measures of each subdomain grouping together to form a unique factor. The other three factors (Factors 5, 6, and 8) were either single-measure unique factors (Factor 8. Health & Fitness: Value, Term 10a) or a combination of two or three subdomains (Factors 5 and 6). There was no indication of a correlational relationship among a set of subdomains at a specific point in time (i.e., no time-dependent factors). These findings support the results of the canonical correlation analyses in that they suggest a much stronger ATPA intraindividual stability with the high school students than that found in the elementary school children.

The Stability of Involvement

As indicated in the introduction, the purpose for collecting the involvement data was to ascertain the degree to which changes in the nature and degree of involvement in physical activity may contribute to attitude instability. However, a comprehensive statistical analysis of the involvement data is now of questionable utility, given that attitudes for this age group have been found to be relatively stable. Nevertheless, analyses of the involvement data could provide supportive explanatory information. Consequently, the involvement data were subjected to a canonical analysis similar to that performed on the attitude scores. In comparison with the results for attitudes (see Table 3), involvement showed even stronger stability over time. The total redundancy for each canonical pairing was approximately 10% greater with the involvement data (e.g., 41% for males Terms 10a–10b, to 55.2% for females Terms 11a–11b). Furthermore, the number of significant canonical coefficients ranged from four to six, with the largest R_C values ranging from .82 (females Terms 10a–10b) to .91 (females Terms 11a–11b). As with attitudes, involvement showed greater stability within Grade 11 than in Grade 10. The obvious conclusion that can be drawn from these findings is that, like ATPA, involvement in physical activity is a fairly stable behavior in young adults. Any instabilities in ATPA over time cannot, on the basis of these data, be attributed to changes in the degree of primary involvement in physical activity.

Attitude-Involvement Relationships

Based on the above results, that is, the relative stability in both ATPA and involvement, our third hypothesis becomes somewhat obscure. It was speculated that a weak ATPA-involvement relationship may be, in part, due to a lack of stability in attitudes and/or involvement. However, with young adults we have shown relatively stable patterns over time in both ATPA and involvement in physical activity. Under these circumstances it would be interesting to examine the attitude-involvement associations for this age group to see if they are stronger than those found with younger children. To this end, canonical correlations were calculated, separately for males and females for each of the four terms, between the ATPA and involvement domains. As can be seen in Table 5, there is no support for any claims regarding even moderately strong attitude-involvement relationships. At best, only 22.8% (females Term 10a) of the variability in the degree of involvement in physical activity can be accounted for by the strength of attitudes held toward participation in physical activity. Thus, even in the presence of stability of both attitudes and involvement, the strength of the attitude-behavior relationship continues to be low. This finding may not be due to the actual absence of such relationships but is probably a function of the measurement techniques employed. If one adopted a theoretical framework along the lines advocated by contemporary attitude-behavior theorists (e.g., Ajzen & Fishbein, 1977;

Table 5. Summary of canonical correlation analyses: Attitude-involvement relationship at each term

Data set	10a	10b	11a	11b
Males				
Total redundancy	7.3%	6.4%	18.0%	
No. of sig. R_c's	1	1	1	0
Largest R_c	.74	.74	.69	.62 ns
Females				
Total redundancy	22.8%	15.6%	7.5%	
No. of sig R_c's	2	1	2	0
Range of sig. R_c's	.62 - .67	.65	.59 - .66	.62 ns

Bentler & Speckart, 1979; Fazio, Powell, & Herr, 1983), stronger relationships may be detected. This could be an interesting and fruitful approach for future inquiry. It would also be interesting to examine the stability of attitudes across the adult lifecycle and to monitor the stability-instability question following significant role transitions such as, divorce, the empty nest, unemployment, retirement, or widowhood.

References

Ajzen, I., & Fishbein, M. (1977). Attitude-behavior relations: A theoretical analysis and review of empirical research. *Psychological Bulletin, 84,* 888-918.

Ausubel, D.P., & Sullivan, E.V. (1970). *Theory and problems of child development* (2nd ed.). New York: Grune & Stratton.

Bentler, P.M., & Speckart, G. (1979). Models of attitude-behavior relations. *Psychological Review, 86,* 452-464.

Carre, F.A., Mosher, R.E., & Schutz, R.W. (1980). *British Columbia physical education assessment: General report.* Victoria: British Columbia Ministry of Education.

Eastgate, C.A. (1975). *Attitudinal differences between female participants and non-participants in a middle school extramural meet.* Unpublished master's thesis, University of Wisconsin, Madison, WI.

Fazio, R.H., Powell, M.C., & Herr, P.M. (1983). Toward a processing model of the attitude-behavior relation: Assessing one's attitude upon mere observation of the attitude object. *Journal of Personality and Social Psychology, 44,* 723-735.

Kenyon, G.S. (1968a). A conceptual model for characterizing physical activity. *Research Quarterly, 39,* 96-104.

Kenyon, G.S. (1968b). Six scales for assessing attitude toward physical activity. *Research Quarterly, 39,* 566-574.

Kenyon, G.S. (1968c). *Values held for physical activity by selected urban secondary school students in Canada, Australia, England, and the United States.* Washington, DC: United States Office of Education.

Krech, D., Crutchfield, R.S., & Ballachey, E.L. (1962). *Individual in society.* New York: McGraw-Hill.

Leventhal, H. (1974). Attitudes: Their nature, growth, and change. In C. Nemeth (Ed.), *Social psychology: Classic and contemporary interpretations.* Chicago: Rand McNally.

Martens, R. (1975). *Social psychology and physical activity*. New York: Harper & Row.

Medinnus, G.R., & Johnson, R.C. (1976). *Child and adolescent psychology* (2nd ed.). New York: Wiley & Sons.

Meyers, C.L., Pendergast, D.R., & DeBacy, D.L. (1978). Interrelationships involving selected physical fitness variables and attitude toward physical activity in elementary school children. In F. Landry & W. Orban (Eds.), *Sports medicine: Electrocardiography and hypertension and other aspects of exercise* (pp. 305-312). Miami, FL: Symposia Specialists.

Rokeach, M. (1968). *Beliefs, attitudes, and values*. San Francisco: Jossey-Bass.

Schutz, R.W., & Smoll, F.L. (1977). Equivalence of two inventories for assessing attitudes toward physical activity. *Psychological Reports*, **40**, 1031-1034.

Schutz, R.W., Smoll, F.L., Carre, F.A., & Mosher, R.E. (in press). Inventories and norms for children's attitudes toward physical activity. *Research Quarterly for Exercise and Sport*.

Schutz, R.W., Smoll, F.L., & Wood, T.M. (1981a). Physical activity and sport: Attitudes and perceptions of young Canadian athletes. *Canadian Journal of Applied Sport Sciences*, **6**, 32-39.

Schutz, R.W., Smoll, F.L., & Wood, T.M. (1981b). A psychometric analysis of an inventory for assessing children's attitudes toward physical activity. *Journal of Sport Psychology*, **4**, 321-344.

Simon, J.A., & Smoll, F.L. (1974). An instrument for assessing children's attitudes toward physical activity. *Research Quarterly*, **45**, 407-415.

Smoll, F.L., & Schutz, R.W. (1980). Children's attitudes toward physical activity: A longitudinal analysis. *Journal of Sport Psychology*, **2**, 144-154.

Smoll, F.L., Schutz, R.W., & Keeney, J.K. (1976). Relationships among children's attitudes, involvement, and proficiency in physical activities. *Research Quarterly*, **47**, 797-803.

19

Motives of Older Adults for Participating in Physical Activity Programs

Helen M. Heitmann
UNIVERSITY OF ILLINOIS–CHICAGO
CHICAGO, ILLINOIS, USA

Among other objectives aimed at improving the physical fitness of the nation, the Surgeon General of the United States has put forth the following objective, "By 1990, 50% of adults 65 years and older should be engaging in appropriate physical activity, (e.g., regular walking, swimming or other aerobic activity)" (U.S. Department of Health and Human Service, 1980). However, as agencies seek to encourage older adults to participate in physical fitness and recreation programs, they often encounter resistance from the target population.

Several surveys in the United States and other countries have revealed a low incidence of vigorous physical activity participation on the part of older adults (Cunningham, Montoye, Metzler, & Keller, 1968; Harris, 1979; Heikkinen & Kayhty, 1977; Hobart, 1975; Kenyon, 1966; McPherson, 1978; President's Council on Physical Fitness and Sport, 1974; Sidney & Shephard, 1977; Wohl & Szwarc, 1981). Participation appears universally to be inversely proportionate to age.

It may be speculated that sport and exercise have been associated with leisure. Pfeiffer and Davis (1971) concluded, after sampling attitudes of adults toward work and leisure, that only 20% of the men and 22% of the women felt leisure was more satisfying than work. McPherson (1978) and Wohl and Szwarc (1981) discussed the process of socialization and pointed out that the values of the social system often color the particular behavior patterns of the population. This would influence the attitudes of people regarding exercise as well as other life style activities.

Studies have revealed a variety of reasons for their participation. Massie and Shephard (1971) surveyed middle-aged Canadian men and determined this group valued physical activity more for aesthetic, cathartic, and social experiences than for health and fitness. Sidney and Shephard (1976) also found elderly men and women to value aesthetic experience highest, followed by health and fitness. Mobily and de Amorin Sa (1982) surveyed 100 elderly Brazilians' (age = 63.93 years) attitudes toward physical activity. They also determined that aesthetic experience was primary followed by health and fitness. Comparing their Brazilian data to the North American data of Sydney and Shephard (1976), they concluded that Brazilian subjects had more positive attitudes toward physical activity than North American subjects.

Telama, Vuolle, and Laakso (1981) determined the motives for physical activity participation of employed adults ($n = 552$), age 27-60 years, in Jyväskyla, Finland. The majority, 80% males and 82% females, selected physical fitness and health as a motive. Those who did select physical fitness and health indicated that they were more concerned with physical fitness than with health.

With conflicting results from various surveys, it was the purpose of this study to identify the motives for participating in physical exercise and recreation programs by older adults in select midwestern U.S. sites. This study was undertaken to capitalize on motivational forces that might encourage participation.

Method

Questionnaire Development

An open-ended questionnaire was given to a sample ($n = 50$) of older adults, ages 50-82, to determine what they believed to be their reasons for participation. Their responses could be classified into six categories: achievement, aesthetics, appearance, coping, health, and social. Descriptive statements were framed for each of the six categories and were presented to a cohort group to assess readability and comprehension of the intended meaning of the statements. The statements were revised to eliminate any ambiguity. External reliability of the instrument was determined with another cohort group ($n = 25$) by a test-retest procedure ($r = .82$), with a one-week testing interval.

Design of the Study

Older adults ($n = 227$; $M = 63$; $SD = 10.27$) participating in physical activity at nine randomly selected sites were asked to force rank the six motives from least (1) to most (6) important. Those who had difficulty reading the questionnaire were read the questions.

Analysis of Data

Data from female subjects were divided into the following age groups: 40-59 ($n = 39$, $M = 49.74$, $SD = 6.52$); 60-69 ($n = 57$, $M = 64.9$, $SD = 2.57$); and 70+ ($n = 52$, $M = 75.42$, $SD = 6.05$). Data from male subjects were divided into the following age groups: 60-69 ($n = 38$, $M = 66.60$, $SD = 2.82$) and 70+ ($n = 41$, $M = 72.44$, $SD = 10.10$).

A series of one-way ANOVA's were utilized to determine differences according to gender. Gender and age groups ($n = 5$) were collapsed and analyzed via a one-way ANOVA. Follow-up Duncan's Mutliple Range Tests were utlized where necessary. The Alpha level was preestablished at 0.05.

Results

Table 1 reports the means and standard deviations of the subjects' responses by gender. A one-way ANOVA revealed the 60-69 male group's mean was higher ($p<.05$) than the 70+ mean for the *Aesthetic* motive. The means of the female subjects yielded significant differences for *Achievement* ($p<.0001$), *Aesthetics* ($p<.001$), *Health* ($p<.0001$), and *Social* ($p< .0001$).

The means and standard deviations of the five groups by age and gender are reported in Table 2. The rankings of the six motives from highest to lowest for both male groups were similar. The order of the rankings was

1. *Health*,
2. *Social*,
3. *Coping*,
4. *Appearance*,
5. *Achievement*, and
6. *Aesthetics*.

Both female groups, age 60-69 and 70+, agreed in their ranking of the motives. The ranking for these older female groups was

1. *Health*,
2. *Social*,
3. *Coping*,
4. *Appearance*,
5. *Achievement*, and
6. *Aesthetics*.

However, the younger females, age 40-59, who were participating in the same classes as the older subjects did differ in their rankings of the motives from the other groups. Their order of ranking was

1. *Health*,
2. *Appearance*,
3. *Achievement*,
4. *Coping*,
5. *Aesthetics*, and
6. *Social*.

The Duncan procedure found significant mean differences between and among the groups by age and sex.

Posthoc analysis of the means of two male groups showed no significant differences for *Achievement*. Among the three female groups, the 40-59 age group mean was significantly higher than for the two older female groups. The 60-69 female group mean was also significantly higher than the mean for the female 70+ age group. The means for the two male groups were significant-

Table 1. Means and standard deviation of motives selected by males and females by gender

Motive	Male (n = 79)		Female (n = 148)	
	M	SD	M	SD
Achievement	3.86	1.54	2.88	1.66
Aesthetic	2.16	1.42	2.36	1.47
Appearance	2.80	1.35	3.36	1.43
Coping	3.65	1.53	3.70	1.46
Health	5.18	1.37	4.93	1.46
Social	3.32	1.39	3.72	1.57

Table 2. Means and standard deviations of motives selected by males and females by age and gender

	Males Age				Females Age					
	60-69 (n = 38)		70+ (n = 41)		40-59 (n = 39)		60-69 (n = 57)		70+ (n = 52)	
Motive	M	SD	M	SD	M	SD	M	SD	M	SD
Achievement	3.71	1.54	4.00	1.55	3.70	1.72	2.91	1.64	2.25	1.36
Aesthetics	2.52	1.50	1.83	1.26	3.18	1.79	2.12	1.36	2.00	1.04
Appearance	2.68	1.44	2.90	1.28	3.74	1.48	3.12	1.38	3.33	1.42
Coping	3.66	1.55	3.66	1.53	3.36	1.56	3.75	1.39	3.88	1.44
Health	5.18	1.45	5.17	1.30	3.97	1.84	5.32	1.10	5.23	1.15
Social	3.24	1.44	3.39	1.36	2.87	1.63	3.77	1.51	4.31	1.31

ly higher than those of the two older female groups. The 40-59 female age group was not statistically different from the two male groups.

A significantly higher mean occurred for *Aesthetics* between the 40-59 female age group and all other groups. The 70+ male age group mean was significantly lower than the younger male group mean as well as the mean for the comparable female age group. However, the 60-69 and 70+ female groups' means for *Aesthetics* also were not significantly different from each other.

The 40-59 female age group mean for *Appearance* was significantly higher than that of all other groups. The males and the 60-69 female age group means were not significantly different. However, the 60-69 male age group was significantly lower than the 70+ female age group for *Appearance*. The *Coping* motive showed no significant differences between group means.

The *Health* motive showed no significant differences between the male and female 60-69 and 70+ groups. However, the 40-59 female age groups' mean was significantly lower than all other groups.

For the *Social* motive no significant differences occurred between the 40-49 female age group mean and the two male age group means. However, the means for these groups were significantly lower than the 70+ female age group mean as was the 60-69 female age group mean. Their mean was also significantly higher than the mean for the 40-59 female age group.

Discussion

Culture and life roles may account for differing motives among and between age and gender groups. Although the subjects in each age group and gender selected *Health* as their first choice, both male age groups selected *Achievement* as their second choice.

Achievement ranked fifth for the oldest female subjects. Perhaps this age group of women has not been socialized to achieve through physical prowess. However, the younger female age group, who differed from the older females on *Achievement*, may be experiencing cultural change regarding the acceptability of achievement through physical prowess. This younger age group is more concerned with *Appearance* and less with *Social* than the older female age groups. The older female age groups are more motivated to participate for social reasons than are their male cohorts. All gender and age group subjects in this sample valued the *Aesthetic* aspect lowest. This is in contradiction to the findings in Brazil (Mobily & de Amorin Sa, 1982) and Canada (Sidney & Shephard, 1976) and more in accord with the Finnish study reported by Heikkinen and Kayhty (1977) and Telama et al. (1981), which reported "good physical fitness" as most important.

The selection of the *Health* motive as primary among all groups may be a reflection of current media attention to the role of exercise in maintaining health. The subjects in earlier reported studies may not have had their attention drawn to the relationship of exercise and health and, therefore, may have been influenced to participate for other cultural reasons.

If it is the intention to lure older adults into participating in physical activity programs it would seem appropriate to understand the differences in motives between and among ages and genders. When designing activity programs for older adults, one must take the range of motives into consideration to insure the appeal of the program. It should also be remembered that group data are descriptive only of the group, not of the individuals within the group. Therefore, the activity leader should seek to identify the motivation of each participant for participating and gear the program to his or her motive as well as to his or her physical needs.

References

Cunningham, D.A., Montoye, H.J., Metzner, H.L., & Keller, J.B. (1968). Active leisure time activities as related to age among males in a total population. *Journal of Gerontology*, **23**, 551-556.

Harris, L. & Associates., Inc. (1979). *The Perrier study: Fitness in America*. New York: Great Waters of France.

Heikkinen, E., & Kayhty, B. (1977). Gerontological aspects of physical activity— Motivation of older people in physical training. In R. Harris & L. Frankel (Eds.), *Guide to fitness after 50* (pp. 191-205). New York: Plenum.

Hobart, C.W. (1975). Active sport participation among the young, the middle-aged and the elderly. *International Review of Sport Sociology*, **10**(3-4), 27-40.

Kenyon, G.S. (1966). The significance of physical activity as a function of age, sex, education and socioeconomic status of northern United States adults. *International Review of Sport Sociology, 1,* 41-54.

Massie, J.F., & Shephard, R.J. (1971). Physiological and psychological effects of training. *Medicine and Science in Sport, 3,* 110-117.

McPherson, B.D. (1978). Aging and involvement in physical activity: A sociological perspective. In F. Landry & W. Orban (Eds.), *Physical activity and human well-being* (pp. 111-125). Miami, FL: Symposia Specialists.

Mobily, K., & de Amorin Sa, H. (1982, Fall). Attitudes of the elderly toward physical activity: A cross-cultural comparison. *Iowa Association of Health, Physical Education, Recreation, and Dance Journal,* 16-18.

Pfeiffer, E., & Davis, G.C. (1971). The use of leisure time in middle life. *Gerontologist, 11*(3, Part 1), 187-195.

President's Council on Physical Fitness and Sport. (1974). National adult physical fitness survey. *Physical Fitness Digest* (Series 4, No. 2). Washington, DC: Author.

Sidney, K.H., & Shephard, R.J. (1976). Attitudes toward health and physical activity in the elderly: Effects of a physical training program. *Medicine and Science in Sports, 8,* 246-252.

Telama, R., Vuolle, P., & Laakso, L. (1981). Health and physical fitness as motives for physical activity among Finnish urban adults. *International Journal of Physical Education, 38*(1), 11-16.

U.S. Department of Health and Human Service, Public Health Service. (1980). *Promoting health/preventing disease: Objectives for the nation.* Washington, DC: U.S. Government Printing Office.

Wohl, A., & Szwarc, H. (1981). The humanistic content and values of sport for elderly people. *International Review of Sport Sociology, 16,* 4, 5-11.

20

Cognitive Processing, Emotional Health, and Regular Exercise in Middle-Aged Men

Abdelwahab M. El-Naggar
UNIVERSITY OF HELWAN
CAIRO, EGYPT

A.H. Ismail
PURDUE UNIVERSITY
WEST LAFAYETTE, INDIANA, USA

A progressive aging of national populations and improvements in the life expectency of the average citizen have directed the interests of applied psychologists to the importance of physical exercise in the elderly. Exercise has been viewed as effective for improving individuals' well-being and the quality of their lives (Morris & Husman, 1978).

Evidence indicates that regular exercise influences not only physiological parameters but also cognitive functioning and personality characteristics of middle-aged and older individuals (El-Naggar & Ismail, 1982; Young, 1979). An obvious extrapolation is that exercise and its concomitant benefits might also postpone age-related psychomotor deterioration (Spirduso, 1980). The purpose of the present study was to investigate whether regular exercise improves the cognitive processing and emotional health of middle-aged men.

Method

Subjects

The subjects were intially 70 men who signed up to participate in the Purdue Adult Fitness Program. Twenty-four of the individuals exercised regularly in the program (at least 70% attendance at no less than 60% of maximum oxygen uptake VO_2 max); they were identified as regular Exercisers. Another 24 individuals failed to exercise regularly in the program (less than 20% attendance); they were identified as regular Nonexercisers. The age of the subjects ranged from 40-65 years.

Physical Fitness Program

The physical fitness program involved 90-minute sessions 3 times a week for 16 weeks. During each session the subjects performed stretching and calisthenics (20 minutes), immediately followed by a few minutes of total relaxation. After the relaxation, progressive walking and/or running took place for about 20-30 minutes for 1-3 miles.

Procedures

The subjects were tested twice during the first and last weeks of pre- and postprogram participation. The tests included measures of physical fitness (PF), cognitive processing (COG), and emotional health (EMO).

Physical Fitness Measures

Physical fitness was measured using the treadmill test and the procedures of Ismail, Falls, and MacLoad (1965), which reveal a single score from six measures. The measures included: submaximal heart rate, percent lean body weight, maximal oxygen uptake ml/kg lean body weight, submaximal volume ventilation kg/body weight, resting diastolic blood pressure, and resting pulse pressure.

Cognitive Processing Measures

The cognitive processing measures included measures of two processes, namely successive (SUC) and simultaneous (SIM), proposed by Das, Kirby, and Jarman (1979). SUC was measured by Successive Numbers Task (SN) (Vernon, Ryba, & Lang, 1978), Digit Span Test (DS), and Trial Making Test Parts A and B (TMA & TMB). SIM was measured by the Space Relations Test (SR) of the Differential Aptitude Test (DAT), and three tests from the Cultural Fair IQ Tests, namely, Classification (CL), Matrices (MA), and Conditions (CO).

Emotional Health Measures

Emotional health was measured using selected factors from the Cattell Sixteen Personality Questionnaire (16PF) and Eysenck Personality Inventory (EPI). The measures were Factor C (FC) dealing with emotional unstable versus emotional stable, Factor E (FE) dealing with submissive versus assertive, Factor M (FM) dealing with practical versus imaginative, Factor N (FN) dealing with simple versus sophisticated, Factor Q2 (FQ2) dealing with group-dependent versus self-sufficient, Factor Q4 (FQ4) dealing with composed versus relaxed, Extraversion (EX) dealing with extraversion versus introversion, and Neuroticism (NE) dealing with neuroticism versus stability.

In order to ascertain the equality of the two groups in the pretest variables, the t-test was used and the results are presented in Table 1. The results showed no significant differences between the two groups in any variable. This indicated the equality of the groups at pretest in all variables.

Table 1. t-Tests between groups means at predata

Variable	Exercisers		Nonexercisers		
	M	SD	M	SD	t
PF	277.76	41.82	280.15	58.89	.16
SN	18.08	2.50	17.72	2.49	.46
DS	21.77	5.12	22.94	2.80	.90
TMA	26.23	9.67	24.94	7.67	.48
TMB	61.53	23.59	67.50	31.59	.74
SR	48.50	10.83	44.89	12.04	1.07
CL	8.13	2.11	7.67	2.66	.67
MA	8.00	2.13	7.22	2.46	1.15
CO	6.90	1.67	6.78	2.37	.21
FC	5.50	1.61	5.06	1.16	1.02
FE	6.40	2.13	5.94	1.98	.74
FM	6.10	1.16	6.39	2.00	.64
FN	5.40	2.37	5.50	1.69	.16
FQ_2	6.33	2.23	6.28	1.93	.09
FQ_4	6.03	1.90	6.39	1.98	.62
EX	11.47	3.49	11.00	4.67	.39
NE	5.43	4.80	7.61	4.89	− 1.51

Results

MANOVA was performed on pre- and posttest results for the Exercisers and Nonexercisers to test the differences between the two groups from pre- to posttests in all variables collectively.

The results of MANOVA (Table 2) showed significant differences between the Exercisers and Nonexercisers from pre- to posttests in all variables collectively ($p<.01$). In order to test which subdomain was more amenable to change from pre- to posttests, the multivariate Hotelling T^2-test was used. The results of the T^2-test between pre- and postmean vectors of COG and EMO subdomains for both groups showed only significant differences between pre- and postCOG mean vector of the Exercisers ($p<.01$).

Table 2. MANOVA and hotelling t^2-test results

Effect	Multivariate F	p
Group differences	2.43	.01

t^2-tests between pre- and postmean vectors of groups

Vector	Exercisers		Nonexercisers	
	T^2	p	T^2	p
Cognition	26.06	.01	16.74	.15
Emotion	9.45	.24	13.60	.18

The univariate paired t-test was applied to the mean differences between pre- and postresults for both groups in all variables independently (Table 3).

The results revealed that only the Exercisers showed significant mean differences from pre- to postresults in PF, and in four tests from the COG variables, namely SN, DS, SR, and CO. The nonexercisers showed no significant mean differences from pre- to posttest results.

Discussion

The results indicated that collectively the Exercisers showed improvements in physical fitness, cognitive processing, and emotional health. The multivariate analyses were able to detect such improvements more effectively than univariate analysis. This indicated that these improvements were dependent and firmly related. Improvement in physical fitness as a result of regular exercise is associated with improvements in cognitive processing and emotional health. Previous studies showed that improvements in cardiovascular functioning following exercise were associated with reports of an increased sense of well-being (Ismail & Trachtman, 1973) and improvements in perceptual psychomotor intelligence function and associate learning (Young, 1979). Some researchers maintained that the unavoidable involvement of the entire brain in physical activity may be an important factor mediating a positive change in mental ability of the elderly (Powell, 1974). Others postulated that increases in oxygen transport capacity, blood circulation, and energy supply to different

Table 3. Paired t-tests of pre- and postdata differences

Variable	Exercisers			Nonexercisers		
	d	SD	t	d	SD	t
PF	24.43	32.55	3.60**	− 3.50	32.28	− .52
SN	1.10	1.61	3.27**	.00	.00	.00
DS	1.86	3.88	2.30**	.17	1.38	.59
TMA	− 1.30	7.08	− .88	− .38	3.96	.46
TMB	− 2.63	20.17	− .63	− 4.44	15.32	− 1.39
SR	1.00	3.93	1.22	.50	3.48	.69
CL	.54	1.47	1.76*	.27	1.54	.84
MA	.33	1.72	− .92	.39	1.41	1.33
CO	.43	1.18	1.75*	.11	1.15	− .46
FC	− .30	1.04	− 1.39	.27	1.05	1.23
FE	− .20	1.25	− .77	.06	1.07	.27
FM	− .20	1.33	− .72	− .05	1.20	.20
FN	− .27	1.49	− .87	− .11	1.39	− .38
FQ²	.07	1.77	.19	.05	.96	.25
FQ⁴	.30	1.22	1.18	− .06	1.07	− .27
EX	− .47	1.86	− 1.21	− .72	2.62	− 1.32
NE	− .36	2.21	− .78	− .28	1.74	− .77

**p<.01.
*p<.05.

parts of the body, including the brain, as a result of regular exercise, may be reflected in cognitive functioning improvements (Young, 1979). Although the precise mechanism is not known, it can be suggested that regular exercise has beneficial effects for cognitive processing and emotional health in middle-aged men.

References

Das, J.P., Kirby, J.R., & Jarman, R.F. (1979). *Simultaneous and successive processes*. New York: Academic Press.

El-Naggar, A.M., & Ismail, A.H. (1982). *Effect of exercise on emotional stability in adult men*. Paper presented at the Midwest Symposium on Exercise and Mental Health, Lake Forest, IL.

Elsayed, M., Ismail, A.H., & Young, R.J. (1980). Intellectual differences of adult men related to age and physical fitness before and after an exercise program. *Journal of Gerontology, 35*, 383-387.

Ismail, A.H., & El-Naggar, A.M. (1982). Effect of exercise on cognitive processing in adult men. *Journal of Human Ergology, 10*, 83-91.

Ismail, A.H., Falls, H.B., & MacLoad, D.F. (1965). Development of a criterion for physical fitness tests from factor analysis results. *Journal of Applied Physiology, 20*, 991-999.

Ismail, A.H., & Trachtman, L.E. (1973). Jogging the imagination. *Psychology Today, 6*, 78-82.

Morris, A.F., & Husman, B.F. (1978). Life quality changes following an endurance conditioning program. *American Corrective Therapy Journal, 32*, 3-6.

Powell, R.R. (1974). Psychological effects of exercise therapy upon institutionalized geriatric mental patients. *Journal of Gerontology, 29*, 157-161.

Spirduso, W.W. (1980). Physical fitness, aging, and psychomotor speed: A review. *Journal of Gerontology, 35*, 850-865.

Vernon, P.E., Ryba, K.A., & Lang, R.J. (1978). Simultaneous and successive processing. An attempt at replication. *Canadian Journal of Behavioral Science, 10*, 1-15.

Young, R.J. (1979). The effect of regular exercise on cognitive functioning and personality. *British Journal of Sport Medicine, 13*, 100-117.

21

Eye Movement Fatigue and Performance Accuracy in Young and Old Adults

Kathleen M. Haywood
UNIVERSITY OF MISSOURI-ST. LOUIS
ST. LOUIS, MISSOURI, USA

Many sports and day-to-day skills (e.g., driving) involve a type of motor response commonly defined as coincidence-anticipation. That is, a performer is required to anticipate the arrival of a person or object at a specified place (a coincidence) and to time a response to that event. In most skills, the greatest amount of perceptual information gathered to make such a judgment comes from the visual sense. The performer is not required to wait passively for the visual information but can actively seek information by moving the eyes. Eye movements position a particular image on the retinal fovea, the area yielding the highest visual acuity. Hence, the performer chooses the images to be viewed with high acuity and, consequently, the images to be viewed with poor acuity because such images fall on the peripheral retina. Performers have eye movement strategies for viewing "visual displays" (Noton & Stark, 1971), and these strategies are related to characteristics of the task, characteristics of the observer, and environmental aspects of the task (Chambers, 1973).

Presumably, there is a relationship between the quality of the visual information gathered and the quality of the performance in skills requiring coincidence-anticipation. Further, visual quality is linked to eye movements. Eye movement recordings taken during skill performance can reflect the effectiveness of information processing (Bard & Fleury, 1981) and might be related to the variability of performance. Of course, other factors might be related to variability of performance as well (e.g., choice delay, response execution), but the relationship between eye movements and skill performance deserves attention. It is commonly assumed that tracking the moving person or object of critical interest (as in the coaching patter, "keep your eye on the ball") yields the best performance. Yet, little systematic investigation of this assumption has been conducted and that done indicates the matter is not so simple (see Haywood, 1984).

The eyes can only "track" a moving object, that is, continually keep its image on the retinal fovea, if it is moving less than about 30 deg/s (Robinson, 1968). This type of eye movement is termed *smooth pursuit*. Faster objects are observed by *saccadic eye movements*, wherein fixations and fast eye movements (during which vision is suppressed) are interspersed. Presumably, the quality of the information obtained during both types of eye movements is enhanced when the two eyes move together but suffers when the eye movements are uncoordinated. The two eyes do not always move together. Bahill and Stark (1975) identified three types of eye movement anomalies that become more prevalent with fatigue. One is a double, or overlapping saccade, significant because a saccade normally is completed before another one begins. Another anomaly is a glissade, a slow drifting movement appended to the end of a fast saccade. The third type of anomaly is a low-velocity, long-duration saccade. Bahill, Ciuffreda, Kenyon, and Stark (1976) recorded a fourth anomaly, a dynamic overshoot, wherein the eye goes beyond its target and returns with a quick saccade. These anomalies can be monocular; that is, they can occur in one eye while the other moves normally. As few as 30 sacccades of 50° can elicit these anomalies. Bahill, Iandolo, and Troost (1980) found that fatigue also affects smooth pursuit eye movements, first by a breakdown of good tracking, then a switch to saccadic movment. Hence, it is clear that with eye movement fatigue anomalies in the movements of the two eyes will occur. These anomalies can affect the quality of visual information gathered, but whether this could account for performance decrements is unknown because eye movement anomalies and task performance have not been studied together.

The purpose of the present study was to determine if eye movement anomalies induced by eye movement fatigue are related to coincidence-anticipation performance. If eye movement anomalies and poor task performance coincide, poor performance may be attributed to the poor quality of visual information obtained. Because variability in coincidence-anticipation performance exists across age groups (Haywood, 1980) and visual inspection strategies vary with subject characteristics such as age, two age groups were tested, young adults and old adults. Eye movement fatigue may be induced sooner in old adults than young adults. If task performance declines in each group with the onset of eye movement anomalies, further evidence of a link between eye movements and performance exists. Moreover, more older adults than younger have been shown to stop "tracking" the moving stimulus in a coincidence-anticipation task during a series of repetitive trials (Haywood, 1982). A possible explanation of this is eye movement fatigue. Older adults have longer eye movement reaction times than younger adults (Haywood, 1982), and this may cause eye movement anomalies to be more detrimental to older adults because there would be less time either to track or to fixate the moving stimulus. It was expected that eye movement fatigue would be evident in eye movement anomalies and uncoordinated movements of the two eyes, that fatigue would have an earlier onset in the old adults than the young adults, and that eye movement anomalies or uncoordinated movements would coincide with poor task performance.

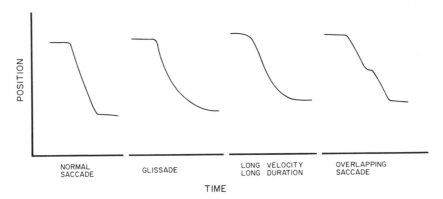

Figure 1. Models of a normal saccade and eye movement anomalies

Method

Subjects

The younger adults who volunteered to participate in this study were undergraduate students at the University of Missouri-St. Louis. The 8 women and 4 men ranged from 18 to 24 years of age, averaging 21.2 years. The older adults were volunteers from the Older Active Adults Program at the same university. These 8 women and 4 men ranged from 56 to 77 years of age, averaging 66.5 years.

Apparatus

A Bassin Anticipation Timer (Lafayette Model 50-575) served as the coincidence-anticipation apparatus. This timer simulates a moving object with sequentially lit LED lamps on a 150 cm runway. The middle of the runway was placed in front of the subject at a distance of 5.2 m so that the light "moved" from the subject's left to the subject's right. The 3 stimulus speeds used were 15.7, 25.8, and 35.1°/s (3, 5, and 7 MPH on the apparatus). Hence, the stimulus was expected to elicit both smooth pursuit and saccadic eye movements. The small visual angle of 16.5° over which the stimulus travels reduces the likelihood of contaminating versional eye movements. The subject was instructed to estimate the arrival of the light at the marked target lamp by pressing a hand-held button with the preferred thumb. Error was recorded in milliseconds early or late.

Eye movements were recorded with an Applied Science Laboratory's Model 200 Eye-Trac output to a Beckman dynograph. This recorder used a photoelectric technique wherein two phototransistors were aimed at the iris-scleral border on each side of the eye and measure the light reflected from either the dark iris or white sclera as the eye moves. The phototransistors were suspended from an empty eyeglass frame or the subject's prescription glasses. The subject was placed in a head restraint to stabilize the head. Only the horizontal movements of *each* eye were recorded.

Procedure

After subjects took a visual screening test and received task instructions, the eye movement recorder was positioned and calibrated. Calibration was checked after every 25 trials. The 138 task trials were presented in a randomized order of stimulus speeds standardized across subjects. The various stimulus speeds required subjects to attend to each trial for accurate performance. Additionally, subjects were instructed to follow the stimulus with their eyes, increasing the likelihood of fatigue in later trials. Subjects completed the 138 trials in less than 15 min.

Experimental Design

Error scores were converted to a percentage of the time each stimulus took to travel the track. This allowed scores to be compared across stimulus speeds. The 138 trials were then blocked into 6 groups of 23 trials each. Initially, an age group by trial block ANOVA with repeated measures on trial block (2 × 6) was conducted on absolute, constant, and variable percent task error. Constant error reflected the direction of the error, early or late, while absolute error ignored the direction. Variable error reflected the variability of error around the subjects' mean constant error. Because the purpose here was to compare performance in fresh and fatigued eye movement states, subsequent analyses involving eye movements were conducted only on Block 1 and Block 6. An age group by trial block ANOVA (2 × 2) was conducted of the number of eye movement anomalies, which were identified by visual inspection of the eye movement record. Eye movement reaction times were measured by hand from the eye movement record. Mean task error and number of eye movement anomalies were also correlated.

Results

Task Performance

Age group by trial block (2 × 6) ANOVAs of absolute, constant, and variable percent error were used to assess task performance. Performance of the age groups was significantly different in terms of absolute error, $F(1, 22) = 5.9$, $p<.03$, and variable error, $F(1, 22) = 15.8, p<.001$. The younger adults were more accurate than the older adults, 8.7 to 11.6%, respectively, and less variable, 9.1 to 13.4%. Performance also differed across trial blocks in terms of absolute error, $F(5, 110) = 2.7$, $p<.03$, and variable error, $F(5, 110) = 4.7$, $p<.001$. Absolute means for Blocks 1 to 6 were 11.8, 9.8, 9.6, 10.1, 9.5, and 9.9% and variable means were 13.9, 11.4, 10.1, 10.3, 11.0, and 10.8%. Performance, then, was less accurate and more variable in the first block but relatively stable thereafter. In no case was the interaction effect significant.

Eye Movement Reaction Times

The eye movement reaction times, that is, the time lag between stimulus movement and movement of the eyes to follow the stimulus, were analyzed for Blocks 1 and 6 to determine whether or not the reaction time lengthened in the later trials. An age group by trial block (2 × 2) ANOVA was conducted. While the mean eye movement reaction time was longer for both groups in Block 6 than Block 1, it was not significantly longer at the .05 level. The younger adults had a significantly shorter reaction time than the older adults, $F(1, 44)$ = 13.6, $p<.001$. Mean values are presented in Table 1.

Eye Movement Anomalies

The number of eye movement anomalies, that is, trials in which the two eyes did not move together throughout, was counted for Blocks 1 and 6. The mean number of anomalies was analyzed in an age group by trial block (2 × 2) ANOVA. Despite the fact that the mean number of anomalies was higher for both groups in Block 6 than Block 1, neither of the main effects nor the interaction effect was significant at the 0.05 level. The mean values are presented in Table 2. As reflected in the high standard deviations, it was noted that a few subjects tended to exhibit a high proportion of the anomalies. When these subjects were identified and their task scores reviewed, it was found that three subjects (two young adults and one old adult: two females and one male) had a mean task error more than one standard deviation above the group mean error. All three subjects had a high number of eye movement anomalies (30, 18, and 13). A Pearson product-moment correlation of mean task error and mean number of eye movement anomalies in Blocks 1 and 6 was calculated. The coefficient was moderate, $r = .37$, but significant at the 0.02 level.

Table 1. Mean eye movement reaction times (msec)

Group[a]	Block 1	Block 6
Younger adults	186 ± 16	198 ± 28
Older adults	240 ± 52	246 ± 74

[a]n = 12 for each group

Table 2. Mean number of eye movement anomalies

Group[a]	Block 1	Block 6
Younger adults	3.3 ± 5.4	4.3 ± 5.1
Older adults	5.2 ± 4.4	6.8 ± 4.2

[a]n = 12 for each group

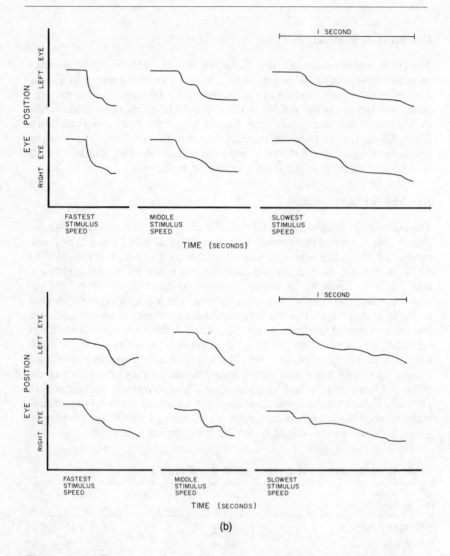

Figure 2. (a) Examples of coordinated eye movements in an older adult, age 71 (b) Examples of eye movement anomalies and uncoordinated eye movements in a younger adult

Conclusion

The present study sought to determine the relationship between eye movement anomalies induced by fatigue and performance on a task involving visual information. The horizontal eye movements of both eyes were recorded during coincidence-anticipation task performance over 138 successive trials. The results of the present study confirmed several aspects of performance noted in previous studies. First, older adults were more variable and less accurate, in terms of absolute error, than the younger adults on the coincidence-anticipation task (Haywood, 1980). Second, the older adults showed a longer eye movement reaction time than the younger adults (Haywood, 1982). In addition, the present study detected no tendency for this latency to significantly lengthen over the trials presented.

In regard to the major purpose of this study, eye movement anomalies were found in Block 1, before subjects would experience eye movement fatigue. Although the mean number of trials with anomalies was higher in Block 6, after 115 trials, it was not significantly so. It is possible that the time to record task performance between trials, although just a matter of seconds, gave subjects a chance to recover and they did not experience significant eye movement fatigue. The eye movements may have to be continuous, or nearly so, to induce fatigue. Fatigue-induced anomalies may also be highly individualistic. Fuchs and Binder (1983) failed to find any evidence of fatigue in three subjects, and recently Bahill, Brockenbrough, and Troost (1981) reported that some subjects fatigue more rapidly than others. Nevertheless, subjects in both age groups exhibited eye movement anomalies, and this provided an opportunity to observe the anomalies and the task performance together.

In several ways, the link between an eye movement anomaly and poor task performance did not prove to be strong. Performance in Block 6 was better than in Block 1 when subjects were familiarizing themselves with the task, whereas the number of anomalies in the two blocks was not significantly different. The older adults performed more poorly on the task than the younger adults, but the difference in the number of anomalies between the age groups was not significant. Even an examination of individual trial scores when an anomaly occurred clearly showed that an anomaly and an excellent score could occur on the same trial. This finding is in general agreement with a previous study (Haywood, 1984), which demonstrated that, at least on the present task, good performance is possible when the two eyes do not either track or periodically fixate (as with saccadic eye movement) the moving stimulus.

On the other hand, evidence shows that a high number of anomalies and poor performance coincide in some subjects. An examination of individual subject means was prompted by the large standard deviations around the group mean number of anomalies. Three subjects were identified who were more than one standard deviation higher than their groups' mean task error and all three showed a high number of anomalies. In fact, these three subjects made 27% of all the eye movement anomalies. A conclusion that the eye movement anomalies caused poor task performance in these subjects is premature, however, because a third, underlying factor (e.g., boredom, inattention, or some aspect of neuromuscular control) could cause both. While the present study found only a moderate relation between eye movement anomalies and task performance ($r = .37$), and this relation is attributable in part to the performance of just a few subjects, further study of this matter is warranted. Identification of the factor(s) causing poor performance in some subset of performers would be of theoretical as well as practical importance. Often breakdowns in performance help identify the critical aspects of perfected skill, and this may eventually help the individuals with that particular problem improve their skills.

References

Bahill, A.T., Brockenbrough, A., & Troost, B.T. (1981). Variability and development of a normative data base for saccadic eye movements. *Investigative Ophthalmology and Visual Science.* **21**, 116-125.

Bahill, A.T., Ciuffreda, K.J., Kenyon, R., & Stark, L. (1976). Dynamic and static violations of Hering's law of equal innervation. *American Journal of Optometry and Physiological Optics,* **53**, 786-796.

Bahill, A.T., Iandolo, M., & Troost, B.T. (1980). Smooth pursuit eye movements in response to unpredictable target waveforms. *Vision Research,* **20**, 923-931.

Bahill, A.T., & Stark, L. (1975). Overlapping saccades and glissades are produced by fatigue in the saccadic eye movement system. *Experimental Neurology,* **48**, 95-106.

Bard, C., & Fleury, M. (1981). Considering eye movement as a predictor of attainment. In M. Cockerill & S. MacGillwary (Eds.), *Vision and sport* (pp. 28-41). Cheltenham, England: Stanley Thorner.

Chambers, A.N. (1973). *Development of a taxonomy of human performance: A heuristic model for the development of classification systems* (Report No. AIR-726-10/69-TR-AA) Washington, DC: American Institute for Research, Washington Office Institute for Research in Psychobiology.

Fuchs, A.F., & Binder, M.D. (1983). Fatigue resistance of human extraocular muscles. *Journal of Neurophysiology,* **49**, 28-34.

Haywood, K.M. (1980). Coincidence-anticipation accuracy across the life span. *Experimental Aging Research,* **6**, 451-462.

Haywood, K.M. (1982). Eye movement pattern and accuracy during perceptual-motor performance in young and old adults. *Experimental Aging Research,* **8**, 153-157.

Haywood, K.M. (1984). Use of the image/retina and eye/head movement visual systems during coincidence-anticipation performance. *Journal of Sports Sciences,* **2** (in press).

Noton, D., & Stark, L. (1971). Eye movements and visual perception. *Scientific American,* **224**, 34-43.

Robinson, D.A. (1968). Eye movement control in primates. *Science,* **161**, 1219-1224.

PART IV

Physiological and Training Perspectives

22

Physiological Aspects of Sport and Physical Activity in the Middle and Later Years of Life

Roy J. Shephard
UNIVERSITY OF TORONTO
TORONTO, ONTARIO, CANADA

There is now a substantial literature on the physiological aspects of physical activity during the late years of life (Shephard, 1978a, 1983; Shephard & Sidney, 1978; Smith & Serfass 1981). The present review considers specifically: (a) problems of methodology, (b) physiological changes associated with aging, (c) interactions between physical activity and the aging process, and (d) implications for the design of activity programs.

Methodological Problems

Sample Selection

Volunteers for exercise studies are generally fit, health-conscious, and nonsmokers (Shephard, 1978b). Selective attrition accentuates this bias in longitudinal studies. Cross-sectional studies are further complicated by cohort effects attributable to the depression, World War II, and postwar migrations.

Data Standardization

Age is usually reported in calendar years, although subjects vary in biological age (Heikkinen, 1979). Anaerobic power, anaerobic capacity, and aerobic

Aging studies within the School of Physical and Health Education are supported by a research development grant from the University of Toronto.

power are usually standardized per unit of body mass. With aging an increased proportion of total body mass becomes attributable to fat. Moreover, absolute values have greater relevance to weight-supported sports and activities that are popular with the elderly. Alternative methods of adjusting for differences of body size also present problems. Hydrostatic estimates of lean tissue mass are invalidated by a decrease in density of lean tissue, while ^{40}K data are complicated by fat-shielding and changes of body potassium (Myhre & Kessler, 1966). Height standardization is made difficult by secular trends to a greater stature (Borkan, Hults, & Glynn, 1983), plus age-related kyphosis and compression of intervertebral discs (Friedlander, Costa, Bosse, Ellis, Rhoads, & Stoudt, 1977).

Intercurrent Disease

Brown and Shephard (1967) noted that only 33 of 62 older female workers were in good health, and 17 of the group had some condition that compromised oxygen transport. In the Canada Fitness Survey (1983), 19% of subjects older than 65 years perceived themselves in sufficient ill-health not to take a fitness test, and 55% were excluded by those conducting the tests. Scores thus depend greatly on medical rejection rates that have varied 15-fold between surveys (Shephard, in press).

Lifestyle Changes

Personal lifestyle interacts with apparent aging. The deterioration of lung volumes is exaggerated by smoking (Niinimaa & Shephard, 1978), whereas oxygen transport, muscular strength, and body composition are all adversely affected by an age-related decrease of habitual activity.

Physiological Changes and Performance

Performance Curves

Performance curves provide some index of physiological aging (Stones & Kozma, 1980, 1982; Riegel, 1981). However, competitive times are very susceptible to environment (Shephard, 1980) and the intensity of selective pressures. As age advances, it becomes progressively less likely that training has been maximal and that the best endowed individuals have participated in a given event (Kavanagh & Shephard, 1977).

Stones and Kozma (1982) concluded that aging affects aerobic events more than anaerobic events. Females also show a more rapid functional loss than males. The change in the men's aerobic events, 1% per year, is similar to that reported for swimmers (Rahe & Arthu, 1975) and coincides with the decrease in aerobic power. However, the change in the women's, 2.5% per year, exaggerates the physiological deterioration.

Oxygen Transport

The aging of maximum oxygen intake $\dot{V}O_2$ max, Shephard, 1977) has been examined by cross-sectional studies, both within a given laboratory (Bink, 1962;

Hollmann & Hettinger, 1976; Bailey, Shephard, & Mirwald, 1976; Shephard, 1977) and in accumulated data (Shephard, 1978a, 1978b; Dehn & Bruce, 1972).

Longitudinal studies have followed smaller and more select samples over shorter intervals (Asmussen, Fruensgaard, & Norgaard, 1975; Hollmann, 1965; Dehn & Bruce, 1972; Åstrand, Åstrand, Hallbäck, & Kilbom, 1973; Robinson, Dill,, Robinson, Tzankoff, & Wagner, 1976; Kasch & Kulberg, 1981; Pollock, Foster, Rod, Hare, & Schmidt, 1982). Changes of habitual activity have frequently confounded the aging response. Thus, Kasch and Kulberg (1981) saw no decrement of $\dot{V}O_2$ max in the first 10 years of a 15-year study, because initially sedentary men had entered a training program. Likewise, Dehn and Bruce (1972) claimed a difference in the rate of aging between athletes and sedentary individuals on the basis of an excessively rapid loss of function by the nonathletes (1.6 ml per kg•min per year); presumably, they became more sedentary over the period of observation.

Cross-sectional studies of male subjects show a loss in $\dot{V}O_2$ max of 0.8 to 1.1% per year (0.34 to 0.51 ml per kg•min). Sedentary women show little change of $\dot{V}O_2$ max prior to 40 years of age, but the total loss over the adult span averages 0.45 to 0.95% per year (Drinkwater, Horvath, & Wells, 1975; Bailey et al., 1976; Shephard, 1977). In both sexes, the loss becomes faster during the sixties, but this may reflect a decrease of habitual activity rather than an acceleration of aging.

Any link in the oxygen transport chain can theoretically limit the performance of an older individual. Gas distribution and pulmonary diffusion often show some deterioration, and an increased proportion of the oxygen intake is diverted to the respiratory muscles (Patrick, Bassey, & Fentem, 1983). Furthermore, mechanical efficiency and thus the yield of work per liter of oxygen decreases. Nevertheless, in the absence of respiratory disease, blood transport continues to be the main determinant of oxygen intake (Shephard, 1977).

A narrowing of maximum arteriovenous oxygen difference is blamed upon a reduction of either tissue enzyme activity (Kraus, 1971) or muscle capillarity (Pařízková, Eiselt, Sprynarová, & Wachtlová, 1971). Evidence for a reducttion of enzyme activity is not very convincing (Timiras 1972). More probably, the narrowed arteriovenous oxygen difference reflects a difficulty in dissipating waste heat, with a larger fraction of total blood flow being directed to the skin (Shephard, 1978a).

The decrease of maximum heart rate accounts for no more than one half of the decrease in oxygen transport. The formula (220 − age, years) implies a 20% reduction of blood transport between 25 and 65 years of age, while the 177 beats•min^{-1} maximum observed by Lester, Sheffield, Trammell, and Reeves (1968) led to a 10% loss at 65 years. Londeree and Moeschberger (1982) found that sedentary Europeans exercising on a treadmill had heart rates of about 170 beats•min^{-1} at 65 years of age. Occasionally, the sinus pacemaker is hypoxic, but oxygen administration does not normally restore a youthful maximum rate. Alternative explanations of the slowing include intrinsic changes in the myocardium (Corre, Cho, & Barnard, 1976), a greater stiffness of the ventricular wall with altered feedback to the cardioregulatory centers (Mirsky, 1979), and a reduced sympathetic drive to the cardiac pacemaker (Shephard, 1978a).

Older subjects sustain stroke volume during a submaximum effort, but their ejection fraction falls as exhaustion is approached (Niinimaa & Shephard, 1978). Possible causes include poorer myocardial perfusion and a reduction of myocardial ATPase activity (Albert, Gale, & Taylor, 1967) with a stiffer ventricular wall, poorer myocardial contractility, and abnormalities of wall motion (Port, Cobb, Coleman, & Jones, 1980). Ventricular mass also decreases (Grimby & Saltin, 1966), while an increase of aortic input impedance (Yin, Weisfeldt, & Milnor, 1981) and a weakening of the skeletal muscles exacerbate after-loading (Shephard, 1978a). Finally, early diastolic filling is limited by a slow rate of ventricular relaxation (Gerstenblith, Frederiksen, Yin, Fortuin, Lakatta, & Weisfeldt, 1977).

Anaerobic Power and Capacity

Vertical sprint speed decreases 45% from 25 to 65 years (Shephard, 1978b). However, creatine phosphate stores decrease only 15% from 21 to 70 years of age (Gronert, 1980). Possibly, sprint performance is also limited by impaired flexibility, unstable knees, poor vision, and fear of stumbling.

Early reports suggested quite low maxima for blood lactate, respiratory gas exchange ratio, and oxygen debt, but in our experience a well-motivated senior citizen can reach a terminal blood lactate of 10-12 mmol, much as in a younger person (Sidney & Shephard, 1977a). Residual discrepancies probably reflect poor motivation, lesser ratio of muscle to blood volume, and slow escape of lactate from the active muscles.

Muscle Strength

Isometric muscle force is fairly well-preserved until about 45 years of age. At 65 years, values are 20% smaller in men and 10% smaller in women (Shephard, 1978a; Hollmann & Hettinger, 1976). Part of this small loss may be motivational; although older individuals sometimes show a loss of lean tissue, the lean mass per cm of height is well-preserved in Master's competitors (Kavanagh & Shephard, 1977). Function is selectively lost in Type II fibres (Grimby, Anianson, Danneskold-Samsoe, & Saltin, 1980). The time to peak tension and the half relaxation time are thus increased, with parallel changes in maximum power, force, and velocity (Davies, White, & Young, 1982).

Petrofsky, Burse, and Lind (1975) suggested that older women have an increased endurance of sustained submaximal muscular contractions, but on simple endurance tests such as sit-ups and push-ups, function deteriorates by 60% over the span of working life (Canada Fitness Survey, 1983).

Bone and Joint Function

Flexibility is impaired by collagen cross-linkage, arthritis, and joint ankylosis. The Canada Fitness Survey (1983) noted that scores for a simple sit-and-reach test decreased by 23% in men and 18% in women through 65 years of age. Muscle and joint stiffness, loss of elastic tissue, and poor periarticular blood supply all increase the risk of injury (Shephard & Sidney, 1978).

Psychomotor Function

A loss of accommodation, a circumscription of the visual field, and a decrease of visual acuity impair responses to visual cues, especially if the light is poor. Disturbances of hearing (both deafness and tinnitus) further reduce the input of sensory information. These limitations are compounded by a slowing of nerve conduction and central processing. Reactions to complex cues are hampered by difficulties in distinguishing signal from noise (Welford & Birren, 1965; Shephard & Sidney, 1978). Elderly tennis players apparently preserve fast reaction times and field independence (Spirduso & Clifford, 1978; Rotella & Bunker, 1978), but it is less clear whether this is a cause or a consequence of their sport participation. Reduced leg lift, poor eyesight, deterioration of balance, and liability to postural hypotension increase the risk of falls during physical exertion (Overstall, Exton Smith, Imms, & Johnson, 1977).

Hormonal Responses

Older subjects have difficulty in maintaining homeostasis, due in part to a deterioration of endocrine function (Weg, 1975). However, catecholamine secretion apparently increases at any given intensity of effort (Palmer, Ziegler, & Lake, (1978).

Interactions Between Training and Aging

Trainability

There is disagreement on the trainability of the elderly (Shephard & Sidney, 1978; Badenhop, Cleary, Schaal, Fox, & Bartel, 1983). Reasons include problems in measuring the training response and in equating initial fitness.

Nervousness of the subject or the investigator may cause symptomatic limitation of an initial test, with a spurious gain of oxygen transport as such fears are overcome. On the other hand, preliminary training may be needed before a maximum test can be performed, so that the early training response is not observed (Sidney & Shephard, 1977a). In submaximal tests, learning and habituation may also reduce heart rates (Shephard, 1977).

The training response depends heavily upon initial fitness (Shephard, 1977). However, proponents of poor trainability have sometimes equated young and elderly volunteers in terms of oxygen transport ($ml \cdot kg^{-1}min^{-1}$), ignoring the fact that any given value implies a higher level of fitness in an older individual.

In sedentary older people, even moderate effort has some training effect (Sidney & Shephard, 1978; Badenhop et al., 1983). The *percentage* training response is generally similar in young and old people, but absolute gains of oxygen transport decrease with aging. Much also depends upon motivation. Faria and Frankel (1977) described a competitive cyclist who had preserved a maximum oxygen intake of 59.9 $ml \cdot kg^{-1}min^{-1}$ to the age of 70 years, and occasional "post-coronary" patients can boost their oxygen transport from 26-27 $ml \cdot kg^{-1}min^{-1}$ to over 60 $ml \cdot kg^{-1}min^{-1}$ (Shephard, 1979).

Characteristics of Training Response

Resting heart rate changes little with training (Sidney & Shephard, 1978). However, systolic blood pressure decreases up to 20 mm Hg through altered pulse wave reflection, habituation, and improved fit of the sphygmomanometer cuff. Blood volume and total hemoglobin increase, while left ventricular ejection time lengthens (Adams, De Vries, Girandola, & Birren, 1977). Muscle biopsies show an augmentation of glycogen stores and aerobic enzyme activities (Suominen, Heikkinen, Liesen, Michel, & Hollmann, 1977).

At any given intensity of submaximal exercise, there are gains of mechanical efficiency, with a lesser increase of systemic blood pressure and thus cardiac work rate (Shephard & Sidney, 1978). ST depression often diminishes at any given heart rate or double product (Sidney & Shephard, 1977b).

Anaerobic power can be increased by an appropriate regimen (Suominen et al., 1977) and it is possible to restore much of the muscle strength lost over the span of working life (Moritani & De Vries, 1980). Sidney, Shephard, and Harrison (1977) demonstrated a 3.3 mm decrease of skinfold readings over the course of a 1-year program of aerobic exercise. The effectiveness of aerobic training in controlling fat is supported by figures of 11-14% body fat for Master's track contestants (Pollock, 1974; Kavanagh & Shephard, 1977).

Other potential dividends of training include improved flexibility (Chapman, De Vries, & Swezey, 1972), increase of collagen turnover (Suominen et al., 1977), and increase of bone mineral content (Smith, Reddan, & Smith, 1981; Sidney et al., 1977; Brewer, Meyer, Keele, Upton, & Hagan, 1983). All of these responses help to reduce the risk of musculoskeletal injuries. Recall and object recognition are improved (Diesfeldt, Diesfeldt, & Groenedijk, 1977), reaction times are speeded (Harris, 1977), and the performance of cognitive tests is upgraded (Stanford, Hambacker, & Fallica, 1974). Training may also increase the growth hormone response to exercise (Sidney & Shephard, 1977c).

Impact Upon the Rate of Aging

There are occasional suggestions that a high rate of energy expenditure accelerates cellular aging (Holloszy, 1983) and predisposes to cancer (Schmid, 1975). Other more widely accepted effects (an increase of HDL cholesterol, an improvement of glucose tolerance, and a reduction of systemic blood pressure) seem likely to increase the quality and/or the quantity of residual lifespan.

Measures of whole-organ function such as maximum oxygen intake apparently show a similar age-related *rate* of loss in athletic and in sedentary individuals (Shephard & Sidney, 1978). Nevertheless, high initial values (Pollock, 1974; Kavanagh & Shephard, 1977) give athletic individuals a significant functional advantage at any given calendar age.

Heart volumes are well conserved in Master's competitors (Pollock, 1974; Kavanagh & Shephard, 1977), but it is less certain whether the enlarged heart of an athlete increases the risk of a cardiac catastrophe once training has ceased (Pyörala, Karvonen, Taskinen, Takkunen, & Kryronseppa, 1967). Both dimensions and function show a slow return to sedentary values after training has stopped (Fardy, Maresh, & Abbott, 1976).

Regular training apparently gives no immunity to musculoskeletal injuries. Over a 1-year period, more than one half of Master's track competitors were prevented from training for a week or more due to injuries (Kavanagh & Shephard, 1977).

Implications for Sport and Physical Activity Programs

Safety

The risk that exercise will induce a fatal cardiac emergency seems relatively greater in a middle-aged person than in an older person (Vuori, Suurnäkki, & Suurnäkki, 1982). Nevertheless, many elderly subjects develop abnormal exercise electrocardiograms (Shephard, 1978a). Given the strong probability that moderate, progressive activity improves the quality of life, such findings are no reason to prohibit physical activity in an asymptomatic senior citizen.

Leg, ankle, and low back injuries are frequent events in the elderly exerciser (Billings, Burry, & Jones, 1977). Specific precautions include the substitution of fast walking for jogging, choice of a load that leaves the subject only pleasantly tired the next day, and avoidance of hard surfaces. Activities to avoid in the gymnasium include traditional knee bends, straight leg lifts from a supine position, hyperextension of the back, and sudden twisting movements (MacCallum, 1980).

Limitations of vision or balance and postural hypotension argue against pursuits where there is a danger of collision, falling, or drowning. Problems of homeostasis also narrow the range of environmental tolerance. Cardiac deaths occur in hot and humid conditions, while cold dry air may provoke both bronchospasm and angina (Vuori, 1977). Poor peripheral circulation increases the risk of frostbite, whereas a low maximum rate of working, poor muscle glycogen reserves, and impaired vasomotor regulation all increase the chances of hypothermia.

Programming

Practical aspects of program design stem from the physiological profile of an older person. At 66 years, 80% of the population can move without difficulty, but by the age of 80 years a high proportion are affected by cardiac or mental problems (Heikkinen & Kähty, 1977). Programs must take into account not only fitness scores but also biological age, social situation, and any medical limitations.

A steady heart rate of 100-120 beats•min^{-1} provides a surprisingly effective training stimulus when a senior citizen begins a reconditioning program (Sidney & Shephard, 1978; Badenhop et al., 1983). Morse and Smith (1981) reported the maximum oxygen intakes as 18-20 and less than 10 ml•kg^{-1}min^{-1} in "young" and "old" recruits to their geriatric exercise program. Plainly, for such individuals walking, recreational swimming, dancing, lawn bowling, and even chair exercises have training value. A good warm-up minimizes the dangers of musculoskeletal problems and cardiac emergencies. The aerobic component of any conditioning program should be progressive, with the participant competing against himself or herself. Slow recovery, poor venous tone, and postural hypotension are all indications for an extended warm-down.

Limitations of coordination, stablity, and the special senses restrict involvment in team sports. Nevertheless, participation can be extended through the introduction of age-specific competitions and simple adjustments to the rules of play.

An Age Ceiling?

Is there an age ceiling, beyond which physical conditioning should be avoided? One study of rats suggested that longevity was extended by regular exercise, but only if this was begun before the 400th day of life (Edington, Cosmas, & McCafferty, 1972). The experiment deserves repetition on further groups of animals, although many Master's athletes certainly started rigorous training after they had passed the equivalent of the 400-day mark, apparently without harmful consequences to their health. Nevertheless, as population age increases, progressively larger proportions of the group are affected by serious pathologies where vigorous exercise is contraindicated. Occasionally, training may worsen ST depression (Vertenten, Miller, & Pollock, 1969), although subjects with abnormal electrocardiograms generally tolerate submaximal training remarkably well (Sidney & Shephard, 1977b).

Despite the 4-5 year advantage of longevity shown by Finnish cross-country ski champions (Karvonen, Klemola, Virkajarvi, & Kekkonen, 1974), no conclusive evidence exists that moderate exercise extends the lifespan of a senior citizen. On the other hand, in the absence of major medical contraindications, no evidence of harm exists. Rather, the quality of the remaining years of life is enhanced. On this basis alone, regular physical activity is well worth recommending to both our friends and our patients.

References

Adams, W.C., De Vries, H., Girandola, R.M., & Birren, J.S. (1977). The effect of exercise training on systolic time intervals in elderly men. *Medicine and Science in Sports, 9*, 68.

Albert, N.R., Gale, H.H., & Taylor, N. (1967). The effect of age on contractile protein ATPase activity and the velocity of shortening. In R.D. Tanz, F. Kavaler, & J. Roberts (Eds.), *Factors influencing myocardial contractility*. New York: Academic Press.

Asmussen, E., Fruensgaard, K., & Norgaard, S. (1975). A follow-up longitudinal study of selected physiologic functions after forty years. *Journal of the American Geriatrics Society, 23*, 442-450.

Åstrand, I., Åstrand, P.O., Hallbäck, I., & Kilbom, A. (1973). Reduction in maximal oxygen intake with age. *Journal of Applied Physiology, 35*, 649-654.

Badenhop, D.T., Cleary, P.A., Schaal, S.F., Fox, E.L., & Bartel, R.L. (1983). Physiological adjustments to higher or lower intensity exercise in elders. *Medicine and Science in Sports and Exercise, 15*, 496-502.

Bailey, D.A., Shephard, R.J., & Mirwald, R.L. (1976). Validation of a self-administered home test of cardiorespiratory fitness. *Canadian Journal of Applied Sports Sciences,* **1,** 67-78.

Billings, R.A., Burry, H.C., & Jones, R. (1977). Low back injury in sport. *Rheumatology and Rehabilitation* (London), **16,** 236-240.

Bink, B. (1962). The physical working capacity in relation to working time and age. *Ergonomics,* **5,** 25-28.

Borkan, G.A., Hults, D.E., & Glyn, R.J. (1983). Role of longitudinal change and secular trend in male body dimensions. *Human Biology,* **55,** 629-641.

Brewer, V., Meyer, B.M., Keele, M.S., Upton, S.J., & Hagan, R.D. (1983). Role of exercise in prevention of involutional bone loss. *Medicine and Science in Sports and Exercise,* **15,** 445-449.

Brown, J.R., & Shephard, R.J. (1967). Some measurements of fitness in older female employees of a Toronto department store. *Canadian Medical Association Journal,* **97,** 1208-1213.

Canada Fitness Survey (1983). *Fitness and lifestyle in Canada.* Ottawa: Government of Canada, Fitness and Amateur Sport.

Chapman, E.A., De Vries, H.A., & Swezey, R. (1972). Joint stiffness: Effects of exercise on young and old men. *Journal of Gerontology,* **27,** 326-333.

Corre, K.A., Cho, H., & Barnard, R.J. (1976). Maximum exercise heart rate reduction with maturation in the rat. *Journal of Applied Physiology,* **40,** 741-744.

Davies, C.T.M., White, M.J., & Young, K. (1982). Contractile properties of leg muscles in relation to dynamic performance of elderly men aged 70 years. *Journal of Physiology,* **327,** 58.

Dehn, M., & Bruce, R.A. (1972). Longitudinal variations in maximal oxygen intake with age and activity. *Journal of Applied Physiology,* **33,** 805-807.

Diesfeldt, H.F., & Diesfeldt-Groenedijk, H. (1977). Improving cognitive performance in psychogeriatric patients. The influence of physical exercise. *Age & Aging,* **6,** 58-64.

Drinkwater, B.L., Horvath, S.M., & Wells, C.L. (1975). Aerobic power of females, ages 10 to 68. *Journal of Gerontology,* **30,** 385-394.

Edington, D.W., Cosmas, A.C., & McCafferty, W.B. (1972). Exercise and longevity: Evidence for a threshold age. *Journal of Gerontology,* **27,** 341-343.

Fardy, P.S., Maresh, C.M., & Abbott, R.D. (1976). A comparison of myocardial function in former athletes and nonathletes. *Medicine and Science in Sports,* **8,** 26-30.

Faria, I., & Frankel, M. (1977). Anthropometric and physiologic profile of a cyclist—age 70. *Medicine and Science in Sports,* **9,** 118-121.

Friedlander, J.S., Costa, P.T., Bosse, R., Ellis, E., Rhoads, J.E., & Stoudt, H.W. (1977). Longitudinal physique changes among healthy white veterans at Boston. *Human Biology,* **49,** 541-558.

Gerstenblith, G., Frederiksen, J., Yin, F.C.P., Fortuin, N.J., Lakatta, E.G., & Weisfeldt, M.L. (1977). Echocardiographic assessment of a normal adult aging population. *Circulation,* **56,** 273-278.

Grimby, G., Anianson, A., Danneskold-Samsoe, B., & Saltin, B. (1980). Muscle morphology and function in 67-81 year old men and women. *Medicine and Science in Sports,* **12,** 95.

Grimby, G., & Saltin, B. (1966). A physiological analysis of physically well-trained middle-aged and older athletes. *Acta Medica Scandinavica,* **179,** 513-526.

Gronert, G.A. (1980). Contracture responses and energy stores in quadriceps muscle from humans age 7-82 years. *Human Biology,* **52,** 43-51.

Harris, R. (1977). Fitness and the aging process. In R. Harris & J. Frankel (Eds.), *Guide to fitness after fifty* (p. 4). New York: Plenum.

Heikkinen, E. (1979). Normal aging: Definition, problems and relation to physical activity. In H. Orimo, K. Shimada, M. Iriki, & D. Maeda (Eds.), *Recent advances in gerontology* (pp. 501-503). Amsterdam: Excerpta Medica.

Heikkinen, E., & Kähty, B. (1977). Gerontological aspects of physical activity—motivation of older people in physical training. In R. Harris & L.J. Frankel (Eds.), *Guide to fitness after fifty* (pp. 191-205). New York: Plenum.

Hollmann, W. (Ed.). (1965). *Körperliches Training als Prävention von Herz-Kreislauf Krankheiten*. Stüttgart, West Germany: Hippokrates Verlag.

Hollmann, W., & Hettinger, Th. (Eds.). (1976). *Sportmedizin—Arbeits und Trainingsgrundlagen* (pp. 1-697). Stüttgart: F.K. Schaltaner Verlag.

Holloszy, J.O. (1983). Exercise, health and aging: A need for more information. *Medicine and Science in Sports and Exercise,* **15**, 1-15.

Karvonen, M.J., Klemola, H., Virkajarvi, J., & Kekkonen, A. (1974). Longevity of endurance skiers. *Medicine and Science in Sports,* **6**, 49-51.

Kasch, F.W., & Kulberg, J. (1981). Physiological variables during 15 years of endurance exercise. *Scandinavian Journal of Sport and Sciences,* **3**, 59-62.

Kavanagh, T., & Shephard, R.J. (1977). The effects of continued training on the aging process. *Annals of the New York Academy of Sciences,* **301**, 656-670.

Kraus, H. (1971). Effects of training of skeletal muscle. In O.A. Larsen & R.O. Malmborg (Eds.), *Coronary heart disease and physical fitness* (pp. 134-137). Copenhagen: Munksgaard.

Lester, M., Sheffield, L.T., Trammell, P., & Reeves, T.L. (1968). The effect of age and athletic training on maximal heart rate during muscular exercise. *American Heart Journal,* **76**, 370-376.

Londeree, B.R., & Moeschberger, M.L. (1982). Effect of age and other factors on maximal heart rate. *Research Quarterly for Exercise and Sport,* **53**, 297-304.

MacCallum, M. (1980). Practical programs for older persons. In R.C. Goode & D.J. Payne (Eds.), *The coming of age of aging* (pp. 83-111). Toronto: Ontario Heart Foundation.

Mirsky, I. (1979). Myocardial mechanics. In R.M. Berne (Ed.), *Handbook of physiology. Section 2. The cardiovascular system* (pp. 497-531). Baltimore: Williams & Wilkins.

Moritani, T. & De Vries, H.A. (1980). Potential for gross muscle hypertrophy in older men. *Journal of Gerontology,* **35**, 672-682.

Morse, C.E., & Smith, E.L. (1981). Physical activity programming for the aged. In E.L. Smith & R.C. Serfass (Eds.) *Exercise and aging. The scientific basis* (pp. 109-120). Hillside, NJ: Enslow.

Myhre, L.B., & Kessler, W. (1966). Body density and potassium 40 measurements of body composition as related to age. *Journal of Applied Physiology,* **21**, 1251-1255.

Niinimaa, V., & Shephard, R.J. (1978). Training and oxygen conductance in the elderly. I. The respiratory system. *Journal of Gerontology,* **33**, 354-361.

Overstall, P.W., Exton Smith, A.N., Imms, F.J., & Johnson, A.L. (1977). Falls in the elderly related to postural imbalance. *British Medical Journal,* (i), 261-264.

Palmer, G.J., Ziegler, M.G., & Lake, C.R. (1978). Response of norepinephrine and blood pressure to stress increase with age. *Journal of Gerontology,* **33**, 482-487.

Pařízková, J., Eiselt, E., Sprynarová, S., & Wachtlová, M. (1971). Body composition, aerobic capacity and density of muscle capillaries in young and old men. *Journal of Applied Physiology,* **31**, 323-325.

Patrick, J.M., Bassey, E.J., & Fentem, P.H. (1983). The rising ventilatory cost of bicycle exercise in the seventh decade: A longitudinal study of 9 healthy men. *Clinical Science,* **65**, 521-526.

Petrofsky, J.S., Burse, R.L., & Lind, A.R. (1975). Comparison of physiological responses of women and men to isometric exercise. *Journal of Applied Physiology,* **38**, 863-868.

Pollock, M.L. (1974). Physiological characteristics of older champion track athletes. *Research Quarterly, 45*, 363-373.

Pollock, M.L., Foster, C., Rod, J., Hare, J., & Schmidt, D.H. (1982). Ten-year follow-up on the aerobic capacity of champion master's track athletes. *Medicine and Science in Sports, 14*, 105. (abstract)

Port, S., Cobb, F.R., Coleman, R.A., & Jones, R.H. (1980). Effect of age on the response of the left ventricular ejection fraction to exercise. *New England Journal of Medicine, 303*, 1133-1137.

Pyörala, K., Karvonen, M.J., Taskinen, P., Takkunen, J., & Kryronseppa, H. (1967). Cardiovascular studies on former endurance athletes. In M.J. Karvonen & A.J. Barry (Eds.), *Physical activity and the heart* (pp. 301-310). Springfield, IL: Thomas.

Rahe, R.H., & Arthur, R.J. (1975). Swim performance decrement over middle life. *Medicine and Science in Sports, 7*, 53-58.

Riegel, P.S. (1981). Athletic records and human endurance. *American Scientist, 69*, 285-290.

Robinson, S., Dill, D.B., Robinson, R.D., Tzankoff, S.P., & Wagner, J.A. (1976). Physiological aging of champion runners. *Journal of Applied Physiology, 41*, 46-51.

Rotella, R.J., & Bunker, L.K. (1978). Field dependence and reaction time in senior tennis players (65 and over). *Perceptual and Motor Skills, 46*, 485-486.

Schmid, L. (1975). Malignant tumors as causes of death of former athletes. In H. Howald & J.R. Poortmans (Eds.), *Metabolic adaptations to prolonged physical exercise* (pp. 85-91). Basel: Birkhauser Verlag.

Shephard, R.J. (Ed.). (1977). *Endurance fitness* (2nd ed.). Toronto: University of Toronto Press.

Shephard, R.J. (Ed.). (1978a) *Physical activity and aging* (pp. 1-353). London: Croom Helm.

Shephard, R.J. (Ed.). (1978b). *Human physiological work capacity* (pp. 1-303). London: Cambridge University Press.

Shephard, R.J. (1979). Cardiac rehabilitation in prospect. In M.L. Pollock & D.H. Schmidt (Eds.), *Heart Disease and Rehabilitation*. Boston, MA: Houghton-Mifflin.

Shephard, R.J. (1980). What can the applied physiologist predict from his data? *Journal of Sports Medicine, 20*, 297-308.

Shephard, R.J. (1983). Physiological aspects of recreation in the older adult. *Recreational Research Review, 9*, 48-66.

Shephard, R.J. (1984). Can we identify those for whom exercise is hazardous? *Sports Medicine, 1*, 75-86.

Shephard, R.J., & Sidney, K.H. (1978). Exercise and aging. In R.S. Hutton (Ed.), *Exercise and sport sciences reviews* (Vol. 6), (pp. 1-57). Philadelphia: Franklin Institute Press.

Sidney, K.H., & Shephard, R.J. (1977a). Maximum testing of men and women in the seventh, eighth, and ninth decades of life. *Journal of Applied Physiology, 43*, 280-287.

Sidney, K.H., & Shephard, R.J. (1977b). Training and electrocardiographic abnormalities in the elderly. *British Heart Journal, 39*, 1114-1120.

Sidney, K.H., & Shephard, R.J. (1977c). Growth hormone and cortisol—age differences, effects of exercise and training. *Canadian Journal of Applied Sport Sciences, 2*, 189-193.

Sidney, K.H., & Shephard, R.J. (1978). Frequency and intensity of exercise as determinants of the response to training in elderly subjects. *Medicine and Science in Sports, 10*, 125-131.

Sidney, K.H., Shephard, R.J., & Harrison, J.E. (1977). Endurance training and body composition of the elderly. *American Journal of Clinical Nutrition, 30*, 326-333.

Smith, E.L., Reddan, W., & Smith, P.E. (1981). Physical activity and calcium modalities for bone mineral increase in aged women. *Medicine and Science in Sports and Exercise,* **13**, 60-64.

Smith, E.L., & Serfass, R.C. (Eds.). (1981). *Exercise and aging: The scientific basis.* Hillside, NJ: Enslow.

Spirduso, W.W., & Clifford, P. (1978). Replication of age and physical activity effects on reaction and movement time. *Journal of Gerontology,* **33**, 26-30.

Stamford, B.A., Hambacker, W., & Fallica, A. (1974). Effects of daily physical exercise on the psychiatric state of institutionalized geriatric mental patients. *Research Quarterly,* **45**, 35-41.

Stones, M.J., & Kozma, A. (1980). Adult age trends in athletic performances. *Experimental Aging Research,* **7**, 269-280.

Stones, M.J., & Kozma, A. (1982). Sex differences in changes with age in record running performances. *Canadian Journal of Aging,* **1**, 12-16.

Suominen, H., Heikkinen, E., Liesen, H., Michel, D., & Hollmann, W. (1977). Effects of 8 weeks' endurance training on skeletal muscle metabolism in 56-70 year old sedentary men. *European Journal of Applied Physiology,* **37**, 173-180.

Timiras, P.S. (Ed.) (1972). *Developmental physiology and aging.* New York: Macmillan.

Vertenten, E., Miller, H.J., & Pollock, M.L. (1969). Development of positive stress electrocardiograms after training. *Circulation,* (Suppl. III), **40**, 208.

Vuori, I. (1977). Feasability of long-distance (20-90 km) ski-hikes as a mass sport for middle-aged and old people. In R. Harris & L.J. Frankel (Eds.), *Guide to fitness after fifty* (pp. 95-142). New York: Plenum.

Vuori, I., Suurnäkki, L., & Suurnäkki, T. (1982). Risk of sudden cardiovascular death (SCVD) in exercise. *Medicine and Science in Sports and Exercise,* **14**, 114-115.

Weg, R.B. (1975). Changing physiology of aging, normal and pathological. In D.S. Woodruff & J.E. Birren (Eds.), *Aging, scientific perspectives and social issues* (pp. 229-256). New York: Van Nostrand.

Welford, A.T., & Birren, J.E. (Eds.). (1965). Behavior, aging and the nervous system. Springfield, IL: Thomas.

Yin, F.C.P., Weisfeldt, M.L., & Milnor, W.R. (1981). Role of aortic input impedance in the decreased cardiovascular response to exercise with aging in dogs. *Journal of Clinical Investigation,* **68**, 28-38.

23

Effect of 8 Weeks Submaximal Conditioning and Deconditioning on Heart Rate During Sleep in Middle-Aged Women

Tomoko Sadamoto, Tokio Fuchi,
Yuhko Taniguchi, and Mitsumasa Miyashita
UNIVERSITY OF TOKYO
BUNKYO-KU, TOKYO, JAPAN

Aerobic physical activity is recommended as part of daily life for a variety of reasons. It is commonly postulated that exercise induces a deeper sleep, especially in persons who have difficulties in relaxing mentally. However, to our knowledge, the longitudinal effects of training on physiological changes during sleep in humans have not been investigated so far, although numerous studies have been concerned with the time courses of nocturnal heart rate (HR), body temperature, blood pressure, brain activity (EEG), and eye movement (EOG) (Miller & Horvath, 1976). These studies comparing asleep HR and EEG have shown that HR is a reliable parameter for evaluating the quality of sleep—a slowing down of HR indicating a deeper sleep stage (Lisneby, Richardson, & Welch, 1976). In the present study, we examined the effect of 8 weeks of submaximal aerobic exercise on asleep HR in sedentary middle-aged women. The middle-aged women were chosen as subjects because there were few previous studies about this group.

The present study was supported by a grant from Otsuka Pharmaceutical Co., Ltd.

Methods

Subjects

Twelve middle-aged healthy women volunteered as subjects. Mean age, height, and total body weight (TBW) were 40.9 ± 1.53 yr, 157.5 ± 1.44 cm, 60.7 ± 3.44 kg (mean ± SE), respectively. Before the investigation the subjects did not participate in any regular physical training for several years. The subjects were fully informed about the nature and purpose of the study before their consent was obtained.

Conditioning Program

The training program consisted of either jogging 3 times per week for 30 min with an HR of about 130 bpm or walking 6 times per week for 50-60 min with an HR of about 120 bpm. Each session of exercise thus amounted to an energy expenditure of 200-300 kcal. The subjects were taught to control their HR during the training bouts every 10 min in order to achieve the desired HR. During the first 8 weeks all the subjects performed their training programs. Subsequently, the subjects were divided in two groups, a control group (the "inactive" group, GI) and a training group (the "active" group, GA), respectively. After the first 8 weeks, GI stopped training while GA continued to train for an additional 8 weeks.

Testing Procedure

Body composition, submaximal work capacity, and blood characteristics were assessed before, between, and after the two 8 week sessions of training. Percentage body fat (% FAT) and lean body mass (LBM) were estimated from hydrostatic weighing methods. A venous blood sample obtained after 12-hr overnight fasting was analyzed for total serum cholesterol (T-CHO), triglycerides (TG), high-density lipoproteins (HDL), and plasma glucose (GPL) by enzymatic methods. After 30 min sitting at rest, submaximal working capacity was measured by an incremental treadmill walking test. The subjects walked for three 4-min periods at speeds of 60, 80, and 100 m/min, respectively. Expired gas was collected in Douglas bags during the last 10 min of the resting period and during the last minute of each exercise. The volume of the expired air was measured in a dry gasometer and the gas fractions of O_2 and CO_2 were determined with an automatic gas analyzer (1H-21A, Sanei Co., Ltd.), which was calibrated against gas cylinders analyzed by Scholander gas analysis. The HR recorded by ECG during the periods when gas was collected were taken as a representative value. Nocturnal HR was measured by a self-contained miniature cumulative counter (Model VHMI-012, Vine Co., Ltd.). The subjects retired between 10 p.m. and 1 a.m. and woke up between 5 a.m. and 8 a.m. Sleeping habits were normal and unchanged throughout the present study. All data were compared statistically using paired t-test. The level of significance was set at $p<0.05$.

Results

Table 1 shows changes in work capacity and blood characteristics during the first 8 weeks of the training period. Oxygen uptake ($\dot{V}O_2$) as well as HR at a given submaximal workload were lowered after the training by 13-22.5% and 7.0-12.4% of the initial level, respectively. The serum lipids (T-CHO and TG) decreased significantly, while HDL increased (see Table 1). Further, the relative $\dot{V}O_2$ to TBW ratio ($\dot{V}O_2$/TBW) also fell significantly ($p<0.01$), although the mean TBW in all subjects decreased significantly by 12% from 66.15 ± 3.18 kg to 58.19 ± 2.84 kg. LBM did not change the initial level during the program. The reduction in TBW was thus caused by a loss of body fat (2.9%).

Figure 1 shows examples of the changes in time course of HR recorded. Each subject showed her own pattern in nocturnal HR. In every case there

Table 1. Changes in oxygen uptake ($\dot{V}O_2$), total cholesterol (T-CHO), triglycerides (TG), HDL cholesterol (HDL), glucose (GPL) before and after 8 weeks of training.

Measurements		Before	After (8)
$\dot{V}O_2$ (ml•min⁻¹)			
Rest	mean	228	196**
	[SE]	11.9	9.2
60 m/min	mean	765	593**
	[SE]	74.7	48.0
80 m/min	mean	909	712**
	[SE]	74.7	52.6
100 m/min	mean	1159	1008***
	[SE]	87.4	87.2
HR (bpm)			
Rest	mean	77.1	68.1***
	[SE]	2.45	1.82
60 m/min	mean	101.0	88.1**
	[SE]	4.41	2.09
80 m/min	mean	109.3	95.8***
	[SE]	4.04	4.16
100 m/min	mean	126.3	114.3**
	[SE]	4.04	4.16
T-CHO (mg/dl)	mean	206.3	184.7*
	[SE]	10.10	9.61
TG (mg/dl)	mean	107.1	73.1**
	[SE]	13.80	6.42
HDL (mg/dl)	mean	45.6	59.9***
	[SE]	2.87	3.90
GPL (mg/dl)	mean	94.7	80.4 NS
	[SE]	8.93	2.89

Before: Before training, After: After 8 weeks of training, *: $p<0.05$, **: $p<0.01$, ***: $p<0.001$.

were periods of irregular variations with increase in minute-to-minute HR. A frequency analysis of HR also indicated that training induced a lower asleep HR (Figure 2). The asleep HR in all subjects decreased significantly from 63.7 ± 2.83 to 59.0 ± 2.35 bpm (mean ± SE). The amount of reduction was positively correlated to the initial TBW or the initial asleep HR ($p<0.05$).

As shown in Table 2, the level of asleep HR in GI returned to the pretraining level after 8 weeks deconditioning when there was no further decrease in GA in spite of continued training for another 8 weeks. Similar changes in GI and GA were found in work capacity and body composition.

Discussion

The present study demonstrated that 8 weeks of aerobic conditioning in middle-aged women induced a deeper sleeping state indicated by a lower asleep HR

Table 2. Changes in asleep heart rate (Asleep HR), oxygen uptake ($\dot{V}O_2$), heart rate (HR), total body weight (TBW) and percentage body fat (% FAT) before and after 8 and 16 weeks of training in active group (GA) and inactive group (GI)

Measurements		GA Before	GA After (8)	GA After (16)	GI Before	GI After (8)	GI After (16)
Asleep HR (bpm)	mean	65.2	57.7	57.7	62.3	60.3	64.6
	[SE]	3.02	2.49	2.45	2.78	2.32	3.35
$\dot{V}O_2$ (ml·min⁻¹)							
Rest	mean	251	206	212	199	187	192
	[SE]	16.1	16.7	18.7	10.0	7.4	9.2
60 m/min	mean	886	677	684	645	509	545
	[SE]	108.3	79.3	69.8	60.0	31.6	21.5
80 m/min	mean	951	791	821	763	597	698
	[SE]	202.6	78.6	58.8	28.7	28.2	14.9
100 m/min	mean	1087	929	1104	980	829	926
	[SE]	222.0	194.8	90.5	27.8	30.2	15.9
HR (bpm)							
Rest	mean	76.8	66.2	66.7	76.8	70.0	72.9
	[SE]	2.98	2.26	3.20	3.74	2.84	2.81
60 m/min	mean	106.5	90.2	89.0	95.5	86.0	92.5
	[SE]	6.65	2.91	3.27	5.38	3.00	2.69
80 m/min	mean	112.2	98.2	98.2	106.3	93.3	105.5
	[SE]	6.00	3.40	3.06	4.55	3.28	3.59
100 m/min	mean	129.2	118.3	114.7	123.3	110.3	124.1
	[SE]	7.18	7.25	3.91	4.11	4.12	2.80
TBW (kg)	mean	67.39	63.32	61.88	53.90	52.76	53.81
	[SE]	5.44	4.44	4.29	2.02	2.04	2.35
% FAT (%)	mean	30.2	28.1	27.9	30.8	28.6	30.3
	[SE]	1.57	1.75	1.29	1.25	1.35	1.27

Before: Before training, After (8): After 8 weeks of training, After (16): After 16 weeks of training.

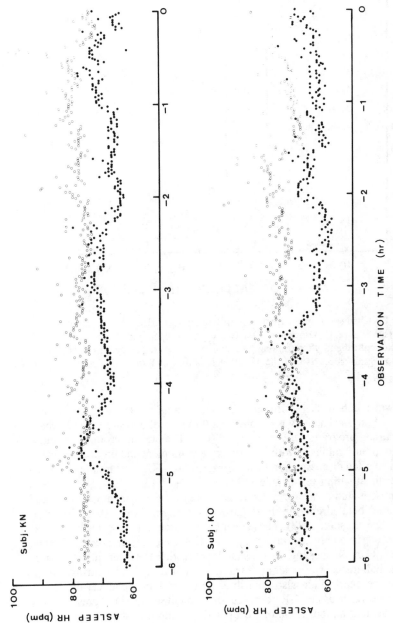

Figure 1. Typical time courses of asleep HR in 2 subjects before and after training. The open and closed circles show asleep HR for every minute during a 6-hour sleep before and after 8 weeks of training, respectively. On the horizontal axis, 0 indicates time of awakening.

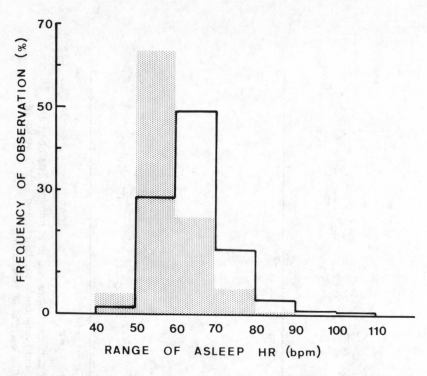

Figure 2. Changes in mean frequency distribution of asleep HR to minute to minute (see Figure 1) before and after training. The open and shaded bars show the results before and after training, respectively. The frequency was obtained after pooling all asleep HR of the 12 subjects before and after the first 8 weeks of training.

with fewer bursts of tachycardia. This pattern in asleep HR was sustained if the level of physical activity was continued (GA) but disappeared after 8 weeks if the training program was discontinued (GI). The present protocol excluded the effect of unfamiliarity with experimental equipment and procedures in the subjects so often discussed as a factor for decreased HR. The training induced bradycardia at sitting rest (Table 1; from 77.1 ± 2.45 to 68.1 ± 0.96 bpm) in the present study was attributed to an increased parasympathetic tone and a decreased beta-adrenergic drive (Brundin & Cernigliaro, 1975; Ekbolm, Kilbom, & Soltysiak, 1973). These changes in autonomic tone also partly explain the observed changes in asleep HR. However, recent studies (Lewis, Nylander, Gad, & Areskog, 1980) stated that resting HR after full autonomic blockage in humans was lower after training, indicating that an intrinsic adaptation of the heart might also contribute to the training bradycardia.

The more stable asleep HR observed after conditioning in the present study may be taken as an indication of a deeper sleep, although there were no concomitant measures of eye movements or EEG in the present study. According to Lisneby et al. (1976), there was an 88.7% correspondence between light sleep (rapid eye movements, REM) and phases of irregular or increased HR. Other studies confirmed this (Miller & Horvath, 1976; Snyder, Hobson, Morrison, & Goldfrank, 1964; Walker, Floyd, Fein, Cavness, Lualhati, & Feinberg, 1978). The effects of the training on pattern of asleep HR or REM sleep have not been studied previously in humans in a longitudinal training study as in the present investigation. However, some studies noted that well-trained athletes showed fewer REM sleep periods compared to normals (Griffin & Trinder, 1978; Walker et al., 1978). In rats, Boland and Dewsbury (1971) found that REM sleep decreased after wheelrunning training. However, two other studies in rats did not yield this result (Hobson, 1968; Matsumoto, Nishisho, Suto, Sadahiro, & Miyoshi, 1968). Thus, the animal studies remain equivocal. On the other hand, the effect of strenuous acute exercise (3-6 days) on asleep HR has been studied in humans to some extent (Roussel & Buguet, 1982; Walker et al., 1978). Both reports agreed that an elevated HR persisted during sleep following exercise. Walker et al. (1978) also found the same result after one day's exercise (177 kcal) at mild intensity in sedentary men. Apart from differences in sex and age of subjects, between the present result and Walker et al.'s results, differences also existed in exercise intensity, duration of training program, and methods of observation. A direct comparison is, therefore, not feasible. The present conclusion that a light exercise conditioning program will enhance the quality of sleep in middle-aged women is, therefore, not contradicted by the above mentioned reports.

References

Boland, B.D., & Dewsbury, D.A. (1971). Characteristics of sleep following sexual activity and wheelrunning in male rats. *Physiology Behavior*, **6**, 145-149.

Brundin, T., & Cernigliaro, C. (1975). The effect of physical training on the sympathoadrenal response to exercise. *Scandinavian Journal of Clinical and Laboratory Investigation*, **35**, 525-530.

Ekbolm, B., Kilbom, A., & Soltysiak, J. (1973). Physical training, bradycardia, and autonomic nervous system. *Scandinavian Journal of Clinical and Laboratory Investigation*, **32**, 251-256.

Griffin, S.J., & Trinder, J. (1978). Physical fitness, exercise, and human sleep. *Psychophysiology*, **15**, 447-450.

Hobson, J.A. (1968). Sleep after exercise. *Science*, **162**, 1503-1505.

Lewis, S.F., Nylander, E., Gad, P., & Areskog, N.H. (1980). Nonautonomic component in bradycardia of endurance trained men at rest and during exercise. *Acta Physiologica Scandinavica*, **109**, 297-305.

Lisneby, M.J., Richardson, P.C., & Welch, A.J. (1976). Detection of cyclic sleep phenomena using instantaneous heart rate. *Electroencephalography and Clinical Neurophysiology*, **40**, 169-177.

Matsumoto, J., Nishisho, T., Suto, T., Sadahiro, T., & Miyoshi, M. (1968). Influence of fatigue on sleep. *Nature*, **218**, 177-178.

Miller, J.C., & Horvath, S.M. (1976). Cardiac output during human sleep. *Aviation Space and Environmental Medicine*, **47**, 1046-1051.

Roussel, B., & Buguet, A. (1982). Changes in human heart rate during sleep following daily physical exercise. *European Journal of Applied Physiology*, **49**, 409-416.

Synder, F., Hobson, J.A., Morrison, D.F., & Goldfrank, F. (1964). Changes in respiration, heart rate, and systolic blood pressure in human sleep. *Journal of Applied Physiology* **19**, 417-422.

Walker, J.M., Floyd, T.C., Fein, G., Cavness, C., Lualhati, R., & Feinberg, I. (1978). Effects of exercise on sleep. *Journal of Applied Physiology, Respiratory, Environmental and Exercise Physiology,* **44**, 945-951.

24

The Effects of Long-Term Physical Training on the Aerobic Power of Middle-Aged and Elderly Japanese

Minoru Itoh, Kazuo Itoh, Tamotsu Yagi, and Chiyoko Takenaka
KYOTO UNIVERSITY
KYOTO, JAPAN

The average life span in Japan is nearly 80 years. Since World War II there has been a 30-year average increase in life span due to changes in lifestyle. At the beginning of the 21st century, 20% of the Japanese population will be over 60 years of age. It will be necessary for middle-aged and older people to improve their physical fitness levels so that they will not impose on the younger generation.

In previous studies using a treadmill and bicycle ergometer we checked the circulorespiratory system of middle-aged and older men and reported on their endurance fitness (Itoh, Itoh, Yagi, & Maeda, 1976). In this study we used ball games (mainly tennis) to interest subjects in training. Subjects trained for 10 years, beginning in 1974. Some subjects could not continue training, but most of them continued for more than 5 years. We will report the conclusions of that training program and the efficiency of long-term physical training using ball games.

Subjects and Method

Subjects were 16 healthy sedentary men, 36-65 years old, as shown in Table 1. The study continued for 10 years. The training period was for 8 months a year, from April to November with a 4-month rest period.

Table 1. Physical characteristics of subjects (before training)

Subject	Age (yr)	Height (cm)	Weight (kg)	Training period	Occupation
K.A.	36	164.9	53.0	1974-1983	Professor
M.S.	42	168.5	64.5	1979-1983	Professor
S.S.	40	170.8	62.0	1976-1981	Office worker
T.A.	43	174.5	56.5	1978-1983	Professor
T.Y.	39	168.0	58.0	1974-1983	Professor
Y.K.	44	165.0	59.7	1976-1983	Office worker
T.F.	41	167.0	52.0	1975-1983	Professor
S.M.	45	166.8	53.2	1974-1983	Professor
M.I.	42	166.5	51.5	1975-1983	Professor
K.H.	46	159.0	53.0	1975-1981	Professor
K.Y.	45	171.0	66.0	1975-1983	Professor
To.Y.	48	164.1	50.3	1975-1983	Professor
M.O.	49	170.0	64.5	1974-1983	Professor
M.T.	51	172.5	68.0	1976-1983	Professor
K.S.	55	163.1	58.0	1974-1982	Professor
S.A.	57	160.3	60.0	1975-1980	Professor

Subjects were measured for 18 physical fitness tests including a $\dot{V}O_2$max test. VO_2max was measured by the treadmill walking method.

To evaluate total physical fitness as a subject aged, the individual physical age (performance age) was calculated by using a tested formula from our previous study (Itoh & Itoh, 1978). Therefore, comparing physical age and chronological age, the subject's training effect was determined.

Training was held regularly for 1-1.5 hours at a time. The first half of the training session included warm-up and skill practice (ground stroke, volley, smash, service, etc.). The latter half was spent on game play (doubles and singles) and cool-down. Sometimes, subjects during training took an ECG test, using a Heartcorder (portable ECG recorder).

Results

Table 2 shows changes in physical fitness performance as a result of long-term training. Every subject trained for more than 5 years. At the same time this table shows the measurement of an individual subject's last training performance. Comparing the data before and after the 5-year training period, most performances increased slightly, but in two tests performances decreased. The average performance age (physical age) remained constant over a 5-year training period. Therefore, physical performance increased, because physical age remained the same. For the untrained individual, physical performance decreases naturally with age (Physical Fitness Laboratory, Tokyo Metropolitan University, 1975).

Table 2. Physical fitness performances before and after long-term training

Items measured		Before training Mean ± SD		after 5 years training Mean ± SD		After latest training Mean ± SD	
Height	(cm)	167.06 ±	4.12	166.77 ±	4.12	167.11 ±	3.88
Weight	(kg)	57.94 ±	5.57	58.25 ±	6.31	58.48 ±	6.17
Chest girth	(cm)	84.25 ±	3.23	84.45 ±	4.48	83.95 ±	2.85
Girth of upper arm	(cm)	25.45 ±	1.86	25.74 ±	2.18	25.26 ±	1.66
Girth of forearm	(cm)	25.01 ±	0.90	25.15 ±	0.81	25.30 ±	0.89
Grip strength (R)	(kg)	45.72 ±	6.43	45.44 ±	6.46	44.30 ±	5.69
Grip strength (L)	(kg)	40.63 ±	5.04	39.81 ±	5.13	39.40 ±	4.58
Back strength	(kg)	114.36 ±	14.85	120.69 ±	18.23	124.38 ±	18.38
Vertical jump	(cm)	49.75 ±	6.89	48.03 ±	6.88	45.33 ±	6.08
One foot balance (closed eye)	(sec)	46.75 ±	39.40	70.45 ±	43.41	84.80 ±	42.89
Standing trunk flexion	(cm)	6.36 ±	6.85	7.42 ±	8.21	5.96 ±	7.87
Resting heart rate	(beats/min)	66.69 ±	5.43	66.81 ±	7.08	67.07 ±	6.23
Blood pressure (high)	(mmHg)	114.75 ±	10.10	119.13 ±	10.29	116.53 ±	11.09
Blood pressure (low)	(mmHg)	74.50 ±	7.05	76.13 ±	6.73	74.00 ±	8.79
Pulse pressure	(mmHg)	40.25 ±	9.59	43.00 ±	9.51	42.53 ±	6.22
Vital capacity	(cc)	3,684.38 ±	496.35	3,613.13 ±	584.17	3,632.00 ±	537.84
Maximum ventilation	(l/min)	67.66 ±	9.31	79.38 ±	11.03	80.51 ±	16.57
Rate of oxygen intake	(%)	3.50 ±	0.47	3.55 ±	0.50	3.54 ±	0.49
Oxygen pulse	(ml)	12.83 ±	2.00	15.20 ±	2.25	15.28 ±	2.42
Max. heart rate	(beats/min)	182.81 ±	8.18	182.63 ±	8.11	181.20 ±	9.51
Recovery ratio	(%)	61.03 ±	7.44	64.71 ±	7.40	66.45 ±	4.66
Max. oxygen intake	(ml/min)	2,342.19 ±	381.22	2,779.56 ±	443.19	2,769.00 ±	454.07
VO₂max/body weight	(ml/kg•min)	40.66 ±	5.90	47.68 ±	5.72	47.78 ±	7.27
Age	(yrs)	46.13 ±	5.82	50.56 ±	5.17	52.67 ±	5.71
Physical age	(yrs)	46.571		45.730		46.724	

The average age of subjects was 51, but physical ages showed a 4-year decrease when compared with chronological ages. Subjects maintained or improved their performances during 5 years of training.

The training duration ranged from 5 to 10 years, with individual subjects beginning in different years. Comparing subject performances before and after training, the results showed no differences or only a slight change. Therefore, about the same physical age was maintained, especially for those who had trained for a prolonged time.

After training, an abnormality was found in subjects M.O. (aged 60) and A.S. (aged 63) in an ECG test. As their symptoms were not serious, they continued to train, with decreased loads. Subjects M.O. and A.S. were not allowed to do an exhaustive treadmill test.

Figure 1 shows each subject's yearly change in $\dot{V}O_2$max. The solid line indicates the training period and the dotted line shows the resting stage. $\dot{V}O_2$max increased during the training period and decreased during the resting term. So, every year there is an increase-decrease effect. In one subject, $\dot{V}O_2$max continued to decrease, but for the majority, the same level was maintained or was slightly increased. This figure shows the change in $\dot{V}O_2$max for seven subjects, all of the other subjects showed the same tendency. $\dot{V}O_2$max is an index of endurance ability. Even when people get older they can maintain or increase past endurance levels through training.

Figure 2 illustrates the change in vertical jump for seven subjects. Vertical jump measures human power. Power decreases inversely as age increases. This decrease cannot be stopped by training. Therefore, endurance performance can be maintained through training, but power performance decreases with age. Balance and agility performances are dependent on the individual. Almost all test data showed an increase in performance results for trained subjects compared to untrained subjects. Through regular training higher performance levels can be maintained.

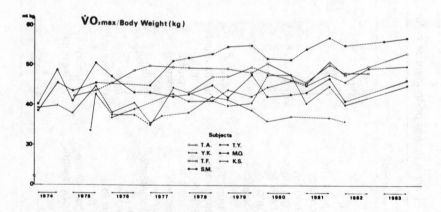

Figure 1. Effects of long-term physical training on $\dot{V}O_2$max

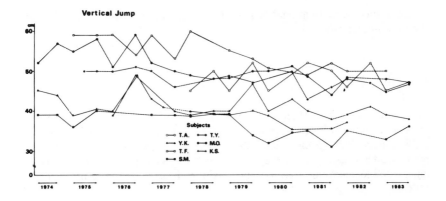

Figure 2. Effects of long-term physical training on vertical jump

Discussion

Usually physical endurance training is examined by walking, running, or bicycling. These forms of exercise are used because subjects can continue to train at a regular tempo and rate.

In this study tennis was chosen as the training load because all subjects were interested in the sport. For all subjects the training load was not consistent. To estimate the total training load, subject heart rates were taken during training, using a Heartcorder. The average heart rate for two beginners during exercise was 143 bpm and 152 bpm. During practices, player movement was recorded on a VTR. The heart rate of two advanced subjects was 10 bpm lower than for beginners. These subjects' real movement time was 42-46 minutes, almost half of the training time. This exercise load was sufficient for endurance training.

. Studies reported on endurance level increases due to training, especially VO_2max in middle-aged and older subjects (Hansen, Tabakin, Levy, & Neddle, 1968; Saltin, Hartley, Kilbom, & Åstrand, 1969; Ribisl, 1969; Pollock et al., 1970). Shindo, Tanaka, and Ohara (1974); Miyashita, Haga, and Mizuta (1974); and Matsui, Miyashita, Kobayashi, and Hoshikawa (1974) performed the same study using Japanese subjects, and they reported the same results. These studies were for a 1-2 year period. Shibayama and Ebashi (1976) reported a 10-year long-term study, using a treadmill wherein two subjects were examined for change in VO_2max. The last few years resulted in a decrease in VO_2max. In this study there was no decrease in VO_2max except for one subject. This was due to differences in exercise loads.

Sinning and Adrian (1968), using basketball training for female students, reported a 12.8% VO_2max increase. Kagaya (1975) found a slight VO_2max increase for volleyball training. By using jumprope, Ogawa, Furuta, Obara, and Tokuyama (1976) reported a 6.3% VO_2max increase. Generally, training by using sport is motivational, and subjects continue for many years because they are interested.

Conclusions

The middle-aged and elderly subjects' (36- to 65-year-old men) required physical training was tennis practice for 1 or 1.5 hours a day, twice a week for 8 months, from spring to autumn every year. Before and after the training periods, an exhaustive test was applied to each subject using the treadmill walking method to determine VO_2max and maximum heart rate. The results were as follows:

1. VO_2max showed a 17.2% increment after 5 years of training.
2. The average maximal heart rate in the exhaustive test was 180 bpm and did not change significantly after the training period.
3. The heart rate during exercise was about 150 bpm so practice was effective training for the circulatory system.
4. Performances in VO_2max increased for each subject, but results in the vertical jump decreased due to age.

From the above results, tennis as a means of training is considered to be effective for the improvement of aerobic power, in middle-aged and elderly men.

References

Hansen, J., Tabakin, B., Levy, A., & Neddle, W. (1968). Long-term physical training and cardiovascular dynamics in middle-aged men. *Circulation, 38*, 783-799.

Hartley, L.H., Grimby, G., Kilbom, A., Nilssen, N.J., Åstrand, I., Biure, J., Ekblom, B., & Saltin, B. (1969). Physical training in sedentary middle-aged and older men. III. *Scandanavian Journal of Clinical Laboratory Investigations, 24*, 335-344.

Itoh, M., & Itoh, K. (1978). The effect of training on the aerobic power of middle-aged and elderly Japanese. *Proceedings of F.I.M.S. Annual meeting in Brasilia.*

Itoh, M., Itoh, K., Yagi, T., & Maeda, K. (1976). Effects of physical training on the aerobic power of the middle and old aged. *Physical activity and human well-being* (Book 4, pp. 445-455). Quebec: Symposia Specialists.

Kagaya, J. (1975). The effects of endurance training on VO_2max for adult women. *Japanese Journal of Physical Fitness and Sports Medicine, 24*, 80-81.

Matsui, H., Miyashita, M., Kobayashi, K., & Hoshikawa, T. (1974). Effects of treadmill walking having intensity of 70% of the maximum oxygen intake on cardiovascular function in middle-aged men. *Report of Research Center in Physical Education, 2*, 197-206.

Miyashita, M., Haga, S., & Mizuta, T. (1974). Improvement in aerobic work capacity of middle-aged and old men. *Report of Research Center in Physical Education, 2*, 174-178.

Ogawa, S., Furuta, Y., Obara, T., & Tokuyama, K. (1976). Effects of rope skipping on aerobic work capacity of middle-aged persons. *Report of Research Center in Physical Education, 3*, 68-75.

Physical Fitness Laboratory, Tokyo Metropolitan University. (1975). *Physical fitness standards of Japanese people*. Tokyo: Fumaido.

Pollock, L.M., Miller, H.S., Janeway, R., Linnerud, A.C., Robertson, B., & Valentina, R. (1970). Effects of walking on body composition and cardiovascular function of middle-aged men. *Journal of Applied Physiology, 30*, 126-130.

Ribisl, P.M. (1969). Effects of training upon the maximal oxygen uptake of middle-aged men. *Int. Z. angew. Physiol., 27*, 154-160.

Saltin, B., Hartley, L., Kilbom, A., & Åstrand, I. (1969). Physical training in sedentary middle-aged and older men. II. *Journal of Clinical Laboratory Investigations, 24*, 323-334.

Shibayama, H., & Ebashi, H. (1976). A study on the effect of long-term physical training of adult men. *Bulletin of the Physical Fitness Research Institute, 34*, 1-9.

Shindo, M., Tanaka, H., & Ohara, S. (1974). Training of 50% VO₂max, 60 min on healthy middle-aged men. *Report of Research Center in Physical Education, 2*, 139-152.

Sinning, W.E., & Adrian, M.J. (1968). Cardiorespiratory changes in college women due to season of competitive basketball. *Journal of Applied Physiology, 25*, 720-724.

25

The Effects of Exercise on Bone Morphometry and Calcium Concentration in the Ovariectomized Rat

Roberta L. Pohlman, Lynn A. Darby, and Andrew J. Lechner
ST. LOUIS UNIVERSITY SCHOOL OF MEDICINE
ST. LOUIS, MISSOURI, USA

Osteoporosis, or decreased total bone mass, is due to the deterioration of cellular activities controlling bone synthesis and degradation with age (Avioli, 1983). Postmenopausal women are especially susceptible to this bone loss with the severity of the condition being correlated with years past menopause rather than total age (Avioli, 1983). Osteoporosis is accelerated with the cessation of estrogen production and thus estrogen is therapeutically prescribed to retard this loss (Avioli, 1983; Lindsay, Hart, Forrest, & Baird, 1980). However, a concern over the close association between certain uterine cancers and estrogen administration has caused many women to seek alternatives.

Exercise may expand the bone calcium pool by increasing bone calcium deposition (Dalen & Olsson, 1974). Although exercise therapy has previously been prescribed for older women, the duration and intensity levels remain largely undefined, and its efficiency in promoting bone calcium retention has been indirectly estimated (Smith, Reddan, & Smith, 1981; Brewer, Meyer, Keele, Upton, & Hagan, 1983).

The rat model provides a useful approximation of human responses and allows for more thorough invasive investigation. Decreased bone calcium was reported in young (21-day-old) as well as mature (1-year-old) sedentary rats within 4 months of ovariectomy (Saville, 1969; Wink & Felts, 1980). Some direct bone measurements have previously been reported in young nonovariectomized exercised rats (Saville & Whyte, 1969), but skeletal calcium has only been estimated after voluntary exercise for mature animals (LeBlanc, Evans, Johnson, & Jhingran, 1983). The purpose of this study was to assess the responses of ovariectomized retired-breeder female rats following a 4-month moderate forced exercise program and to directly measure bone calcium and other appropriate parameters in axial and appendicular skeletal elements.

Method

Female Sprague-Dawley rats (8-9 month retired-breeders, Charles River) were placed into eight groups: ovariectomy (O) or control (C); exercise (E) or sedentary (S); and length of treatment—2 or 4 months. Animals were caged separately at 25°C and were provided food and water *ad libitum*. All rats initially ran on a level calibrated treadmill at 8 m/min for 10-15 min/day for 3 days to acquaint each animal with the treadmill and to remove those animals refusing to run. Exercise duration and running speed were then gradually increased over 8 days for the exercising groups to 1 hour/day, 5 days/week, at a speed of 14.1 m/min and 8° elevation, or 2.62 miles/week.

Under sodium pentobarbital (30 mg/kg, i.p.), body weights and snout-to-anus lengths were obtained, and a 6 ml heparinized blood sample was drawn from the abdominal vena cava. After sacrifice by pneumothorax, left femurs, tibia/fibula complexes, thoracic ribs (T7), and vertebrae (T7) were carefully excised, cleaned, blotted, and weighed. The length and diameter of each bone was measured ($\pm$ 0.02 mm), its volume determined by fluid displacement ($\pm$ 0.01 ml), and its density calculated per gram of fresh weight. Bones were dried to constant weight in a vacuum lyophilizer without freezing the bones to prevent artifactual fractures. Tensile strength of left femurs was measured using an Instron Universal Testing Instrument in which the femurs were pulled longitudinally to the point of failure at a separating speed of 0.25 mm/min (Dickenson, Hutton, & Stott, 1981).

All bones, including femurs, were crushed and rinsed with saline to quantitatively remove saline soluble proteins and calcium. After centrifugation, the pellets were rinsed three times with distilled water, redried, and completely acid hydrolyzed in 5N HC1. Samples of plasma, saline extracts, and neutralized acid hydrolysates were assayed for calcium concentration using cresolphthalein indicator at 575 nm. Plasma alkaline phosphatase activity was measured on a Gilford Instruments System 102 (Gilford Diagnostics) at 405 nm at 30°C in the absorbance mode.

All data were reported as means $\pm$ SEM. Differences among the 2-month and 4-month groups were analyzed using a three-way ANOVA and the Tukey test for unconfounded means, with significance established at the 0.05 level.

Results

Although mature, all animals continued to gain weight during the course of the experiment. Significant treatment differences only existed at 2 months, when sedentary and ovariectomized groups weighed more than their exercise and control counterparts (see Table 1). Whereas proportional growth would yield similar values for $(BW)^{1/3}/SA$ among groups, this ratio increased in the OS groups compared to controls. Again by 4 months, these differences in shape were not evident (see Table 1).

At 2 months, only femoral bone density of the control group was significantly greater than for ovariectomized animals. Within 4 months, femoral density was greater in the control sedentary and exercising animals when compared to their ovariectomized counterparts (see Table 2). Exercise did not appreciably alter the remaining bone morphometrics, whereas ovariectomy did. At 4 months, both tibial/fibular bone densities and vertebral volumes were greater for control groups compared to ovariectomized animals. Rib density was significantly decreased only at 2 months postovariectomy.

Femur and tibial bone [Ca] increased as a result of exercise in both control and ovariectomized animals at 2 months (see Figure 1). This is a first indication of the possible beneficial effects of exercise on this parameter in an ovariectomized animal. However, at 4 months, ovariectomy induced significant losses in most appendicular bones of the sedentary and exercised animals. Thus, ovariectomy at 4 months may have overwhelmed the beneficial effects of exercise observed at 2 months. Axial bone [Ca] decreased at 2 months in the exercised control and the ovariectomized animals when compared to sedentary controls, but within 4 months these bones had either recovered to control [Ca] levels or significantly increased their concentration levels. Four months of exercise, therefore, tended to maintain or to increase bone calcium levels in the ovariectomized animals.

When bone calcium contents, rather than [Ca], are considered (see Table 3), control sedentary and exercised animals demonstrated increased appendicular bone calcium contents when compared to their ovariectomized counterparts. For the axial bones, the effects of exercise, not ovariectomy, were again apparent as increased calcium contents were observed in all 4-month exercised animals.

Table 1. Gross body measurements at sacrifice in exercised and sedentary rats[a]

Group	(n)	BW (g)	SA (cm)	$(BW)^{1/3}/SA$ (g/cm)
CS2	6	339 ± 13	22.9 ± 0.18	0.30 ± 0.003
OS2	8	430 ± 14	23.6 ± 0.19	0.31 ± 0.002
CE2	8	327 ± 10	22.7 ± 0.31	0.30 ± 0.002
OE2	7	387 ± 13	23.2 ± 0.37	0.31 ± 0.002
CS4	7	393 ± 42	23.6 ± 0.41	0.30 ± 0.007
OS4	8	425 ± 16	23.6 ± 0.20	0.31 ± 0.003
CE4	9	385 ± 11	23.8 ± 0.14	0.30 ± 0.002
OE4	7	399 ± 10	23.7 ± 0.26	0.30 ± 0.004

By ANOVA: S2 > E2   O2 > C2
($p < .05$)   O2 > C2
[a]Values presented above and in subsequent tables are $M \pm$ SEM.

Table 2. Bone morphometrics of the appendicular and axial skeleton

Group	(n)	Volume (ml)	Density (g/ml)	Volume (ml)	Density (g/ml)
		Femur		Tibia/fibula	
CS2	6	0.58 ± 0.013	1.62 ± 0.042	0.47 ± 0.014	1.62 ± 0.015
OS2	8	0.59 ± 0.009	1.57 ± 0.024	0.49 ± 0.024	1.57 ± 0.059
CE2	8	0.57 ± 0.016	1.60 ± 0.027	0.48 ± 0.081	1.56 ± 0.031
OE2	7	0.60 ± 0.018	1.54 ± 0.013	0.49 ± 0.018	1.53 ± 0.021
CS4	7	0.62 ± 0.025	1.62 ± 0.039	0.51 ± 0.020	1.60 ± 0.020
OS4	8	0.64 ± 0.013	1.48 ± 0.026	0.53 ± 0.011	1.51 ± 0.032
CE4	9	0.63 ± 0.015	1.62 ± 0.028	0.52 ± 0.008	1.58 ± 0.025
OE4	7	0.60 ± 0.010	1.60 ± 0.017	0.50 ± 0.015	1.58 ± 0.036
By ANOVA: ($p < .05$)		OS4 > OE4 OS4 > CS4	CS4 > OS4 CE4 > OE4 C2 > O2		CS4 > OS4
		Thoracic vertebra		Thoracic rib	
CS2	6	0.10 ± 0.010	1.08 ± 0.09	0.04 ± 0.005	1.78 ± 0.18
OS2	8	0.10 ± 0.008	1.13 ± 0.08	0.07 ± 0.007	1.14 ± 0.11
CE2	8	0.09 ± 0.006	1.21 ± 0.08	0.05 ± 0.005	1.43 ± 0.19
OE2	7	0.09 ± 0.008	1.28 ± 0.08	0.06 ± 0.004	1.30 ± 0.10
CS4	7	0.10 ± 0.009	1.26 ± 0.12	0.06 ± 0.004	1.16 ± 0.13
OS4	8	0.09 ± 0.004	1.35 ± 0.10	0.06 ± 0.005	1.33 ± 0.12
CE4	9	0.11 ± 0.007	1.16 ± 0.07	0.06 ± 0.005	1.45 ± 0.10
OE4	6	0.09 ± 0.008	1.47 ± 0.13	0.09 ± 0.008	1.34 ± 0.16
By ANOVA: ($p < .05$)		C4 > O4	O4 > C4	OS2 > CS2 O2 > E2	C2 > O2

Values for plasma alkaline phosphatase were found to be significantly greater in the ovariectomized animals only at 2 months (see Table 3). Within 4 months plasma [Ca] values were more affected by exercise than ovariectomy (mean for all 4-month exercising animals = 9.0 ± 0.61 mg/dl greater than all 4-month sedentary animals = 6.6 ± 0.82 mg/dl). Exercise and ovariectomy had no significant effects on the tensile strength of the femurs in these mature animals (mean for all 2-month animals = 1.2 ± 0.21 N/m²; mean for all 4-month animals = 1.1 ± 0.25 N/m²).

Discussion

Bone calcium contents and concentrations of these mature female rats increased for all exercise groups when compared to sedentary controls (see Table 3 and Figure 1). Saville (1969) reported axial and appendicular calcium content increases in growing rats after exercise, due to increased bone volume without

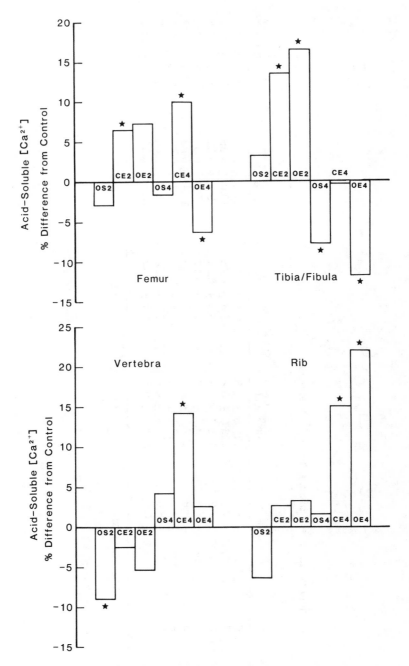

Figure 1. Acid-soluble [Ca²⁺] for the femur, tibia/fibula, vertebra, and rib. All groups were compared with their appropriate 2- or 4-month control group (CS2 or CS4). Bars are recorded as % difference from control with significance (*) at the $p < 0.05$ level.

Table 3. Total calcium contents and plasma alkaline phosphatase values

| Group | (n) | Calcium content (mg) | | | | Alkaline phosphatase (IU) |
		Femur	Tibia/fibula	Rib	Vertebra	
CS2	6	139.1 ± 6.5	101.5 ± 6.5	9.4 ± 0.37	11.0 ± 0.33	47.3 ± 11.0
OS2	7	137.2 ± 7.8	106.0 ± 6.2	8.9 ± 0.46	10.0 ± 0.36	84.4 ± 14.5
CE2	8	148.9 ± 7.2	113.7 ± 4.9	9.3 ± 0.74	9.9 ± 0.55	61.7 ± 7.5
OE2	6	152.5 ± 7.2	118.7 ± 4.3	10.1 ± 0.59	9.8 ± 0.63	70.8 ± 11.3
CS4	6	147.8 ± 8.8	127.1 ± 4.3	9.9 ± 0.99	11.4 ± 0.89	49.1 ± 11.3
OS4	8	146.8 ± 4.2	118.5 ± 4.3	10.4 ± 0.61	11.4 ± 0.50	52.3 ± 5.2
CE4	8	164.9 ± 6.0	129.4 ± 4.9	12.8 ± 0.82	13.9 ± 0.82	49.4 ± 6.2
OE4	7	132.8 ± 3.9	111.3 ± 5.5	11.5 ± 1.02	12.2 ± 0.54	75.1 ± 11.9
By ANOVA: ($p < .05$)		CE4 > OE4	C4 > O4 E2 > S2	E4 > S4	E4 > S4	O2 > C2

a change in density. In the present study, increased calcium concentration together with an increase in bone volume of the four bones better account for the increased calcium contents observed (see Table 3).

Ovariectomy reduced the density of the long bones after 4 months, but not the axial bones (see Table 2), such that the combination of exercise and ovariectomy was either beneficial or detrimental, depending on the bone being assessed. Two months of exercise was apparently beneficial for initiating [Ca] increases in the appendicular bones for both the CE2 and OE2 groups when compared to CS2 (see Figure 1). However, after 4 months, a significant reduction in [Ca] was apparent for the OE4 group in both long bones with minimal change in the CE4 group. Because the loss of bone mass is accelerated in the postmenopausal state (Avioli, 1983), the effects of ovariectomy may have superseded the beneficial effects of exercise in the appendicular bones (OE2 > OE4). Calcium content of the axial bones increased after 4 months of exercise when compared to sedentary animals, and [Ca] increased significantly even with ovariectomy when compared to controls.

Although osteoporosis produces no specific biochemical signal alkaline phosphatase may be elevated, indicative of osteoblastic activity in the acute bone-losing stages (Avioli, 1983). Despite great variability among groups, the 2-month ovariectomized animals had significantly higher values when compared to controls (see Table 3). Alkaline phosphatase activities stabilized by 4 months (CS4 = OS4) but were still greater in the OE4 group when compared to CE4. These data suggest that in the OE4 group, training was retarding bone loss and deposition of bone was increasing. Differences in the rates of mineral loss and remodeling between the axial and appendicular bones may explain the differences in adaptation observed (Wink & Felts, 1980).

As a main effect on bone calcium, all animals benefited from exercise when compared to their sedentary counterparts. Ovariectomization produced significant decreases in [Ca] and contents in the femur and tibia/fibula within 4 months. The moderate exercise program appeared to be of some benefit to the femur, but not the tibia/fibula. In the axial bones, calcium content was increased over time in the OE groups. These encouraging results suggest that calcium losses in the appendicular bones may have stabilized or reversed with a longer training program.

References

Avioli, L.V. (Ed.). (1983). *The osteoporotic syndrome: Detection, prevention, and treatment*. New York: Grune & Stratton.

Brewer, V., Meyer, B.M., Keele, M.S., Upton, S.J., & Hagan, R.D. (1983). Role of exercise in prevention of involutional bone loss. *Medicine and Science for Sports and Exercise,* **15**, 445-449.

Dalen, N., & Olsson, K.E. (1974). Bone mineral content and physical activity. *Acta Orthopaedica Scandinavica,* **45**, 170-174.

Dickenson, R.P., Hutton, W.C., & Stott, J.R.R. (1981). The mechanical properties of bone in osteoporosis. *Journal of Bone Joint Surgery,* **63B**, 233-238.

LeBlanc, A.D., Evans, J.H., Johnson, P.C., & Jhingran, S. (1983). Changes in total body calcium balance with exercise in rats. *Journal of Applied Physiology Respiratory, Environmental Exerercise Physiology,* **55**, 201-204.

Lindsay, R., Hart, D.M., Forrest, C.F., & Baird, C. (1980). Prevention of spinal osteoporosis in oophorectomized women. *The Lancet,* **2**(8205), 1151-1154.

Saville, P.D. (1969). Changes in skeletal mass and fragility with castration in the rat. A model of osteoporosis. *Journal of American Geriatric Society,* **17**, 155-166.

Saville, P.D., & Whyte, M.P. (1969). Muscle and bone hypertrophy. Positive effect of running exercise in the rat. *Clinical Orthopedic Related Research,* **65**, 81-88.

Smith, E.L., Reddan, W., & Smith, P.E. (1981). Physical activity and calcium modalities for bone mineral increase in aged women. *Medicine and Science for Sports and Exercise,* **13**, 60-64.

Wink, C.S., & Felts, W.J.L. (1980). Effects of castration on the bone structure of male rats: A model of osteoporosis. *Calcification of Tissue International,* **32**, 77-82.

26

Observations on Selected Physiological Responses of Older Performers Using Intermittent Gravity Traction

Loarn D. Robertson, Barbara Riley,
and Christine Kauppi
PORTLAND STATE UNIVERSITY
PORTLAND, OREGON, USA

The practice of inverting the body by using gravity boots or an inversion exerciser has attracted over one million users (Klatz, Goldman, Pinchuk, Nelson, & Tarr, 1983). Popular magazines and sales marketing literature extol the many virtues of using inversion techniques, which include improvements to circulation, posture, and back pain relief. Over the past year observations were made on the reactions of men and women exercising on an inversion system while totally inverted and oscillating to a set rhythm under voluntary control, which was called intermittent gravity traction (IGT). The use of rhythmical oscillations of the body has been advocated for older persons in order to improve circulation, to stimulate spinal tissues, and to promote relaxation (Martin, 1982). Yet no objective information was found to help evaluate IGT as a form of exercise. The purpose of this study was to document systemic blood pressure (BP), pulse rate, heart rate (HR), and trunk flexor muscle responses of older subjects performing an IGT exercise protocol. Subjects were 21 paid volunteers and included 14 women and 7 men 35 years and over. The means $\pm$ SDs for age, height, and weight were 43.2 $\pm$ 8.9 yr, 166.6 $\pm$ 7.4 cm, and 64.5 $\pm$

This study was supported by Portland State University Grant #90 050 5801 LRA. The authors are indebted to Dr. John T. Scott, Jr. of the University of Illinois for his advice with the statistical portion of this paper. Finally, our sincere appreciation to the volunteers for their help and interest.

9.8 kg for the sample. Volunteers signed informed consent forms and identified themselves as healthy. Subjects were required to participate on 3 alternate days (D1, D2, and D3) for one week. On D1 standing height, weight,
and sitting systemic BP and pulse rate were taken to obtain baseline records,
and subjects completed an activity questionnaire and a 24-hour inventory.
Twenty-four hour inventories were also completed on D2 and D3. Instruction
and practice of the IGT protocol was provided for each subject on D1. On
D2 standing height and weight were recorded again and electrocardiograms
(ECGs), systemic BP, and pulse rate were taken before, during, and after the
IGT exercise protocol. On D3 systemic BP was taken before, during, and after
the IGT exercise protocol together with electromyograms (EMGs) of the rectus abdominis (RA) and rectus femoris (RF) muscles. Subjects were also asked
to provide, via questionnaire, personal impressions of the IGT protocol.

Methods

IGT Exercise Protocol

Subjects were required to lie supine on the bed of the inversion exerciser with
ankles secured firmly. By using flexion and extension motions of the shoulder
joint, elbows extended, and fingers interlocked, subjects were able to actively
control each oscillation on the inversion exerciser from a foot down (FD) position of $+25°$ to a horizontal (H) position of $0°$, to a head down (HD) position
of $-25°$ and back again. The H position on the inversion exerciser was determined from a spirit level and a Leighton Flexometer, attached to the exerciser, was zeroed at this point. Repeated trials were used to establish the FD
and HD positions ($+25°$ and $-25°$) from the Leighton Flexometer, and blocks
were placed at the appropriate locations together with a mechanical pointer
at the H position. An operator could then visualize the FD, H, and HD positions as subjects oscillated continuously between the blocks to an audible beat
from an electrically controlled metronome. One IGT oscillation took 14.50
sec, and subjects were required to complete 3 sets of 20 oscillations with a
1-minute rest, lying horizontal, following each set on D1, D2, and D3.

Systemic BP and Pulse Rate

Indirect measures of systemic BP and pulse rate were taken with an Astropulse
99 Digital Sphygmomanometer attached to each subject's left arm. BP and
pulse rate were measured 7 times on D2 and D3. Two preexercise BP readings
were taken 5 minutes after quiet sitting (pre-S), and 5 minutes after horizontal
lying on the inversion exerciser (pre-H). Postexercise readings were taken immediately after each IGT exercise set while horizontal (post-1, post-2, post-3).
Two recovery readings were taken 5 minutes following the third IGT set while
still horizontal (rec-H), and 2 minutes after the rec-H reading while seated
(rec-S). Within day reliability coefficients for systolic and diastolic BP and
pulse rate mean values for 10 subjects (pre-S) were 0.92, 0.90, and 0.61 (r
.05, 8 = .63). Using paired t-tests no significant differences ($p > .05$) were
found between test-retest within-day means for both systemic BP and pulse rate.

ECG

Standard procedures were used in preparing and connecting V6 and ground leads for each subject. Samples of heart activity were taken at rest in the H position before and after each IGT exercise set, and after 5 minutes of recovery. In addition, samples were taken during oscillations 16, 17, and 18 of each IGT set. Visualization of FD, H, HD, H, and FD positions within each oscillation were made by the ECG operator and corresponding reference marks made on the ECG record with an event marker. HR activity was analyzed within 4 phases constructed from referenced positions and these were: (1) FD-H, (2) H-HD, (3) HD-H, and (4) H-FD. Calculations of HR were made from displacements between R wave maximum amplitudes (Winsor, 1977). The average number of beats per minute (bpm) for oscillations 16, 17, and 18 was calculated for each phase for each set and used for later statistical analyses.

EMG

Standard procedures were used in preparing and connecting bipolar silver-silver chloride surface electrodes over the right lower RA and RF muscles of each subject. ECG artifact could not be eliminated from EMG records. In order to differentiate between ECG artifact and EMG, subjects were asked to contract and relax RA and RF muscles prior to the IGT protocol. The presence of EMG was established when continuous amplitudes greater than 1 mm above the isoelectric line were found. EMG records were inspected for evidence of EMG activity from samples taken while subjects lay at rest in the H position before and after each IGT exercise set, after 5 minutes of recovery following the IGT protocol, and within the 4 IGT phases (FD-H, H-HD, HD-H, and H-FD) described above for oscillations 16, 17, and 18 within each set. Average proportions of EMG activity were calculated within each IGT phase for each set across oscillations 16, 17, and 18 and all subjects and used for later descriptive purposes.

Statistical Procedures

Of interest were pre- and postIGT changes to systemic BP and pulse rate over trials. In addition, ECG and EMG records were analyzed for changes in HR and evidence of trunk flexor muscular activity during IGT exercise. Two-way analysis of variance and trend analysis were applied to systemic BP, pulse rate, and HR. Tukey (HSD) tests were used to identify significant mean differences across trials when significant F-ratios were found. EMG records were inspected for evidence of RA and RF muscular activity during IGT exercise. Statistical significance was set at the 0.05 level.

Results

Mechanical problems and irregular physiological responses from some subjects resulted in incomplete data for some variables. Systemic BP and pulse rate data collected on D2 were used for analysis. Two-way ANOVAs indicated significant differences ($p < .01$) between systemic systolic and diastolic BP trial means. Posthoc *t*-tests showed that the mean systolic value for Trial 1 (pre-S) was significantly larger ($p < .05$) than Trials 3, 4, and 5 (post-1, post-2, and post-3) means and was still significantly larger than Trial 6 (rec-H) mean (Table 1). There was a 10.7% drop in systolic BP between pre-S and post-2 representing the greatest mean change. Tests on mean differences for diastolic BP showed that Trial 1 (pre-S) was significantly larger ($p < .05$) than Trials 3 and 4 (post-1 and post-2) (Table 1). In addition, Trial 7's (rec-S) mean was significantly larger ($p < .05$) than Trials 3, 4, 5, and 6 (post-1, post-2, post-3, and rec-H) means. There was a 12.3% change between rec-S and post-2 representing the greatest mean difference in diastolic BP. *F*-ratios for pulse rate were not statistically significant ($p > .05$), perhaps due to the poor reliability of the procedure.

ECG

Percentage mean differences between the 3 IGT sets showed only small differences (0.6-3.2%) between the same phases (FD-H, H-HD, HD-H, and H-FD). Therefore, Set 2 was chosen as representative of IGT exercise HR responses and further statistical analysis was carried out on data from this set. The two-way ANOVA indicated that there were significant ($p < .01$) differences between trial means (pre-H, FD-H, H-HD, H-FD, post-2, rec-H). Of the exercise HR means only Trials 4's (HD-H) mean was not significantly greater ($p > .05$) than pre-, post-, or recovery HR means (Table 2). Trial 2 (FD-H) showed a significantly higher ($p < .05$) HR mean than all other means and was 19% higher than the lowest HR response found at rec-H. Generally, the exercise HR means for each set rose and fell about 10 bpm per oscillation.

Orthogonal comparisons analysis on systemic BP, pulse rate, and HR revealed significant ($p < .01$) quadratic effects for trial means indicating strong curvilinear trends for the trials (Edwards, 1967).

EMG

No activity greater than 1 mm was found during pre-, post-, or recovery IGT exercise stages for any subject. No consistent electrical activity was found for RF within the study sample. Careful inspection of EMG records for RA re-

Table 1. Systemic systolic and diastolic BP for pre-, post-, and recovery IGT[+] exercise ($n = 15$)

	Trials[Δ]						
	1	2	3	4	5	6	7
Systolic blood pressure (mm Hg)	116.4* ±4.5	108.8 ±4.9	105.7 ±4.1	105.2 ±4.5	106.9 ±4.9	106.5 ±4.5	111.8 ±3.3
Diastolic blood pressure (mm Hg)	75.6* ±2.7	70.9 ±3.9	68.8 ±3.9	68.4 ±3.9	70.3 ±2.5	70.3 ±3.1	76.8* ±3.9

Values are $M \pm SE$
[Δ]1 = pre-S, 2 = pre-H, 3 = post-1, 4 = post-2, 5 = post-3, 6 = rec-H, 7 = rec-S
[+]intermittent gravity traction
*$p < 0.05$

vealed consistent patterns of electrical activity between each IGT exercise phase for each set. Figure 1 shows the average proportions of electrical activity for RA for each phase within Set 2. Toward the end of the FD-H phase (last 16%)

Table 2. HRs before, during and after IGT+ exercise ($n = 18$)

	Trials△						
	1	2	3	4	5	6	7
Heart rate (BPM)	67.8 ±2.8	77.2* ±2.9	71.2* ±2.7	67.9 ±2.3	72.2* ±2.5	67.9 ±2.3	64.8 ±2.1

Values are $M \pm SE$
△1 = pre-H, 2 = FD-H, 3 = H-HD, 4 = HD-H, 5 = H-FD, 6 = post-2, 7 = rec-H
+intermittent gravity traction
*$p < 0.05$

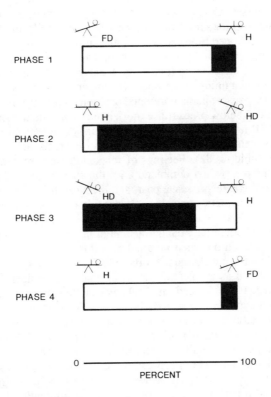

Figure 1. EMG pattern of muscular activity for the rectus abdominis between intermittent gravity traction phases. Positions between phases are: FD-H—foot down to horizontal; H-HD—horizontal to head down; HD-H—head down to horizontal; and H-FD—horizontal to foot down. Shaded areas represent average (for 18 subjects) amount of EMG activity (expressed as a percentage) for each phase.

a burst of abdominal activity was seen that was probably due to necessary control over increasing momentum of the exerciser initiated by the arm motions from the FD position. From H to HD most of that phase (91%) showed continuous electrical activity corresponding to increased stretch of the abdominals as the head was lowered under control of the arms to the HD position. From HD to H electrical activity was observed over 71% of that phase and was thought to be a concentric contraction required to help initiate and sustain reverse momentum of the exerciser toward the H position. The final phase H-FD showed, on average, electrical activity over the last 9.1% of that phase, which we suspect was due to those subjects who were required to flex the trunk slightly in order to achieve the FD position.

Discussion

The rapid changes to HR during IGT exercise suggests that reflex activity may be responsible for those changes. Alterations to blood flow dynamics as described by Asmussen, Christensen, and Nielsen (1940) and Guyton (1966) combined with baroreceptor stimulation (Lamb & Roman, 1961) may be associated with the aforementioned reflex activity. Both sympathetic and parasympathetic reflexes have been intimately associated with inactive head-up and head-down tilting (Lamb & Roman, 1961), with the latter reflex being of considerable importance in maintaining homeostasis (Heiniger & Randolph, 1981). Post-IGT exercise responses, in the horizontal position, show systolic and diastolic mean values at or below preexercise (horizontal) levels demonstrating steady control over BP in the horizontal position. Further, the mean recovery HR response falls below pre- or post-IGT exercise levels approaching sinus bradycardia (Dubin, 1982). Feelings of relaxation were reported by nearly 80% of the sample, which combined with the steady, or slightly lowered, systemic BP and HR responses at post- and recovery from IGT exercise suggests that parasympathetic control is dominant. In contrast, recent inactive inversion studies by Klatz et al. (1983) and LeMarr, Golding, and Crehan (1983) suggest rapid and potentially dangerous initial increases in systemic BP with no immediate adaptation when inverted at $-90°$.

The use of inversion techniques for those with certain types of hypertension has been advocated as a potential means of control (Heiniger & Randolph, 1981; Steingard, 1983). Indeed, medical advice to the lay public suggests that those with mild hypertension may derive no benefits from long-term drug use and that exercise, as part of an overall change in lifestyle, may play a more prominent part in restoring normal responses (DeVries, 1982; Sheehan, 1983). Perhaps reductions in overall systemic BP for those with essential hypertension may be found with continued extensive use of IGT or at least provide limited relief to hypertension. If, as Heiniger and Randolph suggest, chronic hypertension is in part due to lack of appropriate stimulation of the carotid sinus, IGT may provide more acceptable levels of stimulation compared to those experienced during inactive total body inversion (Klatz et al., 1983; LeMarr et al., 1983).

The regular patterns of electrical activity for the RA suggest that IGT may offer a potential source of exercise stimulus for those with weakened abdominals. For those with low back syndrome a popular method for isolating RA muscles during a sit-up is to perform posterior pelvic tilt with flexed knees and hips in a supine position without foot support (Caillet, 1976). The practice of performing sit-ups with legs straight in the supine position is thought to develop an increased lordotic curve due to the lines of pull of the hip flexor muscles and resulting anterior inclination of the pelvis combined with the physiological advantage offered by the initial length of the hip flexors (Kelley, 1982). Straight leg sit-ups are, therefore, considered to be risky (Kelley, 1982) due to potential weakening of low back structures. Because this study found no consistent RF muscular activity in the supine position during IGT, the potential for low back misalignments due to RF activity may be minimized.

It is necessary to echo the words of some physicians (Klatz et al., 1983; Steingard, 1983) who worry about potential risks to members of the public who have early or silent heart conditions and who wish to engage in inversion activities. In this study two subjects were found to be present with premature ventricular contractions (PVCs) during ECG analysis. One subject demonstrated runs of trigeminy in response to IGT exercise considered pathological (Dubin, 1982). In another study (Lamb & Roman, 1961) heart arrhythmias and sinus bardycardias were noted in 215 of 224 subjects who were exposed to $+g$ (foot down) followed by $-g$ (head down) body tilting. Most arrythmias were considered harmless and were detected during a period of cardiac slowing (head down), and one subject demonstrated runs of bigeminy during this cardiac-inhibited phase (Lamb & Roman, 1961). In this study PVCs were observed in all phases of IGT exercise but then disappeared after 5 minutes of recovery.

The evidence presented in this study tentatively suggests that active IGT may provide some older performers with a sense of reduced effort combined with mild abdominal exercise and reductions to or maintenance of both BP and HR immediately following exercise.

References

Asmussen, E., Christensen, E.H., & Nielsen, M. (1940). The regulation of circulation in different postures. *Surgery,* **8**, 604-616.

Caillet, R. (1976). *Low back pain syndrome*. Philadelphia: Davis.

DeVries, H.A. (1982). On exercise for relieving anxiety and tension. *Executive Health,* **18**, 12.

Dubin, D. (1982). *Rapid interpretation of EKGs*. Tampa: Cover.

Edwards, A. (1967). *Statistical methods*. New York: Holt, Rinehart & Winston.

Guyton, A.C. (1966). *Textbook of medical physiology*. Philadelphia: Saunders.

Heiniger, M.C., & Randolph, S.L. (1981). *Neurophysiological concepts in human behavior—The tree of learning*. St. Louis: Mosby.

Kelley, D.L. (1982). Exercise prescription and the kinesiological imperative. *Journal of Health, Physical Education, Recreation and Dance,* **53**, 18-20.

Klatz, R.M., Goldman, R.M., Pinchuk, B.G., Nelson, K.E., & Tarr, R.S. (1983). The effect of gravity inversion procedures on systemic blood pressure, intraocular pressure and central retinal arterial pressure. *Journal of the American Osteopathic Association,* **82**, 853/111-857/115.

Lamb, L.E., & Roman, J. (1961). The head-down tilt and adaptability for aerospace flight. *Aerospace Medicine, 32,* 473-486.

LeMarr, J.D., Golding, L.A., & Crehan, K.D. (1983). Cardiorespiratory responses to inversion. *The Physician and Sports Medicine, 11,* 51-57.

Martin, R.M. (1982). *The gravity guiding system.* Pasadena, CA: Gravity Guidance.

Sheehan, G. (1983). Easing the pressure. *Runners World, 18,* 93.

Steingard, P.M. (1983). Importance of documenting effects of gravity inversion procedures. *Journal of American Osteopathic Association, 82,* 817/63.

Winsor, T. (1977). The electrocardiogram in myocardial infarction. *Clinical Symposia, 29,* 3-29.

27

The Physical Fitness Ages of Middle-Aged and Old People in Relation to Motor Fitness

Eitaro Nakamura
KYOTO UNIVERSITY
KYOTO, JAPAN

Yasuko Hatasa
SEIAN WOMEN'S COLLEGE
KYOTO, JAPAN

The purpose of health administration for the aged is not to extend their life span but to prevent diseases and to suggest ways that will enable them to spend their daily lives actively (Shephard, 1978; Schettler, 1972). In this regard, it is very important to understand the rate of deterioration of physical fitness with age. The present study was undertaken in an attempt to characterize the prediction of "Physical Fitness Age" as an index of aging with special reference to physical fitness.

Methods

Subjects

The subjects were 453 healthy men (ages 20-69). Seventy-nine of these subjects participated in a training program on the basis of calisthenics and jogging twice a week for a period of 3 to 5 years at a YMCA.

Test Items and Procedures

Analysis of the literature relating to the physical fitness tests for middle-aged and old people resulted in the empirical selection of test items that best fit in estimating physical fitness age. The nine tests selected for use in this study are as follows:

1. grip strength (right hand);
2. grip strength (left hand);
3. back strength;
4. vital capacity;
5. standing trunk flexion;
6. one foot balance—eyes closed;
7. vertical jump;
8. side step; and
9. sit-ups—time limit.

These tests were administered to the subjects according to the procedures of the Adult Physical Fitness Test by Meshizuka and Nagata (1969) and Matsushima (1968). Scores for these 9 tests were the better of two trials.

Mathematical Model

The groundwork for the study will be found in a previous article giving the mathematical expression for the assessment of biological age (Furukawa et al., 1975). For the generation of a reference value of aging with special reference to physical fitness, a linear regression given by the following form was used:

$$y_i = a_o + \sum_{j=1}^{k} a_j x_{ij}, \, i = 1, 2, \cdots, n$$

where y_i is the estimated age of the subject i and x_{ij} stands for the scores of motor fitness test j of the subject, while a_j $(j = 0, 1, \cdots, k)$ are unknown parameters to be estimated, and n is the sample size.

Results

Figure 1 shows the age regression for the nine motor fitness tests and height and weight. In order to compare tests with different units of measurements, all curves, being drawn through the mean test score of each age group, have been plotted as percentage deviations from the mean values of the 20-24 age group. The curves, except for those of height (1) and weight (2), decreased remarkably as age advanced. However, the rates of change with age varied greatly for different tests.

In order to select the variables applicable to the estimation of physical fitness age from the nine motor fitness tests, a multiple regression analysis based on "stepwise regression" procedures was completed for all combinations of the nine motor fitness test variables (Table 1). This table revealed that the multiple correlations did not increase after the three best independent variables were combined. Therefore, a multiple regression equation for estimating

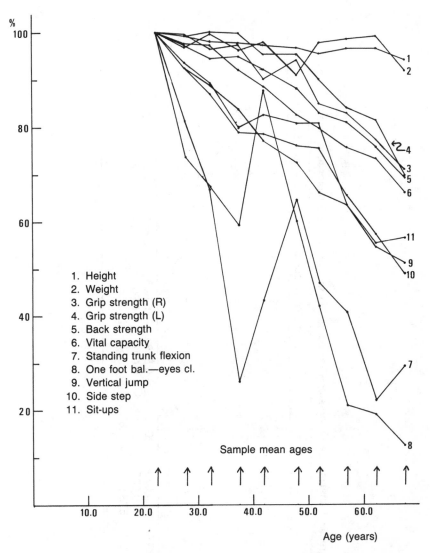

Figure 1. Declines in height, weight, and the 9 motor fitness test scores with age. (Values were adjusted so that the mean value of the 20-24 age group equaled 100%.)

chronological age was calculated with the three variables. The obtained multiple regression equation was

$$Y_{age} = 93.984$$
$$- 0.958 \text{ (vertical jump, in cm)}$$
$$+ 0.070 \text{ (back strength, in Kg)}$$
$$- 0.482 \text{ (side step, in number of times/20 sec).}$$

Table 1. Result of multiple regression analysis based on stepwise regression applied to the 9 motor fitness test variables

Tests	Variables selected								
Grip strength (R)							+	+	+
Grip strength (L)								+	+
Vital capacity						+	+	+	+
Standing trunk flexion				+	+	+	+	+	+
One foot bal.—eyes cl.					+	+	+	+	+
Vertical jump	+	+	+	+	+	+	+	+	+
Back strength		+	+	+	+	+	+	+	+
Side step			+	+	+	+	+	+	+
Sit-ups									+
R	0.847	0.870	0.877	0.879	0.880	0.881	0.881	0.881	0.880
R increase		0.023	0.007	0.002	0.001	0.001	0.000	0.000	-0.001
F-ratio	946.6	578.8	411.8	312.5	252.9	211.8	181.8	158.8	140.8

The multiple correlation between chronological age and a combination of three independent variables was 0.88 ($p < 0.01$), and the standard error of estimate was 6.2 years.

Figure 2 presents the relationship between chronological ages and physical fitness ages in the 374 ordinary subjects. Of the 374 subjects, 297 (79.4%) were scattered between the upper and lower dotted lines (45° standard line ± 1.0 *SD*).

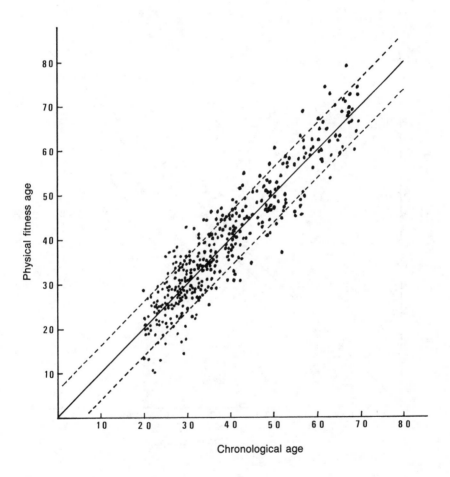

Figure 2. Relationship between physical fitness ages and chronological ages in the 374 ordinary healthy men. The values of physical fitness age were corrected so that the mean physical fitness ages for the groups equaled to the mean chronological ages. (The upper and lower dotted lines correspond to ± 1.0 *SD*.)

Figure 3 presents the relationship between chronological ages and physical fitness ages in the 79 trained subjects. Of the 79 trained subjects, 55 (69.6%) were scattered below the 45° standard line. The mean physical fitness age was 40.8 years, while the mean chronological age was 44.3 years. The mean physical fitness age was 3.5 years younger than the chronological age ($p < 0.01$, with paired t-test).

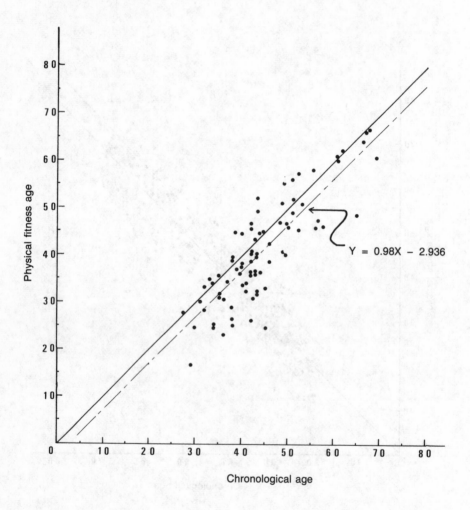

Figure 3. Relationship between physical fitness ages and chronological ages in the 79 trained subjects. (The dotted line is the regression line of physical fitness ages on chronological ages.)

Discussion

It is indisputable that after the middle twenties, various human functional capacities and physical fitness decrease on the average with advancing age (Åstrand, 1956; Shock, 1967; Wessel, Small, Van Huss, Heusner, & Cederquist, 1966; Meshizuka & Nagata, 1969). However, the rate of change in these functions and physical fitness with age varies among functions and subdomains of physical fitness (Shock, 1967; Meshizuka & Nagata, 1969). In this study, it was observed that several tests such as the vertical jump, side step, vital capacity, and sit-ups were remarkable age-related variables. However, the rate of change with age varies greatly for different tests, and the individual variations were rather great even in the same age group. As is apparent from Figure 1, there is no single index of aging if the rate of aging is defined as the slope of the regression of a test against age. Therefore, in order to devise an appropriate index of aging, it will be necessary to combine a number of age-related variables.

In the present study, an index was devised to summarize the age-related variables concerning physical fitness in a form that can provide a comparison with the standard at one's chronological age. Chronological age was adopted as the dependent variable on the basis of the Furukawa et al.'s proposal (1975), because it was expected to simulate the reference value of aging when the normal subject was concerned. The multiple correlation between a combination of the selected three variables (vertical jump, back strength, and side step) and chronological age was 0.88 ($p < 0.01$) and the standard error of estimate was 6.2 years. The estimation of physical fitness age was found to be fairly good. Therefore, the physical fitness age estimated from the multiple regression equation or the difference between physical fitness age and chronological age seemed to have favorable characteristics as one of the aging indices. However, longitudinal observations of the same subjects, as Dehn and Bruce (1972) and Shock (1967) pointed out, should be used to confirm the validity of this estimation method because cross-sectional observations never evaluate age changes in an individual.

There is little question that physical activity improves physical fitness. During the period of old age, an enhanced level of physical activity will enable the aged to spend daily life actively and increase the duration of the good years (Shephard, 1978; Shock, 1967). However, it is still not clear that physical activity can alter the rate of aging. In order to obtain one of the resolutions to this problem, the 79 trained subjects between 20 and 69 years in age were tested with respect to the correlation with aging for the physical fitness age estimated by the formula for ordinary healthy subjects. The estimated physical fitness age was significantly lower than chronological age. However, a statistically reliable difference between the two slopes of regression was not determined. But, the line was below that of the ordinary subjects by about 3 years. This indicates that trained subjects are younger than untrained subjects with respect to physical fitness.

References

Åstrand, P.-O. (1956). Human physical fitness with special reference to sex and age. *Physiological Reviews, 36*, 307-335.

Dehn, M.M., & Bruce, R.A. (1972). Longitudinal variations in maximal oxygen intake with age and activity. *Journal of Applied Physiology, 33*, 805-807.

Furukawa, T., Inoue, M., Kajiya, F., Inada, H., Takasugi, S., Fukui, S., Takeda, H., & Abe, H. (1975). Assessment of biological age by multiple regression analysis. *Journal of Gerontology, 30*, 422-434.

Matsushima, S. (Ed.). (1968). *Adult physical fitness test*. Tokyo: Daiichi-Hoki.

Meshizuka, T., & Nagata, A. (1969). Adult physical fitness test and physical fitness status of Japanese adults. *Research Journal of Physical Education, 13*, 287-296.

Schettller, G. (Ed.). (1972). *Alterskrankheiten*. Stuttgart: Georg Thieme Verlag.

Shephard, R.J. (1978). *Physical activity and aging*. London: Croom Helm.

Shock, N.W. (1967). Physical activity and the "rate of aging." *Canadian Medical Association Journal, 96*, 836-840.

Wessel, J.A., Small, D.A., Van Huss, W.D., Heusner, W.W., & Cederquist, D.C. (1966). Functional responses to submaximal exercise in women 20-69 years. *Journal of Gerontology, 21*, 168-181.

28

Exercise Training in Elderly Persons: Do Women Benefit as Much as Men?

Dennis M. Davidson
UNIVERSITY OF CALIFORNIA
IRVINE, CALIFORNIA, USA

Catherine Reith Murphy
CARDIAC TREATMENT CENTERS, INC.
HARRISBURG, PENNSYLVANIA, USA

The effects of physical training in young persons have been well documented. These include: (a) the ability to exercise at a higher work rate; (b) lower heart rate and systolic blood pressure values at a given submaximal work rate; and (c) a loss of body fat (which may be counterbalanced by a gain in lean body mass). These principles apply equally to persons in the cardiac rehabilitation setting (Davidson, 1983). However, until recently, little has been written about such changes in elderly healthy persons who undertook physical training (Sidney & Shephard, 1978; Schocken, Blumenthal, Port, Hindle & Coleman, 1984). Even fewer reports have appeared regarding the effects of cardiac rehabilitation in elderly populations.

The purpose of this investigation was to assess the efficacy of a standardized cardiac rehabilitation program in men and women, aged 65 and older, who were recovering from a myocardial infarction (MI) or coronary artery bypass surgery (CABS). Three null hypotheses were chosen:

Supported in part by a Preventive Cardiology Academic Award from the National Institutes of Health (NIH HL 01243-01).

1. There will be no significant gains in male and female participants during the 12-week training period as measured by the following three outcome variables: maximal oxygen uptake (in METs); heart rate-systolic blood pressure product at a submaximal workrate; and body weight change.
2. There will be no significant differences between men and women in absolute and percentage changes in the three outcome variables.
3. There will be no significant correlation within this elderly population between the three outcome variables and age.

Subjects and Methods

We asked 19 hospital-based cardiac rehabilitation programs throughout the United States to review their records for the preceding 12 months and report data on each of their participants, aged 65 and older, who had completed: (a) a 12-week training program within the preceding 12 months; and (b) a symptom-limited treadmill test before and after program participation.

Participants at each center were required to follow a common training protocol. Features of this protocol included an initial exercise prescription based upon the program entry treadmill test; circuit interval exercise training three times weekly for 12 weeks (intensities ranging between 65% and 75% of measured peak heart rate on the entry treadmill test); exercise period duration (exclusive of warmup and cooldown) increasing progressively from 21 minutes during the first week to 45 minutes during week 12; and adjustment of the individual's exercise prescription during the 12-week program to maintain training heart rates within the target range.

Using these criteria, 74 men and 21 women qualified for inclusion. Preliminary analyses were done on these 95 persons, with results indicated below.

We then applied stricter exclusion criteria to the group of 95, requiring that (a) both entry and exit exercise evaluations be done using the same exercise test protocol, and (b) there was no change throughout the study period in either the type or dosage of the following medications: digoxin, diuretics, nitrates, or beta-adrenergic blocking agents. The more stringent criteria resulted in a final study population of 36 men and 8 women, whose baseline characteristics are listed in Table 1.

Variables of interest in our subsequent analyses included the follwing data extracted from program and exercise test records: age, gender, diagnoses, height, weight, medications, program entry and exit times, and, from the exercise tests, oxygen uptake, heart rate, and blood pressure values at submaximal and peak work rates. From these observations, the heart rate-systolic blood pressure product was computed at submaximal and peak work rates. The absolute and percentage changes of all observed and derived variables were calculated.

Data analyses were accomplished using the Statistical Package for the Social Sciences (Nie, Hull, Jenkins, Steinbrenner, & Bent, 1975) programs on the University DEC-10 computer. Variables with independent value in predicting the outcome variables were determined with a stepwise multiple regression

Table 1. Baseline population characteristics

Variable	Men	Women
Number of subjects	36	8
Age (years)	67.9	67.6
Height (inches)	68.8	63.1
Weight (pounds)	170.0	132.1
Diagnosis		
Myocardial infarction	27/36	6/8
Bypass surgery	9/36	2/8
Weeks entered after		
cardiac event	6.3	6.7
Digoxin use	9/36	1/8
Beta-blocker use	12/36	4/8
Diuretic use	13/36	5/8
Nitrate use	11/36	2/8

program and analysis of variance testing. The probabilities that observed differences occurred by chance were calculated and are reported herein as "p" values.

Results

In the larger sample (74 men, 21 women), both men and women made significant gains in maximal oxygen uptake during the 12-week training period. The men improved from 5.68 MET to 8.34 MET, a 46% increase ($p<.02$), while the women improved from 5.53 MET to 6.71 MET, a 25% improvement ($p<.05$). The difference between men and women in improvement was significant ($p<.01$). Similarly, heart rate-systolic blood pressure ("rate-pressure") product decreased a mean of 19.6% in men ($p<.01$) and 10.2% in women ($p<.10$). Again, the difference between men and women was significant at the $p<.05$ level. Finally, men lost a mean of 2.53 lb, while women gained a mean of 1.29 lb. Of 74 men, 49 (66%) lost weight, compared to only 7 of the 21 women (33%). This difference between men and women was significant ($p<.05$).

Upon testing the rigor of these findings by imposing stricter exclusion criteria, the differences between men and women persisted. As noted in Table 2, the 36 men increased their maximal oxygen uptake 54.1% ($p<.001$), while the women improved by 20.6% ($p<.05$). This intergender difference was significant at $p<.001$.

At a mean submaximal work rate of 3.5 MET, men decreased their rate-pressure product 20.4% ($p<.05$), compared to the mean change in women of 10.5% ($p = .3$). The difference in responses between men and women for this parameter was significant ($p<.01$). Men lost an average of 2.1 lb (-1.2%), while women gained a mean of 0.3 lb ($+0.8\%$), an intergender difference significant at $p<.05$.

Table 2. Changes in outcome variables after training

Variable	Men		Women		Difference Men-Women
Max. O$_2$ uptake (MET)					
Initial	5.72		6.75		
Final	8.17				
Difference	2.45	(54%)	1.00	(21%)	p<.001
Submax. rate-pressure					
Initial	11991		13879		
Final	9480		12421		
Difference	2511	(21%)	1458	(10%)	p<.01
Weight					
Initial	170.0		132.1		
Final	167.9		132.4		
Difference	−2.1	(−1%)	0.3	(+0.1%)	p<.05

Univariate Correlations

Univariate correlations coefficients of the three outcome variables with age are shown in Table 3 for men, women, and the two genders combined. While most relationships showed almost no correlation, men did show a negative correlation ($r = -.26$) of maximal oxygen uptake change with age.

Stepwise Multiple Regression Analyses

Gender was the most important predictive variable of change in maximal oxygen uptake, accounting for 14.1% of variance. The maximal oxygen uptake on the first test was also independently predictive of change in that parameter, adding another 7.2% in explanation of variance. Finally, addition of age to the other two variables raised the cumulative explanation of variance to 27.7%. When dichotomized by age into a group below 70 years and those 70 and older, women showed no difference (a change of 1.0 MET in both groups). In contrast, younger men had slightly higher improvement in maximal oxygen uptake (2.65 MET), compared to 1.57 MET in older men. The differences between the two groups of men was not statistically significant, however.

When submaximal rate-pressure product was used as the outcome variable in the stepwise regression analysis only the rate-pressure product on the first test emerged as independently predictive, accounting for 41.8% of the variance in men. No variables were significantly predictive in the 8 women.

Table 3. Univariate correlations age versus outcome variables

Variables	Men	Women	Both
Max. O$_2$ uptake	−.26	.138	−.19
Submax. rate-pressure	.138	−.146	.096
Weight	−.01	.02	−.009

Examination of precent body weight change, with gender as a potentially predictive variable, allowed direct comparison of men and women by the stepwise program. Two variables emerged as predictive: (a) week of entry into the program (earlier enrollees lost more weight) and (b) beta-adrenergic blockade use (users lost less weight). These two variables accounted for 13.9% and 7.6% of variance, respectively.

Discussion

Houston, Fair, and Davidson (1980) studied 14 women and 14 men matched for age ($M = 56$), cardiovascular risk factors, and type and severity of disease, who participated in a YMCA gymnasium-based cardiac rehabilitation program. After 3 months of participation, treadmill testing revealed that men had improved 1.0 MET compared to 0.5 MET for women. Men had increased body weight by 0.6 lb, compared to a gain of 8.6 lb in women. Men reduced their serum cholesterol and triglyceride levels by 2.0 and 13.0 mg/dl, respectively, while women's values increased 24.7 and 71.3 mg/dl.

Our findings are consistent with this earlier study, despite the differences in age and program. In the present study, women did make significant improvements in maximal oxygen uptake, but less impressive changes in submaximal rate-pressure product. In all three major outcome variables, women did not improve as much as men. We saw no consistent correlation of age with the outcome measures in this group of subjects, all of whom were 65 or older.

We interpret these findings to confirm the utility of cardiac rehabilitation programs for persons 65 and older. We also conclude that women do less well on an absolute and percentage change basis than men during participation in traditional cardiac rehabilitation programs. Perhaps the woman of "coronary-age" (65 and older) finds the traditional orientation towards jogging, treadmill, and bicycle exercise less attractive than does a man of the same age. Perhaps there is less motivation for women to "achieve" higher levels of fitness in such a program.

To further explore these differences, we recommend separate exercise classes for women, with a different orientation and atmosphere. If introductory sessions could be devoted to reestablishing flexibility and motor strength, aerobic dance or equivalent activities could then be offered. Such a sequence may be more attractive and enjoyable for women and improve both motivation and adherence.

References

Davidson, D.M. (1983). Recovery after cardiac events. In R.L. Frye (Ed.), *Clinical Medicine* (Vol. 20) (Chapter 6). Philadelphia. Lippincott.

Houston, N., Fair, J. & Davidson, D.M. (1980). Differences in responses to exercise training in men and women with cardiac disease. *Circulation, 32*, III-172.

Nie, N.H., Hull, C.H., Jenkins, J.G., Steinbrenner, K., & Bent, D.H. (1975). *SPSS: Statistical package for the social sciences* (2nd ed.). New York: McGraw-Hill.

Schocken, D.D., Blumenthal, J.A., Port, S., Hindle, P., & Coleman, R.E. (1984). Physical conditioning and left ventricular performance in the elderly: Assessment by radionuclide angiography. *American Journal of Cardiology, 53*, 359-364.

Sidney, K.H., & Shephard, R.J. (1978). Frequency and intensity of exercise training for elderly subjects. *Medicine and Science in Sports, 10*, 125-131.